Immunology of the Female Genital Tract

Ernst Rainer Weissenbacher
Monika Wirth • Ioannis Mylonas
William J. Ledger • Steven S. Witkin

Immunology of the Female Genital Tract

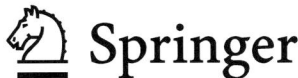 Springer

Ernst Rainer Weissenbacher
Klinik und Poliklinik für
Frauenheilkunde
Klinikum
der LMU München - Großhadern
München
Germany

Monika Wirth
Olching
Germany

Ioannis Mylonas
Ludwig-Maximilians-Universität
München
Germany

Klinik für Geburtshilfe
und Frauenheilkunde
Klinikum Innenstadt
München
Germany

William J. Ledger
Department of Obtetrics
and Gynaecology
Weill Cornell Medical Center
New York, NY
USA

Steven S. Witkin
Division of Immunology
and Infectious Diseases
Weill Cornell Medical College
New York, NY
USA

ISBN 978-3-642-14905-4   ISBN 978-3-642-14906-1   (eBook)
DOI 10.1007/978-3-642-14906-1

Library of Congress Control Number: 2013956431

Springer Heidelberg New York Dordrecht London
© Springer-Verlag Berlin Heidelberg 2014

Printed on acid-free paper

Springer-Verlag GmbH Berlin Heidelberg is part of Springer Science+Business Media
(www.springer.com)

Contents

Introduction

The mucosal immune system in the female reproductive tract has evolved to meet the unique requirements of dealing with colonization with commensal microorganisms, sexually transmitted bacterial and viral pathogens, allogeneic spermatozoa, and the immunologically distinct fetus. It is now established that the mucosal immune system is a distinct and separate component of the host's immune apparatus and differs from the lymphoid tissues in peripheral sites. Furthermore, despite some common features, the female genital tract mucosal system displays some distinct characteristics, which outlines its special role. Analysis of the female genital tract indicates that the key cells of the innate and adaptive immune systems are present and functionally responsive to antigens; however, there is a certain degree of compartmentalization within the tract. The identification of TLRs in the fallopian tubes, uterus, cervix, and vagina; the presence of ECs, macrophages, DCs, NK cells, and neutrophils throughout the reproductive tract; and the responsiveness of these cells to selected PAMPs indicate that the female reproductive tract has evolved to meet the challenges of STDs while at the same time supporting an immunologically distinct fetal placental unit. To meet these diverse challenges, the innate and adaptive immune systems in the female genital tract are precisely regulated not only by a network of cytokines and chemokines but also by the sex hormones estrogen and progesterone. The mechanisms that regulate this mucosal immune system are still only incompletely understood. This is due to the complexities and interactions of the female immune and endocrine systems as well as to difficulties of conducting experiments in this field.

During the last decade, there has also been an increasing need for further investigation in this area due to the rising prevalence of sexually transmitted diseases (STDs), among them the pandemics caused by the human immunodeficiency virus (HIV). Progress is being made in understanding how immune responses can best be stimulated at the genital tract mucosal level. On the basis of this information, the attempt to construct new mucosal vaccines specifically targeted to the genital tract is one of the ambitious goals of research in this field. Also, the blossoming of the field of reproductive medicine, with the tremendous increase in the number of infertile couples seeking to undergo assisted reproduction, has led to advances in characterizing immunological mechanisms and disturbances related to ovulation, conception, and pregnancy maintenance.

Understanding the specialty of the genital tract immune system is of critical importance, because STDs are and will continue to be a major health problem worldwide. Despite extensive efforts, only limited success has been achieved in dealing with a growing list of STDs. The role of immune factors in the control of genital viral and bacterial infections appears complex and needs further study, also with respect to the development of vaccines. Despite the recognition that innate immunity, as the first line of defense, and adaptive immunity, especially Th1 immune responses, play a critical role in preventing infection and in limiting viral

E.R. Weissenbacher et al., *Immunology of the Female Genital Tract*,
DOI 10.1007/978-3-642-14906-1_1, © Springer-Verlag Berlin Heidelberg 2014

replication, factors such as antimicrobials and TLRs that contribute to the mucosal response in the female genital tract have only recently begun to receive attention. Further studies are also needed to elucidate the relationship between mucosal immunity, the hormonal environment, and response to pathogen challenge.

More data must be collected on the mechanisms of immune evasion by several pathogens such as HSV, *N. gonorrhoeae*, and *Chlamydia*. While considerable information can be obtained from animal experiments, important differences in the physiology of reproduction and the immune system result in the need for studies in humans. Further knowledge on female tract immunology will also impact on immunological approaches to contraception, immunological infertility, and the immunological aspects of pregnancy. This will introduce new options not only for diagnostics but also for treatment of pregnancy complications such as preeclampsia, preterm birth, and early pregnancy loss as well as infertility.

The objective of this book is to systematically review and discuss recent advances in immunology of the female genital tract. The emphasis hereby lies on the evaluation of studies concerning the basics of female reproductive immunology, research on immunology of the most important genital infections and vaccination strategies, immunological principles at the fetomaternal interface during normal pregnancy and its complications, and immunological data on infertility and immunocontraception.

The second chapter in this book gives a brief introduction to the basic principles of human innate and acquired immunity and mucosal immunology, while the third aims to define the mucosal immune system in the female reproductive tract. The focus thereby is on identification of what is known about the humoral and cellular factors of this particular mucosal immune system and definition of the regulatory influences of sex hormones and cytokines. The unique immunological characteristics of the female genital tract are then considered with respect to the design of mucosal vaccines for protection against microbial disease.

The fourth chapter deals with the most important infections of the female genital tract and describes the latest results regarding innate and adaptive immune responses and vaccine development for each infection. These are the following:

- Viral infections
  - *Herpes simplex virus (HSV)*
  - *Human immunodeficiency virus (HIV)*
  - *Human papillomavirus (HPV)*
- Bacterial infections
  - *Neisseria gonorrhoeae*
  - *Chlamydia trachomatis*
  - *Bacterial vaginosis (BV)*
- Mycoses
  - *Candida albicans*
- Parasites
  - *Trichomonas vaginalis*

Finally, the fifth chapter reports on different important areas of immunology in reproductive medicine. Pregnancy involves maternal tolerance of the semiallogenic histoincompatible fetus and is characterized by the enhancement of the innate immune system and suppression of the adaptive immune response, probably with progesterone as the important regulator. In contrast to normal pregnancy, improper immune responses and an unbalanced cytokine network may characterize implantation failures, pregnancy loss, and obstetric complications. These are the presence of elevated Th1/Th2 cell ratios, high concentrations of Th1 cytokines, elevated NK cell cytotoxicity and levels, and emergence of various autoantibodies. Immunological approaches need to be investigated and evaluated further with respect to widening of treatment options by modification of immune responses.

After describing immunological principles at the fetomaternal interface during normal pregnancy and labor, different disturbances in maternal–fetal interactions and their immunological background are discussed. These are:

- Preeclampsia
- Preterm labor/preterm birth
- Fetal growth retardation
- Early pregnancy loss

Furthermore, the topic of infertility is further elucidated from an immunological point of view. Remarks on the latest developments in immunocontraception conclude this chapter.

Contents

The immune system has evolved to provide appropriate defense systems at various levels of innate (nonspecific) and acquired (specific) immune responses. Innate immunity is the ancient part of the host defense mechanisms and lies behind most inflammatory responses. Acquired immunity can provide specific recognition of foreign antigens, an immunological memory of infection, and pathogen-specific adaptor proteins. However, the adaptive immune response is also responsible for allergy, autoimmunity, and the rejection of tissue grafts.

In most cases, components of both systems interact to create an appropriate immune response to an infectious agent. But it is not only the protection from penetration by foreign or modified cells but also the elimination of old and deficient cells which characterizes a functioning immune system.

2.1 Concepts of Innate and Specific Immunity

The term immunity derives from the Latin word *immunitas*, which stands for the privilege of the Roman senators to be protected from legal punishment or exempted from certain public duties. Initially, immunity was described as protection against illness, especially infectious illness. In modern times immunity has been more exactly defined as reactions of the body against foreign or altered self substances.

2.1.1 The Innate Immune Response to Infectious Agents

Recognized as the first line of defense, innate immunity consists of different mechanisms which are already available before exposition with pathogens or unknown molecules and do not need prior activation or induction. Innate immune responses do not change in type or magnitude if there is more than one encounter with the same antigen, and differences between unknown substances cannot be distinguished. In the following, a short overview of the different factors of innate immunity is given (Table 2.1).

E.R. Weissenbacher et al., *Immunology of the Female Genital Tract*,
DOI 10.1007/978-3-642-14906-1_2, © Springer-Verlag Berlin Heidelberg 2014

Table 2.1 Factors of the innate immune system

Mechanical and chemical barriers

Skin, mucosal surfaces

Enzymes (lysozyme), peptides (defensins), fatty acids, acidic pH, etc.

Cellular factors

Mononuclear phagocytes (blood monocytes/tissue macrophages)

Granulocytes

Dendritic cells

Mast cells

Natural killer cells

Humoral factors

Complement

Acute-phase proteins

Interferons

M. Wirth 2006, Personal communication

Table 2.2 Localization of phagocytic cells

Localization	Phagocytic cells
Blood	Monocytes
	Neutrophils (eosinophils. basophils)
Lung	Alveolar macrophages
Liver	Kupffer cells
Brain	Microglia
Bone	Osteoclasts
Kidney	Mesangial cells in glomeruli
Joint	Synovial A cells

M. Wirth 2006, Personal communication

Preventing microorganisms from gaining access to the body is achieved by mechanical barriers such as the skin and surface epithelia. These are also equipped with additional chemical features including fatty acids in the skin, low pH in the stomach, or antibacterial enzymes in saliva, for example. Once the pathogen has crossed the epithelial barrier, cellular effector mechanisms involving granulocytes and mononuclear phagocytes are activated to eliminate the intruder by phagocytosis.

To recognize foreign structures that are not normally found in the host, the innate immune system relies on conserved germline-encoded receptors that recognize conserved pathogen-associated molecular patterns (PAMPs) found in groups of microorganisms. These are essential conserved products produced by microorganisms but not by the host, such as lipopolysaccharide (LPS) in the outer membrane of gram-negative bacteria and peptidoglycan membrane components of gram-positive bacteria. Recognition of these molecular structures allows the immune system to distinguish infectious nonself from noninfectious self.

Among receptors for PAMPs which are expressed by cells of the innate immune system, Toll-like receptors (TLRs) are of major importance. Signaling through TLRs in response to PAMPs leads to recruitment, differentiation, and activation of other immune cells and production of antimicrobial factors that kill invading microbes as well as link innate and acquired immunity. Studies have found 10 different subtypes of mammalian TLRs. Among the cells that bear innate immune or germline-encoded recognition are mononuclear phagocytes, dendritic cells (DCs), mast cells, granulocytes, natural killer (NK) cells, and epithelial cells.

2.1.1.1 Cellular Factors

Phagocytic cells are located at strategically important locations in the organism (Table 2.2) and are all derived from pluripotent stem cells of the bone marrow.

Monocytes circulating in blood vessels and macrophages in other tissues like the lung, liver, and lymph nodes as well as granulocytes are capable of killing microorganisms. After activation by cytokines, especially interferon-γ (IFN-γ), macrophages produce toxic effector molecules such as reactive oxygen intermediates (ROI) and reactive nitrogen intermediates (RNI) which are interactively able to kill the pathogen. RNI have proved to be the most effective defense mechanism in murine macrophages but also an increasing amount of studies supports RNI production by human macrophages. Lysosomal enzymes within the phagosome or depletion of intraphagosomal iron function as other mechanisms of phagocytic cells to kill intracellular pathogens.

The group of granulocytes consists of neutrophils, eosinophils, and basophils, but the uptake and intracellular killing of microorganisms is in the first place the task of neutrophils. By expressing Fc receptors for immunoglobulin (Ig)

Fig. 2.1 Components and effector mechanisms of the complement system (Adapted from Janeway CA Jr., Travers P. Immunologie. 2nd ed. Heidelberg: Berlin: Oxford; Spektrum Akademischer Verlag; 1997)

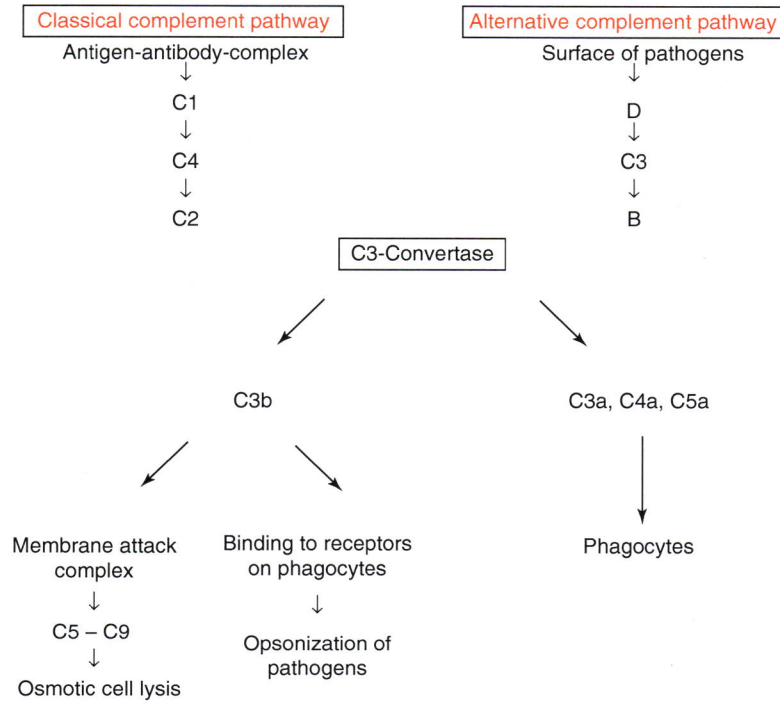

G (CD16) and receptors for activated complement factors (C3b), neutrophils can phagocyte pathogens coated by antibodies or complement factors. Neutrophils are able to release azurophil granule with myeloperoxidase and lysozyme, specific granule with lactoferrin or alkaline phosphatase as well as superoxide radicals, which leads to an inflammatory reaction of tissue. Extracellular killing of large parasites such as helminths is performed by eosinophils. They also provide surface receptors for complement factor C3b and release their granule with major basic protein (MBP), cationic protein, and anti-inflammatory enzymes. Basophils play an important role in allergic reactions and in immune responses against parasites where they release mediators such as histamine or heparin and chemotactic factors and therefore induce an anaphylactic reaction. They have surface receptors for both IgE and activated complement factors C3a and C5a.

Other cellular components of the innate immunity are NK cells which are large granular lymphocytes comprising 5–10 % of circulating peripheral lymphocytes. They express surface receptors for IgG (CD16) as well as T cell markers such as CD8 and are able to mediate antibody-dependent cellular cytotoxicity (ADCC). Thereby, they are able to destroy target cells such as malignantly transformed cells or virus-infected cells by binding these antibody-loaded cells to the Fc receptor of NK cells via the Fc region of the antibody.

2.1.1.2 Humoral Factors

The complement system is a multicomponent triggered enzyme cascade (Fig. 2.1). Activation results in direct killing of viruses and bacteria as well as marking microorganisms for ingestion by phagocytic cells.

Complement activation can start via the classical pathway with Igs in complex with antigens binding to complement protein C1. The alternative pathway beginning with the binding of complement factor C3b on different activated bacterial surfaces is initiated in the absence of antibodies and therefore is a more rapid humoral mechanism. A third pathway, the lectin pathway, is initiated by the binding of mannose-binding lectin (MBL) to carbohydrate patterns on microorganisms. This activates MBL-associated serine proteases to cleave C2 and C4, generating the C3 convertase C4bC2a and cleavage of C3. All pathways lead to the splitting and activation of factor C3 whose activated fragments enable the opsonization of antigens on bacteria surfaces. The terminal components C5–C9 form a membrane attack complex which enables the osmotic lysis of the pathogen.

Other humoral factors of the innate immune system involve IFNs and acute-phase proteins. IFN-α produced by leukocytes and IFN-β synthesized by fibroblasts and other cell types block viral replication in virus-infected cells. C-reactive protein as the most common representative of acute-phase proteins promotes the binding of complement to bacteria and facilitates their phagocytosis.

2.1.2 Specific Acquired Immunity

Following interaction of the intruding microorganism with effector mechanisms of the innate immune system, components of the specific or acquired immune system are activated. Acquired immunity is characterized by recognition of specific antigenic determinants. The following responses to the same antigen are specific and quantitatively and qualitatively different from the primary response. This specificity is achieved through the use of clonally distributed antigen receptors, i.e., surface Ig on antibody-producing B lymphocytes and T cell receptors (TCR) on the surface of T lymphocytes. Another feature of the adaptive immune system is that it develops memory which allows a faster response of specific effector cells when encountering the relevant antigen a second time.

Responding to antigens is either realized by producing specific antibodies (humoral immunity) or direct specific-lymphocyte contact with host cells expressing foreign antigenic peptides (cell-mediated immunity). The cell-mediated response needs the cooperation of different subclasses of T cells, macrophages, and perhaps NK cells. Humoral responses involve the interaction of B cells, T cells, and antigen-presenting cells (APCs).

Table 2.3 MHC classes with examples for encoding proteins

MHC class Ia	HLA-A, HLA-B, HLA-C
MHC class Ib	HLA-E, HLA-F, HLA-G
MHC class II	HLA-DP, HLA-DQ, HLA-DR
MHC class III	Complement components, TNF-α, TNF-β

M. Wirth 2006, Personal communication

2.1.2.1 The Major Histocompatibility Complex

T and B lymphocytes need a system to distinguish between "self" and "nonself," which is the function of the major histocompatibility complex (MHC). This group of genes encodes for several proteins, also called human leukocyte antigens (HLA) (Table 2.3). MHC class I molecules, which include HLA-A, HLA-B, and HLA-C, are expressed by all nucleated cells whereas MHC class II molecules including HLA-DR, HLA-DP, and HLA-DQ are expressed by APCs and B and T lymphocytes.

2.1.2.2 B Lymphocytes

After the process of B-cell differentiation in the bone marrow, each mature B cell bears a surface receptor, an Ig, which is different in its antigen specificity from all other B cells. These mature but naive B cells circulate in the blood, lymph, and secondary lymphoid organs waiting to encounter antigen. By interaction with antigen, B cells differentiate into antigen-specific memory B cells and effector plasma cells which generate large amounts of soluble versions of the membrane-bound Ig.

This clonal selection hypothesis explains why subsequent responses to the same antigen are more effective and long-lasting than the initial response. In the first encounter with antigen, a primary antibody response is generated; later, a reencounter with the same antigen causes a more rapid secondary response, producing high levels of antibodies with a strong affinity for the target antigen. This process is also exploited in prophylactic vaccination.

The primary humoral immune response involves generation of IgM class antibodies, whereas the secondary and all subsequent responses to the same antigen may be of IgG, IgE,

Table 2.4 The different classes of immunoglobulins

	IgG	IgA	IgM	IgD	IgE
Form	Monomer	Monomer Dimer	Pentamer Hexamer	Monomer	Monomer
Subclasses	G1,G2,G3,G4	A1. A2	–	–	–
Percent of Ig	75–85	7–15	5–10	0.3	0.019
Binds to	Macrophages NK cells Neutrophils	Lymphocytes	Lymphocytes	–	Mast cells Basophils B cells
Complement fixation	Classical	Alternative	Classical	–	–
Cross placenta	Yes	–	–	–	–

M. Wirth 2006, Personal communication

or IgA subclasses, depending on specific location. Proliferation and differentiation of B cells as well as Ig isotype class switching are driven by cytokines, especially by interleukins (IL)-4 and -5. The differences between the Ig subclasses are shown in Table 2.4. In addition to their unique role as antibody-producing plasma cells, B cells have the capacity to present antigen to T lymphocytes. Upon binding of antigen to membrane-bound Ig, antigen–antibody complexes are internalized and degraded. Antigen-derived peptides are then introduced to MHC-II-dependent pathways and can be presented to peptide-specific CD4+ T cells.

2.1.2.3 T Lymphocytes

In contrast, T cells only recognize antigen when it is presented by appropriate MHC molecules on APC such as DCs or macrophages. During their differentiation in the thymus, T lymphocytes learn to recognize MHC molecules and develop the cluster of differentiation (CD) 4 and 8 surface receptors which mark them as CD4+ T helper cells or CD8+ cytotoxic T cells (CTL). Antigenic peptides presented to T cells by MHC class I molecules stimulate the CD8+ T cells whose primary function is to destroy intracellular pathogens. Peptides presented by MHC class II molecules stimulate the CD4+ T cells which are able to eliminate both intracellular and extracellular pathogens. They produce various cytokines required for the activation of leukocytes and are therefore also termed T helper (Th) cells.

Activation of T cells requires signaling mediated through both the TCR and costimulatory receptor–ligand interactions which involve the costimulatory molecules CD80 (B7.1) and CD86 (B7.2) on APCs. These can bind to T cell surface molecule CD28 and CD125 (CTLA-4).

As CD4+ Th cells produce different cytokines upon antigenic stimulation to activate B cells and macrophages, they can be divided into the three subpopulations of Th1, Th2, and Th17 cells. Th1 cells are characterized by secretion of IFN-γ and IL-2; Th2 cells produce IL-4, IL-5, and IL-10; and Th17 cells release IL-17. Th2 cells are therefore important for the induction of humoral immune responses by controlling B-cell activation, Th1 cells initiate cell-mediated immune responses by activating macrophages by IFN-γ and CD8+ T cells by IL-2, and Th17 cells activate neutrophils (667, Table 2.5). The differentiation of these subsets from Th0 precursor cells is driven by cytokines, especially by IL- 12/IL-18 and IL-4, respectively.

A fourth category of T cells, regulatory T cells (Tregs) with the phenotype CD4+ CD25+, usually secretes IL-10 and tumor growth factor-β (TGF-β). Cells with this phenotype are thought to recognize self-antigens and function to prevent autoimmunity, but they also regulate responses to exogenous antigens and have been implicated in chronic and immunopathologic viral infections.

CTLs are able to eliminate virus-infected cells or tumor cells by lysis or apoptosis. Cytotoxicity is mediated by pore-forming proteins (perforins) and enzymes (granzymes) that perforate the target cell. CTLs can also trigger apoptosis,

Table 2.5 The role of Th1, Th2, and Th17 cells in immunity

Activation of cytotoxic T cells → protection against viruses	B-cell maturation → protection against extracellular microbes, virions, and helminths
Macrophage activation → protection against intracellular microbes	Ig class switch to IgE (mast cell, basophil, eosinophil) → protection against helminthes
Ig class switch to IgG (complement activation/opsonization) → protection against extracellular microbes	Ig class switch to IgG (neutralization) → protection against virions, toxins
Th1 activation → protection against all microbes and viruses	Ig class switch to IgA (mucosa) → protection against many pathogens
	Eosinophil activation → protection against helminths

Adapted from Kaufmann SHE, Kabelitz D. The immune response to infectious agents. In: Kaufmann SHE, Kabelitz D, editors. Immunology of infection. Methods in microbiology, vol. 32. 2nd ed. London: Academic Press; 2002. p. 1–20

i.e., programmed cell death, in target cells through receptor–ligand interaction. Upon activation, CTLs are induced to express Fas ligand (FasL) which interacts with the corresponding receptor Fas expressed on virus-infected target cells.

The division of the immune system into innate and specific immunity (Table 2.6) does not mean the strict separation of both when encountering pathogens. Instead, it is required that both systems closely cooperate and that components of both activate each other. Over the recent years, it has become increasingly clear that the two systems cannot be seen separately and that the innate immune system is even instrumental for the development of the adaptive immune response.

2.2 Mucosal Immunology

The immune system can be divided into two compartments that display considerable functional independence: on the one hand, the systemic compartment represented by the bone marrow, spleen, and lymph nodes and, on the other hand, the mucosal compartment represented by lymphoid tissues in mucosae and external secretory glands. Numbers and types of cells involved in immune responses and their soluble products, primarily antibodies, are remarkably different in the mucosal and systemic compartments of the immune system, which are now further elucidated.

A distinct immune system at mucosal surfaces in humans was first presumed during the times of Paul Ehrlich in the nineteenth century. Further anatomical and biological studies of a common mucosa-associated immune system go back to the 1970s where Tomasi described the function of secretory (S)-IgA and cellular immune mechanisms as components of a mucosa-associated immune system.

Several hundred square meters comprise the surface areas of mucosal membranes where antigens from ingested food or inhaled air and resident pathogens represent the most important exogenous stimulants. Due to the high antigen load of mucosal surfaces, the mucosal immune system exhibits immunological hyporesponsiveness or unresponsiveness to most antigens. On the other hand, it must also be capable of inducing effective cell-mediated and antibody-mediated immune responses toward selected antigens. To meet this task, mucosal surfaces possess a unique immune system that tightly controls the balance between responsiveness and nonresponsiveness (tolerance). Besides mechanical barriers, humoral factors such as lysozyme, peroxidase, and specific antibodies as well as cellular mechanisms contribute to the protection of mucosal surfaces (Table 2.7).

Immune responses generated by organized lymphoid structures in the mucosa-associated lymphoreticular tissue (MALT) result in the development of B cells capable of producing antigen-specific Igs that can reach the draining lymph nodes and other mucosal tissues where they differentiate into plasma cells. A second major outcome of the entry of antigen and antigen presentation by DCs is the activation and differentiation of T cells that can subsequently

Table 2.6 The concepts of innate and specific acquired immunity

	Innate immune system	Adaptive immune system
General characteristics	First line of defense	Specific recognition of foreign antigens
	No specificity and no adaptation following antigen exposure	Immunological memory
		Responsible for allergy. autoimmunity, rejection of tissue grafts
Physical and chemical barriers	Skin	Immune systems of skin and mucosal membranes
	Mucosal membranes	Antibodies in secretions
Circulating molecules	Complement	Antibodies
Cellular factors	Macrophages/monocytes	Lymphocytes
	Granulocytes	
	Natural killer cells	
Soluble mediators effective on other cells	Cytokines like α- and β-interferons, tumor necrosis factor (derived from macrophages)	Cytokines like γ-interferons (derived from lymphocytes)
Receptors	Genes encoded in germline DNA	Encoded in gene segments
	No gene rearrangement	Rearrangement necessary
Recognition	Conserved molecular patterns (PAMPs)	Details of molecular structure (proteins. peptides)
Self-nonself discrimination	Perfect (selected over evolutionary time)	Not perfect (selected in individual somatic cells)
Response	Immediate activation of effectors	Delayed activation of effectors

Adapted from Janeway CA Jr., Travers P. Immunologie. 2nd ed. Heidelberg: Berlin: Oxford; Spektrum Akademischer Verlag; 1997

Table 2.7 Protection of mucosal surfaces

Mechanical barriers and peristalsis
Desquamation of epithelial cells with attached microorganisms
Humoral factors: Mucin, acids, lysozyme, lactoferrin, peroxidase system antimicrobial proteins, interferon-α. Complement specific antibodies: IgA $\gg$ IgG > IgM
Cellular factors: Phagocytic cells, T cells, NK cells

Adapted from Kutteh et al. Reproductive Immunology. Ann Arbor: Blackwell Science; 1996. p. 28–51

migrate out of the MALT and reach mucosal as well as peripheral non-mucosal tissues.

The mucosal immune system is structurally and functionally divided into sites for antigen uptake and processing at inductive sites on the one hand and effector sites engaging lymphocytes, granulocytes, and mast cells on the other hand. Besides the nasal-associated lymphoreticular tissue (NALT), the gut-associated lymphoreticular tissue (GALT) is the prototype of MALT and possesses APCs, T lymphocytes, and IgA-committed B cells.

2.2.1 S-IgA as the Major Ig Subclass in the Mucosal Immune System

Igs of all isotypes have been detected in various human external secretions. The predominant Ig isotype in normal human serum is IgG, followed by IgA and IgM. In contrast to serum, the major isotype in human excretions such as saliva, tears, bile, urine, and milk is IgA. IgA is the most important subclass of Igs that can actively and efficiently be secreted through epithelia. Due to the size of mucosal surfaces, the total amount of daily IgA production was quantified as 66 mg/kg body weight, which is more than twice the concentration of IgG. Approximately 1,500 mg/day IgA is produced systemically in the bone marrow, lymph nodes, or spleen but twice as much IgA is released in the mucosal immune system.

Most of the serum IgA is found in a monomeric form with two heavy and two light chains whereas S-IgA is mainly polymeric with presence of a J chain and secretory component (SC). IgA is produced by plasma cells in the lamina

Table 2.8 Effector functions of secretory and serum IgA

	Secretory-IgA	Serum IgA
Molecular form	Polymeric	Monomeric
Subclass	IgA1 ≥ IgA2	IgA1 >>> IgA2
SC- mediated transport into secretions	Yes	No
J-chain expression	Yes	Mostly no
Origin of precursor cells	Bone marrow, no circulation	Peyer's patches, IgA cells in circulation
Neutralization of antigens	Yes	Yes
Inhibition of bacterial adherence	Yes	?
Loss of bacterial plasmid	Yes	?
Inhibition from antigen uptake from mucosa	Yes	No
Enhancement of innate factors	Yes	Yes (?)
Suppression of inflammatory effects (phagocytosis, lysis, NK cell activity, etc.)	Yes	Yes

Adapted from Kutteh et al. Reproductive Immunology. Ann Arbor: Blackwell Science; 1996. p. 28–51

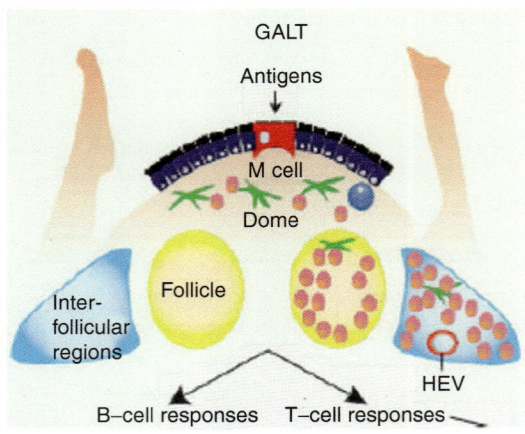

Fig. 2.2 Inductive site of the GALT (Neurath MF, Finotto S, Glimcher LH. The role of Th1/Th2 polarization in mucosal immunity. Nat Med. 2002;8:567–73)

almost exclusively polymeric forms of approximately equal proportions of IgA1 and IgA2 are found. Furthermore, specific antibodies to viral antigens, including HIV, are often found in the IgA1 subclass, whereas IgA2 antibodies in external secretions are associated with specificity for common structural microbial antigens as LPS and lipoteichoic acid.

propria and combined with the SC, a glycoprotein expressed on the surface of mucosal epithelial cells (ECs). This protein then handles the active transport of polymeric IgA into the intestinal lumen where IgA is released by proteolytic cleavage again. Investigations concerning the origin of S-IgA have demonstrated that it is produced locally at mucosal sites and is not derived to a significant degree from the circulation.

The two different molecular forms of IgA also show different effector functions, which is illustrated in Table 2.8.

IgA can also be divided into two subclasses IgA1 and IgA2 which differ in primary structure, carbohydrate composition, and their sensitiveness to bacterial proteases. Neisseria gonorrhoeae, for instance, is a producer of extra cellular proteases, specific for IgA which constitutes its most important phatogen factor, which is specific for IgA1. In serum, monomeric IgA1 predominates over IgA2 whereas in external secretions

2.2.2 Inductive Sites of the Mucosal Immune System: GALT

The primary inductive sites for mucosal immune responses are organized lymphoid aggregates such as Peyer's patches in the wall of the intestine or tonsils in the uppevr respiratory tract. The Peyer's patches of the GALT consist of a follicle-associated epithelium with specialized ECs known as membranovus epithelial (M) cells, a subepithelial dome overlying B-cell follicles, and interfollicular regions enriched in T cells (1528, Fig. 2.2). Following ingestion, antigens and microorganisms are transported from the gut lumen to the dome region through specialized M cells where they encounter APCs such as DCs leading to cognate interactions between APCs and T cells. DCs can also migrate to the interfollicular regions which are enriched with T cells and containing high endothelial venules (HEV) and efferent lymphatics to initiate immune responses upon antigen uptake. DCs as the APCs bind bacterial products with their TLRs, process antigen as relative imma- ture cells, and then migrate to the T cell region and present antigen to naive T cells. There they have the properties of mature and immunogenic DCs with high surface expression of costimulatory molecules such as CD40, CD80, and CD86 and adhesion molecules such as CD44.

After antigen uptake via M cells, B cells are induced to switch into IgA-secreting cells. Following IgA switch and affinity maturation, B cells migrate from the Peyer's patches to the mes- enteric lymph node via efferent lymphatic vessels and finally to the lamina propria where they undergo terminal differentiation to plasma cells. Peyer's patches are an enriched source of IgA pre- cursor cells capable of lodging in the recipient's gut as well as in other glands and mucosal tissue. Depending on the type of antigen and the duration of stimulation, ingestion of pathogens induce local and systemic immune responses with parallel appearance of specific S-IgA in saliva, milk, and tears, for example. The production of IgA is there- fore induced in lymphoid follicles such as the Peyer's patches from where the cells recirculate through lymph and blood to diffusely populate other mucosal tissues and exocrine glands where terminal differentiation into IgA plasma cells under the influence of locally produced cytokines occurs.

This provides the mucosal immune system with the ability to induce responses at sites that are distant from the immediate inductive envi- ronment, or even in different mucosal tissues. This has led to the concept of generalized func- tioning of mucosal tissues with some cross talk between them. Substantial dissemination of primed immune cells from GALT to exocrine effector sites beyond the gut is also the rationale for many desired oral vaccines.

2.2.3   Effector Sites of the Mucosal Immune System, in the Example of the GALT

Following induction in the MALT, mature lymphocytes leave the inductive sites and migrate to the effector sites such as the lamina propria where they can induce proinflammatory as well as suppressive immune responses. Effector mecha-

nisms that protect mucosal surfaces include CTLs and effector CD4+ T cells for cytokine production and IgA response. Lamina propria T cells are mainly CD4+ Th cells (60–70 %), the majority of which also express the TCR, just as in peripheral blood. However, lamina propria T cells are in a more activated state than blood lymphocytes and have a mature or memory phenotype, indicated by the surface markers CD44, CD62, and CD45RO+.

Cytotoxic CD8+ T cells account for about 30–40 % of T cells in the lamina propria. They con- trol the level of viral infection and have a cellular memory. A more restricted T-cell population, the intraepithelial lymphocytes (IEL), mainly CD8+ T cells, may play a role in maintenance of epithelial integrity and in class switching to IgA. Cytologically, they are T lymphocytes but their function is equiva- lent to NK cells of the innate immunity.

Besides an inflammatory phenotype T cells can adopt immunosuppressive function. These cells have been termed Treg cells, and it is cur- rently not clear if these cells are identical cell types or different immunoregulatory cells. Treg cells can actively inhibit activation or differentia- tion of other T cells and also express the CD25 marker besides their CD4 marker. Treg cells have been shown to produce large amounts of IL-10 and/or TGF-β, and their immunosuppressive properties are most likely explained by the ability of these cytokines to inhibit APC function and to mediate direct antiproliferative effects on T cells.

Another task which is presumably performed by T cells is the constant distinguishing of harm- less antigens in food and on commensal bacteria from pathogenic microbes. Oral tolerance is defined as the induction of a state of systemic immune nonresponsiveness to orally administered antigen upon subsequent antigen challenge. This mechanism seems to prevent the development of an immune reaction or allergy against intestinal intraluminal antigens. T cells appear to be the major target of tolerance and the reduction in anti- body responses after antigen exposition is due to the reduction in T helper activity rather than to a tolerization of B cell directly. In addition to active suppression by Treg cells, tolerance is also main- tained by deletion and anergy of T cells specific for luminal antigens. Deletion of specific T cells occurs by apoptosis whereas anergy of mucosal T

Table 2.9 Cytokine help for the regulation of mucosal immunoglobulin response

Th subset	Cytokine production	Effect on IgA response
Th1	IL-2	Synergizes with IL-5/TGF-β $\rightarrow$ IgA synthesis
	IFN-γ	Ig switch to IgG2a
	Lymphotoxin β	Development of Peyer's patches
Th2	IL-4, IL-5	Differentiation to plasma cells
	IL-6	IgA synthesis
	IL-10	IgA synthesis
Th3	TGF-β	IgA isotype switching
TR1	IL-10, TGF-β	Suppression of immune responses
		Downregulation of Th1

Adapted from Wittig BM, Zeitz M. The gut as an organ of immunology. Int J Colorectal Dis. 2003;18:181–7

cells is believed to be induced when cells are stimulated without proper costimulatory molecules.

2.2.4   Cytokine Regulation of the Gut Mucosal Immune Response

The differentiation into Th cells and Treg cells in the mucosa results in secretion of proinflammatory cytokines such as IFN-γ and TNF-α by Th1 cells; Th2 cells secrete IL-4, IL-5, IL-6, IL-10, and IL-13 and promote IgA expression, Treg cells secrete TGF-β, and Treg produce predominantly IL-10 (Table 2.9). Several reports suggest that the level and type of costimulation a naive T cell receives influences whether Th1, Th2, or Th17 cells develop. Further, different types of APCs may selectively trigger either Th1 or Th2 responses; however, the same APC cell can function equally well for inducing a Th1 or Th2 response.

Further Reading

Concepts of Innate and Specific Immunity

Aagaard-Tillery KM, Silver R, Dalton J. Immunology of normal pregnancy. Semin Fetal Neonatal Med. 2006;11:279–95.

Abbas AK, Lichtman AH, Pober JS. Immunologie. Bern/Göttingen/Toronto/Seattle: Verlag Hans Huber; 1996.

Akira S. Mammalian Toll-like receptors. Curr Opin Immunol. 2003;15:5–11.

Bellati F, Visconti V, Napoletano C, Antonilli M, Frati L, Panici PB, Nuti M. Immunology of gynecologic neoplasms: analysis of the prognostic significance of the immune status. Curr Cancer Drug Targets. 2009;9:541–65.

Dawson RD. Modern concepts of humoral and cellular immunity. In: Bronson RA, Alexander NJ, Anderson D, Branch DW, Kutteh WH, editors. Reproductive immunology. Ann Arbor: Blackwell Science; 1996. p. 3–27.

Finlay BB, Cossart P. Exploitation of mammalian host cell functions by bacterial pathogens. Science. 1997; 276:718–25.

Heine H, Lien E. Toll-like receptors and their function in innate and adaptive immunity. Int Arch Allergy Immunol. 2003;130:180–92.

Hughes A. Evolution of the host defense system. In: Kaufmann SHE, Sher A, Ahmed R, editors. Immunology of infectious diseases. Washington: ASM Press; 2002. p. 67–78.

Jablonowska B, Selbing A, Palfi M, Ernerudh J, Kjellberg S, Lindton B. Prevention of recurrent spontaneous abortion by intravenous immunoglobulin: a double blind, placebo-controlled study. Hum Reprod. 1999;14:838–41.

Adapted from Janeway CA Jr., Travers P. Immunologie. 2nd ed. Heidelberg: Berlin: Oxford; Spektrum Akademischer Verlag; 1997.

Janeway Jr CA, Medzhitov R. Innate immune recognition. Annu Rev Immunol. 2002;20:197–216.

Kaufmann SHE, Kabelitz D. The immune response to infectious agents. In: Kaufmann SHE, Kabelitz D, editors. Immunology of infection. Methods in microbiology, vol. 32. 2nd ed. London: Academic Press; 2002. p. 1–20.

Kaufmann SHE, Kabelitz D. The immune response to infectious agents. In: Kaufmann SHE, Kutteh WH, Mestecky J, editors. The concept of mucosal immunology. In: Bronson RA, Alexander NJ, Anderson D, Branch DW, Kutteh WH, editors. Reproductive immunology. Ann Arbor: Blackwell Science; 1996. p.28–51.

Lieu PT, Heiskala M, Peterson PA, Yang Y. The roles of iron in health and disease. Mol Aspects Med. 2001; 22:1–87.

Medzhitov R, Biron CA. Innate immunity. Curr Opin Immunol. 2003;15:2–4.

Naccasha N, Gervasi MT, Chaiworapongsa T, Berman S, Yoon BH, Maymon E, et al. Phenotypic and metabolic characteristics of monocytes and granulocytes in normal pregnancy and maternal infection. Am J Obstet Gynecol. 2001;185:1118–23.

Neurath MF, Finotto S, Glimcher LH. The role of Th1/Th2 polarization in mucosal immunity. Nat Med. 2002;8:567–73.

Neutra MR, Kraehenbuhl JP. Regional immune response to microbial pathogens. In: Kaufmann SHE, Sher A,

Ahmed R, editors. Immunology of infectious diseases. Washington: ASM Press; 2002. p. 191–206.

Roitt I. Essential immunology. 8th ed. Oxford: Blackwell Science; 1994.

Rouse BT, Suvas S. Regulatory T cells and infectious agents: détentes cordiale and contraire. J Immunol. 2004;173:2211–5.

Saito S, Nakashima A, Ito M, Shima T. Clinical implication of recent advances in our understanding of IL-17 and reproductive immunology. Expert Rev Clin Immunol. 2011;7:649–57.

Schöllmann C, Stauder G, Schäffer A, Schwarz G, Rusch K, Peters U. Grundlagen der Immunologie. Ein Repetitorium. Germering: Forum Medizin; 2004.

Talmage DW. The acceptance and rejection of immunological concepts. Annu Rev Immunol. 1986;4:1–11.

Tomasi TB. The immune system of secretions. Englewood Cliffs/New York: Prentice-Hall; 1976.

Watts C. Capture and processing of exogenous antigens for presentation on MHC molecules. Annu Rev Immunol. 1997;15:821–50.

Mucosal Immunology

Abbas AK, Lichtman AH, Pober JS. Immunologie. Bern/Göttingen/Toronto/Seattle: Verlag Hans Huber; 1996.

Cheroutre H. IELs: enforcing law and order in the court of the intestinal epithelium. Immunol Rev. 2005;206:114–31.

Dawson RD. Modern concepts of humoral and cellular immunity. In: Bronson RA, Alexander NJ, Anderson D, Branch DW, Kutteh WH, editors. Reproductive immunology. Ann Arbor: Blackwell Science; 1996. p. 3–27.

Heller F, Duchmann R. Intestinal flora and mucosal immune responses. Int J Med Microbiol. 2003;293:77–86.

Kaufmann SHE, Kabelitz D. The immune response to infectious agents. In: Kaufmann SHE, Kabelitz D, editors. Immunology of infection. Methods in microbiology, vol. 32. 2nd ed. London: Academic Press; 2002. p. 1–20.

Kutteh WH, Mestecky J. The concept of mucosal immunology. In: Bronson RA, Alexander NJ, Anderson D, Branch DW, Kutteh WH, editors. Reproductive immunology. Ann Arbor: Blackwell Science; 1996. p. 28–51.

Kutteh WH, Prince SJ, Hammonds KR, Kutteh CC, Mestecky J. Variations in immunoglobulins and IgA subclasses of human uterine cervical secretions around the time of ovulation. Clin Exp Immunol. 1996;104: 538–42.

Liu YJ, Kanzler H, Soumelis V, Gilliet M. Dendritic cell lineage, plasticity and cross-regulation. Nat Immunol. 2001;2:585–9.

Lutz MB, Schuler G. Immature, semi-mature and fully mature dendritic cells: which signals induce tolerance or immunity? Trends Immunol. 2002;23:445–9.

Maloy KJ, Powrie F. Regulatory T cells in the control of immune pathology. Nat Immunol. 2001;2:816–22.

Mestecky J, Fultz PN. Mucosal immune system of the human genital tract. J Infect Dis. 1999;179 Suppl 3: S470–4.

Mestecky J, Russell MW. Immunoglobulins and mechanisms of mucosal immunity. Biochem Soc Trans. 1997;25:457–62.

Naccasha N, Gervasi MT, Chaiworapongsa T, Berman S, Yoon BH, Maymon E, et al. Phenotypic and metabolic characteristics of monocytes and granulocytes in normal pregnancy and maternal infection. Am J Obstet Gynecol. 2001;185:1118–23.

Neurath MF, Finotto S, Glimcher LH. The role of Th1/Th2 polarization in mucosal immunity. Nat Med. 2002;8:567–73.

Revaz V, Nardelli-Haefliger D. The importance of mucosal immunity in defense against epithelial cancers. Curr Opin Immunol. 2005;17:175–9.

Roitt I. Essential immunology. 8th ed. Oxford: Blackwell Science; 1994.

Rouse BT, Suvas S. Regulatory T cells and infectious agents: détentes cordiale and contraire. J Immunol. 2004;173:2211–5.

Salamonsen LA, Butt AR, Hammond FR, Garcia S, Zhang J. Production of endometrial matrix metalloproteinases but not their tissue inhibitors is modulated by progesterone withdrawal in an in vitro model for menstruation. J Clin Endocrinol Metab. 1997;82: 1409–15.

Schöllmann C, Stauder G, Schäffer A, Schwarz G, Rusch K, Peters U. Grundlagen der Immunologie. Ein Repetitorium. Germering: Forum Medizin; 2004.

Talmage DW. The acceptance and rejection of immunological concepts. Annu Rev Immunol. 1986;4:1–11.

Tomasi TB. The immune system of secretions. Englewood cliffs/New York: Prentice-Hall; 1976.

Watts C. Capture and processing of exogenous antigens for presentation on MHC molecules. Annu Rev Immunol. 1997;15:821–50.

Wittig BM, Zeitz M. The gut as an organ of immunology. Int J Colorectal Dis. 2003;18:181–7.

General Immunology of the Genital Tract

Contents

The female genital tract was long neglected as a subject of studies but its importance in the human immune system has increasingly been recognized in recent years. Advances in female genital tract immunology may have implications for other related research fields such as the immunology of genital infections and the immunology of pregnancy. Especially the continuously rising number of STDs indicates the need for further investigations in this field.

It is now established that the mucosal immune system is a distinct and separate component of the host's immune apparatus and differs from the lymphoid tissues in peripheral sites which contribute to the antibody isotypes found in the blood circulation. Furthermore, regulation of the mucosal immune system is different from that of the systemic immune system. The mucosal immune system can be divided into discrete inductive sites where antigens or vaccines are endocytosed, processed, and presented to B and T cells and separate effector areas where immune cells actually function.

Protection against potential pathogens in the female reproductive tract is provided by a variety of measures that can be grouped into the two broad categories of innate and adaptive immunity. The innate immune system differs from the adaptive immune system in the cells involved, the type and specificity of receptors for antigen, and the immediacy and nature of the response to antigenic challenge. Recognized as the first line of defense, the innate immune system functions to prevent and control the invasion of pathogens. It has evolved to recognize foreign structures, the so-called PAMPs, via pattern-recognition receptors of the host expressed on cells of the innate immune system, the TLRs. Signaling through TLRs in response to PAMPs involves a number of adapters and other molecules that lead to recruitment of immune cells as well as the production of intracellular and secreted antimicrobial factors that both kill invading microbes and link innate and acquired immunity. Adaptive immunity encompasses pathogen-specific defense mechanisms.

Of the mucosal surfaces in the body, the female reproductive tract has unique requirements for the regulation of immune protection because it must deal with sexually transmitted bacterial and viral pathogens, allogeneic spermatozoa, and the immunologically distinct fetus. The immune system of the female genital tract is the least understood part of the mucosal immune system with respect to the origin of its immune cells, the role of tissue CTL responses, the induction of antibody responses, and the contribution of serum-derived versus mucosally produced antibodies. Although it is considered a part of the common mucosal immune system, it offers some distinct features indicative of its special role.

3.1 Distinct Features of the Genital Mucosal Tissue

Mucosal surfaces have evolved to handle potential pathogens against a background of selective physiological functions. The mucosal immune system of the female genital tract has developed to meet the unique requirements of dealing with the presence of a resident population of bacteria in the vagina as well as with the presence of sexually transmitted pathogens. It also has to deal with bacteria and semen, allogeneic spermatozoa, and long-term exposure of an immunologically distinct fetus.

- The lower genital tract in women is comprised of four discrete anatomical regions:
- The introitus, which is covered by a keratinized stratified squamous epithelium resembling skin
- The vaginal mucosa, which is covered by an aglandular nonkeratinized stratified squamous epithelium
- The ectocervix, which is covered by a mucosal layer histological similar to that of the vagina
- The endocervix, which consists of simple columnar epithelium with numerous glands

The transformation zone represents an abrupt transition between the ectocervix and endocervix. The susceptibility of these regions to infectious microorganisms differs. The transformation zone is the main target of high-risk human papillomavirus (HPV) infection whereas *Candida albicans* and Trichomonas vaginalis colonize the vagina, and the cervix is susceptible to infection by Chlamydia trachomatis and Neisseria gonorrhoeae. Among the tissues of the female reproductive tract, the upper genital tract consisting of the endometrium, myometrium, fallopian tubes, and ovary needs to be investigated as well. Separate compartments have evolved to meet the different challenges and are precisely regulated by the endocrine system.

The reproductive tract has various systems of defense against the risk of infection, which are complementary and synergistic. These defenses comprise nonimmune strategies, namely, passive factors such as pH, mucus, and epithelial

Table 3.1 Comparative characteristic features of humoral compartments of the human genital and intestinal tract

	Genital tract	Intestinal tract
Dominant Ig isotype	IgG ≥ IgA	IgA >>> IgG
Hormonal regulation	+++	–
Contribution of Ig from the circulation	++ (50 %)	– (1 %)
Inductive site for local and generalized humoral responses	– to +	++
Effector site	+	++
Expression of homing receptors on lymphocytes and ligands on ECs	LFA-1, ICAM-1, VCAM-1, α4β1	CCR9, CCR10, CCL25, CCL28, MAdCAM-1 α4β7, αEβ7
Response after intranasal immunization	++	+
Dominant function	Resident commensal flora in vagina vs exposure to sexually transmitted pathogens	Induction of effective cell-mediated and antibody-mediated immune responses toward selected antigens
	Acceptance of histoincompatible sperm/ allogeneic fetus	Oral tolerance

Adapted from Lamm ME, Mestecky J. Immunology and immunopathology of the genitourinary tract: an overview. In: Mestecky J, Lamm ME, Strober W, Bienenstock J, McGhee JR, Mayer L, editors. Handbook of mucosal immunology. Oxford: Elsevier Academic Press; 2005. p. 1575–7 and Mestecky J, Moldoveanu Z, Russell MW. Immunologic uniqueness of the genital tract: challenge for vaccine development. Am J Reprod Immunol. 2005;53:208–14

barrier on the one hand as well as active factors such as secretion of humoral soluble factors on the other. Innate immune strategies are also involved in rapid protection before specific antigenic stimulation. Following these initial immunological strategies of defense, acquired and antigen-specific immunity is induced along with associated humoral responses with S-IgA/ IgM and locally produced IgG as well as cellular immune responses. The latest knowledge of these lines of defense will be reviewed here.

Although the genital tract is considered to be a component of the mucosal immune system, it displays several distinct features not shared by other mucosal tissues or the systemic compartment. Differences include the endogenous microbial flora, the predominance of IgG, hormonal fluctuations that may modify mucosal immunity, and the need to be tolerant of sperm and to a developing fetus but also the ability to respond to sexually transmitted bacterial and viral pathogens.

Despite the fact that the genital and intestinal tracts share a common embryologic origin and remain in anatomical proximity, these two compartments display distinct immunological features that reflect their very different physiological functions (Table 3.1).

A major difference between the genital tract and the intestinal tract is the compartmentalization of the genital mucosa: part of the genital mucosa is generally believed to be sterile, lacking the presence of a microbial flora. The female reproductive tract can thus be divided into two compartments, the vagina and ectocervix, which host a commensal flora with predominantly lactobacilli in most women that may play an important part in host defense, and the endocervix, uterus, and fallopian tubes, which are sterile, lacking the presence of a microbial flora.

Sterility in the endocervix depends on the hormonal phases of the menstrual cycle, which will be discussed in further detail later. The epithelium of the vagina and ectocervix therefore is required to provide a strong barrier whereas the epithelium of the uterus and endocervix is less afflicted by microorganisms. A sophisticated barrier function is also provided by the cervical mucus that filters bacteria but allows sperm to ascend to the uterus. The endocervix, uterus, and fallopian tubes respond to bacteria with distinct patterns of cytokines and chemokines.

Several basic characteristics of mucosal immunity in the intestine and respiratory tract are absent in the genital tract. Mucosal lymphoid nodules and M cells for antigen uptake overlaying organized lymphoid tissue like in the intestinal tract are missing in the reproductive tract. There are lymphoid aggregates in the basal layers of the uterus but their presence and distribution strongly varies under hormonal influence. Besides lymphoid aggregates, the genital tract mucosa contains APCs such as macrophages and DCs as well as genital ECs. Due to the specialized functions of the genital tract immune system, it seems reasonable to assume that this system hosts unique regulatory cells. Both pregnancy and infection are associated with increased numbers or alterations of function of T cells which is discussed later.

The mucosal immune system of the female genital tract is under strong hormonal control that regulates the transport of Ig, the levels of cytokines, the distribution of various cell populations, and antigen presentation in the genital tissues during the reproductive cycle. In addition to protecting against infectious agents, it must adapt to a spectrum of physiological events that includes semen deposition, fertilization, implantation, pregnancy, and parturition. A balance is maintained by sex hormones throughout the menstrual cycle to respond to the challenges of bacteria, yeast, and viruses without interfering with events that surround conception. The hormonal influence on the ability to respond to antigen is considerable, because vaginal immunization only in the follicular, but not in the luteal, phase gave strong local IgA antibody responses. Also the ability to present antigen is a property that is under strong hormonal control.

Although sometimes disputed, several studies have revealed that human urine, seminal plasma, and cervicovaginal washings collected at various stages of the menstrual cycle contain IgG rather than IgA as the dominant isotype. In contrast to the predominance of IgA-producing cells in most mucosal tissues, the endocervix was found to contain a high proportion of IgG-secreting cells whose product, IgG, reaches the cervical fluid by a currently unknown mechanism.

3.2   Functions and Regulations of Innate Immune Responses in the Human Reproductive Tract

While much attention has been paid to innate immune function in other mucosal tissues like the lung and intestine, few studies have investigated presence and function of the innate immune system in the female reproductive tract. What is becoming more clear is that the innate immune system is present throughout the reproductive tract and functions in synchrony with the adaptive immune system to provide protection in a way that enhances fetal survival while protecting against potential pathogens.

The focus of this section is on the different cells of the innate immune system defining the role of ECs, macrophages, DCs, neutrophils, and NK cells throughout the female reproductive tract; their functions and regulation during the menstrual cycle; and the ways in which these cells communicate with the adaptive immune system.

3.2.1   Epithelial Cells in Mucosal Immunity

The epithelium of the endocervix, uterus, and fallopian tubes is composed of polarized ECs connected by tight junctions. This single cell layer was initially thought to reside in a sterile environment that was only infrequently exposed to bacteria constitutively present in the ectocervix and vagina. However, studies demonstrate that polarized ECs of the reproductive tract are exposed to bacteria at a frequency not previously appreciated. Nevertheless, routine histological analysis has determined that the uterus and fallopian tubes have a relatively low incidence of chronic infections.

Once thought to function only by providing a physical barrier between the lumen and internal tissue, mucosal ECs are now known to be a part of the mucosal immune system, protecting against the microorganisms present throughout the reproductive tract. They function as sentinels that recognize antigen and also produce antimicrobial molecules that leads to either killing or inactivation of the pathogen. They have the ability to signal to underlying immune cells when pathogenic challenge exceeds their protective capacity. Estradiol and progesterone regulate epithelial cell proliferation, apoptosis, secretions, and effects on pathogenic microbes. Finally, uterine ECs are involved, through their cytokine and chemokine secretions, in normal physiological processes such as menstruation and receptivity.

3.2.1.1 Epithelial Cells as a Mechanical Barrier

Throughout the reproductive tract, ECs form an uninterrupted physical barrier between the lumen and underlying cell layers. This aims at preventing opportunistic and pathogenic microbes from infiltrating the body. However, they also permit the transport of sperm or ovum to the site of fertilization and implantation or support the conceptus through gestation.

Each site of the female reproductive tract has an unique morphological form of ECs. Whereas the vagina and the lower part of the cervix are lined with stratified squamous ECs, the uterus and fallopian tubes as well as the upper part of the cervix have a columnar epithelium. For the integrity of these cell formations, the presence and maintenance of tight junctions are essential. Paracellular permeability is regulated by these apical epithelial intercellular junctions which form a regulated, semipermeable barrier and act as a fence that segregates protein components of the apical and basolateral plasma membrane domains. Built of several different proteins, tight junctions seal off the lumen from the basolateral compartment. However, this barrier is continuously regulated by calcium, cytokines, leukocytes, and, above all, hormones.

When established in culture, ECs from the female genital tract form polarized monolayers with distinct luminal and basolateral surfaces. They also establish an electrochemical gradient and a transepithelial resistance (TER) which illustrates the tightness of the epithelial barrier. Interestingly, estradiol significantly decreased TER (and therefore EC layer integrity) within 24 h when incubated with polarized uterine ECs from mice, whereas other sex hormones had no effect. ICI 182,780, an estradiol receptor (ER) antagonist, neutralized this effect, whereas incubation with progesterone, cortisol, aldosterone, and dihydrotestosterone had no effect on uterine epithelial TER. This demonstrated that epithelial monolayer integrity is directly influenced by estradiol via ER, which suggests a cycle dependency.

3.2.1.2 Stromal Cell Regulation of Epithelial Cell Function

Stromal cells and ECs in the genital tract act as a single unit with each cell type, producing factors to regulate each other. The stroma is critically important for endometrial function by influencing epithelial development and differentiation. Conversely, ECs influence stroma cell function through soluble factors and cell–cell contact. Stromal cells from neonatal tissues are able to change the phenotype of adult epithelium. Regional differentiation in the reproductive tract epithelium is therefore directed by the inductive capability of the stroma. Uterine stromal cells also communicate with ECs via soluble factors to maintain epithelial barrier function, i.e., TER, and secretory activity. Previous studies showed that human uterine stromal cells modulate the barrier function of ECs by decreasing TER.

Also stromal cells influence the release of the cytokines TNF-α and TGF-β by ECs. Mouse uterine ECs, which reach confluence as indicated by high TER, release TGF-β into the basolateral compartment and TNF-α into the apical lumen. When brought together with mouse uterine stromal cells in culture, the release of TNF-α by ECs decreased whereas the amount of released TGF-β was not affected. This indicated that uterine stromal cells communicate with ECs via soluble factors to maintain uterine barrier function and epithelial secretory activity. They produce soluble factors that regulate EC TER and release of TNF-α without effecting TGF-β release.

The proliferation of ECs due to estrogen is also dependent on underlying stromal cells and their release of mediators. Several studies

suggested that estrogen regulation of EC proliferation is mediated indirectly by uterine stroma.
Also mediated by uterine stroma is the effect of
estradiol on EC TNF-α release. While estradiol
treatment on ECs alone led to a significant
decrease in TER, the amount of released TNF-α
did not change. But when ECs were cocultured
together with stromal cells and treated with estradiol, apical TNF-α release was significantly
decreased. However, the amount of released
TGF-β was not altered by estradiol. Estradiol
directly influences epithelial electrical integrity
whereas its effect on TNF-α release is dependent
on the presence of uterine stromal cells. Estradiol
acts through the ER to regulate uterine growth
and functional differentiation. Epithelial ER is
neither necessary nor sufficient for estradiol-
induced uterine epithelial proliferation. Instead,
estradiol induction of epithelial proliferation
appears to be a paracrine event mediated by
ER-positive stroma.

Stromal fibroblasts release soluble factors
such as hepatocyte growth factor (HGF), insulin-
like growth factor (IGF), and keratinocyte growth
factor (KGF) as mediators of estrogen-induced
proliferation of uterine ECs. HGF, a mesenchy-
mal growth factor, is expressed by uterine stromal cells and mediates EC proliferation via HGF
receptor. HGF was shown to increase TER so that
it was concluded that stromal cells act through
HGF receptors on ECs to increase TER. At the
same time, HGF was shown to decrease apical
TNF-α release. Both effects could be blocked by
incubating epithelial and/or stromal cells with
anti-HGF or anti-HGF receptor antibody. HGF
receptor, which is located at the basolateral surface of ECs, seems to mediate the effect of HGF
on TER and TNF-α release. Moreover, as neutralization of stromal media failed to affect
TNF-α secretion, these results suggest that other
growth factors, in addition to HGF, affect EC
cytokine production.

3.2.1.3 Production of Antimicrobial Molecules

To encounter microbial pathogens, the genital
tract ECs produce soluble innate immune factors
with microbicidal effects. Among these secre-

tions of ECs that inhibit the growth of pathogens
are the enzymes lysozyme and lactoferrin, defensins, secretory leukocyte protease inhibitor
(SLPI), and the tracheal antimicrobial peptide
(TAP), among other peptides.

3.2.1.3.1 Defensins

Defensins, also called "natural antibiotics," are
small cationic peptides with proven effectiveness
against bacteria, fungi, and some viruses and
contribute to mucosal immune responses at epithelial sites. Defensins are abundant in microbicidal granules of polymorphonuclear leukocytes
and epithelia, including human intestinal Paneth
cells and bovine tracheal epithelium. Human
defensins can be divided into two classes, the α-
and β-defensins, which are both expressed in ECs
and granulocytic leukocytes. The crucial step in
defensin-mediated antimicrobial activity and
cytotoxicity is the permeabilization of target
membranes; they kill pathogens by creating pores
in their membranes. ECs at mucosal surfaces,
and especially in the genital tract, produce human
β-defensin (HBD)-1 and HBD-2. HBD-1 is an
essential part of epithelial secretions in the genitourinary tract and present in the epithelial layers
of the vagina, cervix, uterus, and fallopian tubes
as well as in vaginal secretions. The highest concentrations of HBD-1 were noted in the urine of
pregnant women, intermediate concentrations in
nonpregnant women, and the lowest concentration in men. Exposure to microbial products,
microtrauma, and hormonal influences may regulate HBD-1 synthesis. HBD-2 was originally isolated from psoriatic skin lesions and is inducibly
expressed in inflamed skin lesions and lung tissues upon treatment with bacterial LPS and cytokines. Its expression is increased by infection or
inflammation sites, for example, in the endometrium. HBD-2 is a potent chemoattractant of
human neutrophils.

The expression of these defensins seems to be
regulated by cycle-associated changes in sex hormones and influenced by contraceptive use.
HBD-1 expression was highest during the secretory phase while HBD-2 expression peaks during
menstruation. The use of the oral contraceptive
pill downregulated expression of both HBD-1

and HBD-2, which may among other factors contribute to altered susceptibility to infection. Concerning HBD-3 and HBD-4, it was shown that HBD-3 messenger ribonucleic acid (mRNA) expression in the human endometrium is highest during the secretory stage of the menstrual cycle, and HBD-4 mRNA expression peaks in the proliferative phase. Expression is altered due to hormonal contraceptive use which may contribute to differential infection rates in oral contraception users relative to nonusers. HBD-3 is also upregulated during infection, allowing an increased immune response.

Concerning the α-defensins, leukocytes express human neutrophil peptides (HNP) 1–4 whereas human defensin (HD)-5 and HD-6 are expressed mainly by intestinal cells. HD-5 has been detected in female genital tract epithelia with variable expression in the upper genital tract but also in the lower genital tract. It was also found in cervicovaginal lavages (CVL), with its highest concentration during the secretory phase of the menstrual cycle. In addition to their bactericidal activity, defensins also have multiple functions in innate immunity. For example, β-defensins are chemotactic for immature DCs and memory T cells by binding to the chemokine receptor CCR6. Uterine ECs also produce CCL20/macrophage inflammatory protein (MIP) 3α, a chemokine ligand of CCR6, which has significant homology to defensins and has been shown to have antimicrobial activity.

3.2.1.3.2 SLPI

SLPI is a neutrophil elastase inhibitor which also has antibacterial and antiinflammatory properties. It is produced not only by macrophages but also by uterine and cervical ECs and is active against a variety of pathogens including gram-positive and gram-negative bacteria and HIV-1.

King showed that the primary site of SLPI synthesis in the endometrium is the glandular epithelium and that secretory peaks are higher in the progesterone-dominated late secretory phase than in the proliferative phase of the menstrual cycle. Expression of endometrial SLPI has been shown to be upregulated by estrogen in the rat and by progesterone in the human. Studies also demonstrated that uterine SLPI production in premenopausal women was significantly higher than in postmenopausal women. These results confirm that expression of SLPI varies in cervical mucus during the different stages of the menstrual cycle and with menstrual status. Furthermore, SLPI concentrations increase in amniotic fluid during gestation and labor. This may be to modulate proinflammatory paracrine interactions needed for the maintenance of pregnancy and limit those occurring at parturition within the uterus. There is also a positive correlation between SLPI expression and implantation as well as early pregnancy which could be a benefit due to its antibiotic action and antiinflammatory effects of inhibiting elastase and nuclear factor-κB (NF-κB). NF-κB is a transcription factor that induces production of inflammatory cytokines in response to pathogens.

3.2.1.3.3 Surfactant Proteins A and D

Previous studies have demonstrated the essential role of surfactant protein A (SP-A), a member of the collectin family of proteins, in protecting the respiratory system from infections. SP-A has been identified in two layers of vaginal epithelium which makes SP-A an essential component of the host defense system in the genital tract as well. SP-A can facilitate phagocytosis by opsonizing bacteria, fungi, and viruses. It can also modulate proinflammatory cytokine production by phagocytic cells and provides a link between innate and adaptive immunity by promoting differentiation and chemotaxis of DCs. SP-D, originally detected in alveolar cells type II, has also been demonstrated in cells lining the epithelium and secretory glands in the vagina, cervix, uterus, fallopian tubes, and ovaries. The endometrial presence of SP-D varied according to stage of menstrual cycle with highest concentrations in the secretory phase. SP-D may play a role in preventing intrauterine infection at the time of implantation and during pregnancy.

3.2.1.4 Cytokine and Chemokine Production

In the reproductive tract, growth factors and cytokines are synthesized in abundance at almost every level. There is evidence that they are not only regulators of immune function but also local modulators of steroid hormone action. Cytokines are small secreted proteins regulating immunity, inflammation, and hematopoiesis by acting either on the cells that secrete them (autocrine action), on nearby cells (paracrine action), or on distant cells (endocrine action). Although still considered a subclass of cytokines, chemokines are developing their own identity. Their hallmark is their ability to induce chemotaxis, but they are also involved in cellular proliferation and differentiation, angiogenesis, and inflammation. The known chemokines form a large subsets of cytokines and basically consist of four families, CC, C, CXC, and CXXXC, and their corresponding receptors (-R) and ligands (-L). The CC chemokines are functionally and structurally different from the CXC chemokines, stimulating multiple cell types such as monocytes, lymphocytes, basophils, and eosinophils. In contrast, most of the CXC chemokines are specifically chemotactic for neutrophils with only minor effects on other cells.

Cytokines are the mediators of communication between ECs as the first line of defense and other immune cells. They are produced by ECs, macrophages, T lymphocytes, and epithelial cells and act through different receptors in the reproductive tract to regulate differentiation, maturation, and recruitment of lymphocytes. Cytokine and adhesion molecule expression are also decisive for endometrial growth in preparation for fertilization, implantation, and successful pregnancy but also for the renewal of the uterus during each menstrual cycle.

Several studies described the production of numerous cytokines including granulocyte–macrophage colony-stimulating factor (GM-CSF), granulocyte colony-stimulating factor (G-CSF), TNF-α, IL-1, IL-6, leukemia inhibitory factor (LIF), and TGF-β and of chemokines such as MIP-1β, monocyte chemoattractant protein-1 (MCP-1), RANTES (regulation upon activation, normal T cell expressed and secreted), and IL-8 by endometrium ECs. They are constitutively produced by the polarized ECs, preferentially secreted apically, and contribute to the resident and temporary populations of immune cells in the subepithelial layers of the endometrium, for example, by recruiting neutrophils, monocytes, and T cells. Besides HBD-2, another chemokine of uterine ECs, MIP3α/CCL20, attracts B cells, memory T cells, and immature bone marrow-derived DCs. Its levels were significantly increased together with levels of TNF-α by the presence of *Escherichia coli* and PAMPs. Chemokines could also account for the influx of leukocytes and lymphocytes that form lymphoid aggregates observed during the secretory phase of endometrium. IL-8 and MCP-1 among others are produced by endometrial, myometrial, and trophoblast cells which also display specific roles in endometrial angiogenesis, apoptosis, proliferation, and differentiation. IL-8 takes part in cervical ripening and parturition and is also found at high levels in the peritoneal fluid of women with endometriosis. Besides mesothelial cells that form the majority of the peritoneal cells, macrophages and endometrial cells are potential sources of this chemokine. There are menstrual cycle-dependent changes in IL-8 mRNA in the endometrium. IL-8 mRNA levels in the late secretory and early to mid-proliferative phase samples are higher than the level observed in the middle of the cycle. IL-8 may modulate the timely recruitment of neutrophils and lymphocytes into the endometrium.

Endometrial, stromal and epithelial cells produce IL-6 in response to hormones and other activators. Besides its role in inflammation and cell differentiation of immunocompetent cells, IL-6 also regulates ovarian steroid production, folliculogenesis, and embryo implantation. Endometrial stromal cell IL-6 is induced by IL-1β or IL-1α, TNF, platelet-derived growth factor (PDGF), and IFN-γ. IL-6 inhibits the proliferation of human endometrial stromal cells, dependent on cell density, which suggests that IL-6 may play a role in epithelial–stromal interaction in the uterus. IL-6 fluctuations during the menstrual cycle reflect an inverse relationship with estrogen action; IL-6 levels are high during the secretory phase and low during the proliferative phase. Interestingly, IL-6 has no effect on the growth of endometrial stromal cells from the proliferative phase, but it inhibits proliferation of endometrial stromal cells from the secretory phase.

Concentrations of cytokines and chemokines vary in the endometrium during physiological processes as well as in pathological conditions. Many cytokines such as GM-CSF, TNF-α, TGF-β, and LIF show temporal release patterns and are regulated by sex hormones. Four different patterns of cytokine expression related to the menstrual cycle were identified in CVL obtained from healthy ovulating women:

- LIF, RANTES, and MIP-1α are detectable at menses only.
- IL-8, IL-6, TGF-β, and IL-1β are detected throughout the cycle but at highest levels at menses.
- M-CSF and epidermal growth factor (EGF) are found throughout the cycle but peak during the late proliferative phase.
- IFN-γ and TNF-α are detectable in a subpopulation of women during non-menses stages of the cycle and may be associated with inflammatory events.

Progesterone withdrawal results in upregulation of MCP-1 and IL-8, leading to chemotaxis and activation of monocytes and neutrophils. A correlation between high levels of IL-6, IL-8, and MCP-1 and amniotic microbial infections has been found in cervicovaginal fluids and amniotic fluids from women in preterm labor. However, low cervicovaginal concentrations of IL-6 and IL-8 were found in patients with chorioamnionitis in early pregnancy. The conclusion was that low concentrations of multiple cytokines indicated a broad immune hyporesponsiveness that could create a permissive environment for infection whereas high levels correlated with a dangerous infection.

Among other cytokines, GM-CSF, which regulates granulocyte and macrophage proliferation, is released by ECs of the pregnant and nonpregnant uterus in mice. They also demonstrated that GM-CSF synthesis and release by uterine EC cultures is stimulated by estrogen and moderately inhibited by progesterone. GM-CSF can synergize the effect of IL-8 of attracting neutrophils. TNF-α plays a dominant role in inflammatory processes and has been demonstrated in both normal pregnancies and conditions of pregnancy loss. It is also promoted by estrogen in uterine

mast cells whereas studies in macrophages suggested that TNF-α expression is unaffected by estrogen but inhibited by progesterone. TGF-β seems to regulate cellular proliferation, migration, differentiation, and protein expression. Diethylstilbestrol, a synthetic estrogen, was shown to increase TGF-β mRNA expression and protein for TGF-β1, TGF-β2, and TGF-β3 in the immature mouse uterus.

3.2.1.5 Regulation of Ig Secretions into the Lumen

At genital tract mucosal surfaces, the polymeric Ig receptor (pIgR), a transmembrane glycoprotein in ECs, is responsible for transporting polymeric IgA across ECs. The secretory component (SC), as the external part of the pIgR, is synthesized by ECs and tends to accumulate in the apical compartment, especially in the endocervix and ectocervix. It binds polymeric IgA at the basolateral surface of ECs and builds a receptor–ligand complex which is internalized and transported to the apical surface. There the ectoplasmic portion of the receptor is cleaved from the transmembrane and cytoplasmic component.

The female sex hormones estradiol and progesterone influence the local production and Ig transport in ECs in the reproductive tract. During the estrous cycle and after the administration of estradiol in rats, IgA, SC, and IgG accumulations are stimulated in the uterine lumen and are inhibited in cervicovaginal secretions (CVS).

In the uterus, estradiol increases vascular permeability, which results in serum transudation of IgA and IgG into the uterine tissues. In contrast, movement of IgA and IgG in CVS is inhibited by estradiol and progesterone. Estrogen was found to increase expression of pIgR and SC expression and therefore IgA transport into the lumen when ECs were cultured with IL-4 and IFN-γ. IgG, however, moves down a concentration gradient from the blood to the uterine lumen under the influence of estrogen.

Ig levels in cervical mucus correspond to hormonal fluctuations during the human menstrual cycle. Peak concentrations of IgA and IgG occur approximately 1 day before the estradiol peak around ovulation and decrease from the time of ovulation in cervical mucus secretions of nor-mal ovulating women. The decrease of Ig levels could represent an effect of dilution secondary to the increased volume of cervical mucus and estradiol produced at the time of ovulation. When compared with women on birth control pills, the mean peak of IgA detected was about one-third less in normal ovulating women. This supports the general agreement that reproductive hor-mones enhance immunity.

3.2.1.6 Antigen Presentation

As mentioned previously, the role of APCs throughout the body as well as at mucosal sur-faces is central to the generation of immune pro-tection. An effective immune response requires that exogenous antigen is internalized, processed, and returned to the cell surface of APCs in asso-ciation with MHC class II for recognition by CD4+ T cells. It can also stimulate MHC class I-restricted T cell activation after uptake by APCs via a phagocytic pathway. After antigen presenta-tion, lymphocyte effector functions including cytokine production, cytotoxicity, and antibody synthesis are activated.

By analogy to a primary immune response in MALT, antigen reaching the submucosa of the vagina is taken up by APCs, which then migrate to draining lymph nodes. Once in the lymph nodes, the APCs stimulate B and T lymphocytes, including memory subpopulations, that enter the bloodstream via the efferent lymph and thoracic duct. These T and B lymphocytes migrate to the genital tract and, on exposure to the antigen, par-ticipate in a secondary immune response.

Experiments that investigated mixed cell sus-pensions from throughout the genital tract found cells capable of presenting foreign of antigen to autologous T cells independent menstrual status. Isolated uterine ECs expressed MHC class II anti-gen and were able to process and present tetanus toxoid to T cells, as well as cells from the baso-lateral subepithelial stroma. This was supported by the finding that preparations of endometrial ECs without being contaminated with profes-sional APCs such as DCs or macrophages pre-sented tetanus toxoid to autologous T cells. ECs also had the ability to express CD1d and CD40

which shows that these cells interact with CD8+ T cells. In addition to MHC class II molecules, CD40 and CD1d proteins are another family of antigen-presenting molecules that bind bacterial and lipid antigens for presentation to T cells.

In contrast to the intestinal tract, the mucosal immune system of the female genital tract is under the hormonal control of:
(a) The sex hormones estrogen and progester-one, which regulate the transport of Igs, the levels of cytokines, the distribution of vari-ous cell populations, and antigen presenta-tion in the genital tissues during the reproductive cycle.
(b) Soluble factors from stromal cells. Isolated uterine and vaginal cells from ovariecto-mized rats treated with estrogen were incu-bated with sensitized T cells.

ECs from animals treated with estrogen pre-sented more antigen than did ECs from saline con-trols. In contrast, uterine stromal and vaginal cells from estrogen-treated animals presented fewer antigens than the saline control group. Estradiol enhances antigen presentation by ECs of rat uter-ine at a time when uterine and vaginal stromal anti-gen presentation is inhibited. More recent studies demonstrated that stromal antigen presentation is regulated by cytokine production by ECs. In response to estrogen, uterine ECs produce TGF-β which suppresses underlying APCs in the stroma.

It can be concluded that uterine ECs as well as APCs in the uterine stroma and vagina are capable of presenting antigen which initiates an immune response in the female reproductive tract. Moreover, sex hormones play a principal role in regulating antigen presentation in the genital tract.

3.2.1.7 TLRs on Epithelial Cells

As mentioned above, TLRs are a family of inte-gral membrane receptors which can stimulate cytokine and chemokine production after ligand recognition. First, a Drosophila toll receptor made up of a type 1 transmembrane protein with a cyto-plasmic protein was described. Then, a human homologue of this receptor was similar to the IL-1 receptor. The Drosophila toll and human TLR both act through the NF-κB pathway. The ten known TLRs in humans comprise a family of

Table 3.2 Toll-like receptors and examples for their ligands

Receptor	Ligand	Origin of ligand
TLR1	Lipopeptides	Bacteria/ mycobacteria
	Soluble factors	*Neisseria meningitides*
TLR2	Lipopeptides	Various pathogens
	Lipoteichoic acid	Gram-positive bacteria
	Peptidoglycan	Gram-positive bacteria
	Zymosan	Fungi
	Lipoarabinomannan	Mycobacteria
TLR3	Double-stranded RNA	Viruses
TLR4	Lipopolysaccharide	Gram-negative bacteria
	Taxol	Plants
	Fusion protein	RS virus
TLR5	Flagellin	Bacteria
TLR6	Diacyl lipopeptides	Mycoplasma
	Lipoteichoic acid	Gram-positive bacteria
	Zymosan	Fungi
TLR7	Single-stranded RNA	Viruses
TLR8	Single-stranded RNA	Viruses
TLR9	CpG-containing DNA	Bacteria and viruses
TLR10	?	?
TLR11	?	Uropathogenic bacteria

Adapted from Akira S, Takeda K. Toll-like receptor signaling. Nat Rev Immunol. 2004;4:499–511
? Unknown

structurally related receptors that recognize specific products of pathogens referred to as PAMPs as well as endogenous ligands associated with cell damage. Just as TLRs are conserved from one species to another, PAMP ligands are repeated in a high variety of pathogenic microbes. An overview of TLRs and their ligands is shown in Table 3.2.

Stimulation of different TLRs induces distinct patterns of gene expression which not only leads to the activation of innate immunity but also instructs the development of antigen-specific acquired immunity. TLRs are expressed mainly on immune cells such as lymphocytes, macrophages, and neutrophils and on APCs, but low levels of expression have also been observed on fibroblasts and endothelial and epithelial cells.

Human uterine EC lines express TLRs that are capable of recognizing specific structural components of bacterial, fungal, and viral pathogens. The expression of TLRs in ECs from the vagina, ectocervix, and endocervix has been reported. mRNA for TLR1, TLR2, TLR3, TLR5 and TLR6, but not TLR4, was observed in both whole endometrium and separated endometrial ECs. Both whole endometrial samples and purified epithelium lacked detectable TLR7, TLR8, and TLR10. Since B cells are the predominant cell type for expressing TLR10, the absence of TLR10 is consistent with data, suggesting that B cells are rare in the endometrium. Constitutive expression of TLR1–TLR6 was observed throughout the female genital tract. They also described the differential expression of TLR2 and TLR4 in human reproductive tract tissue. TLR2 mRNA levels were highest in fallopian tube and cervical tissues, followed by endometrium and ectocervix. In contrast, TLR4 expression declined along the tract with highest levels in the fallopian tubes and endometrium. TLR4 is expressed in primary endometrial ECs but not in cervicovaginal epithelium. This is maybe because gram-negative bacteria in the upper genital tract are likely to be associated with infection whereas bacteria are usually found as commensal organisms in the lower genital tract. Another study showed that TLR1–TLR9 were expressed by the uterine EC line EEC1 and that PAMP agonists of TLR2, TLR4, and TLR9 stimulated expression of IL-6, IL-8, and MCP-1. However, it is not known if changes in sex hormones affect TLR expression.

More recently, studies were undertaken to examine the expression of TLRs on human primary uterine ECs and to determine if exposure to the TLR agonist poly(I:C) would induce an antiviral response. The ligand for TLR3, dsRNA, is produced by virtually all viruses at some point in their life. When investigating exposure of poly(I:C), a synthetic dsRNA which binds TLR3 to uterine ECs, the expression of the proinflammatory cytokines IL-6, G-CSF, GM-CSF, and TNF-α and of the chemokines IL-8, MCP-1, and MIP-1β as well as of MIF and HBD-1/HBD-2, was induced. Also the uterine ECs initiated an antiviral response when inducing IFN-β and

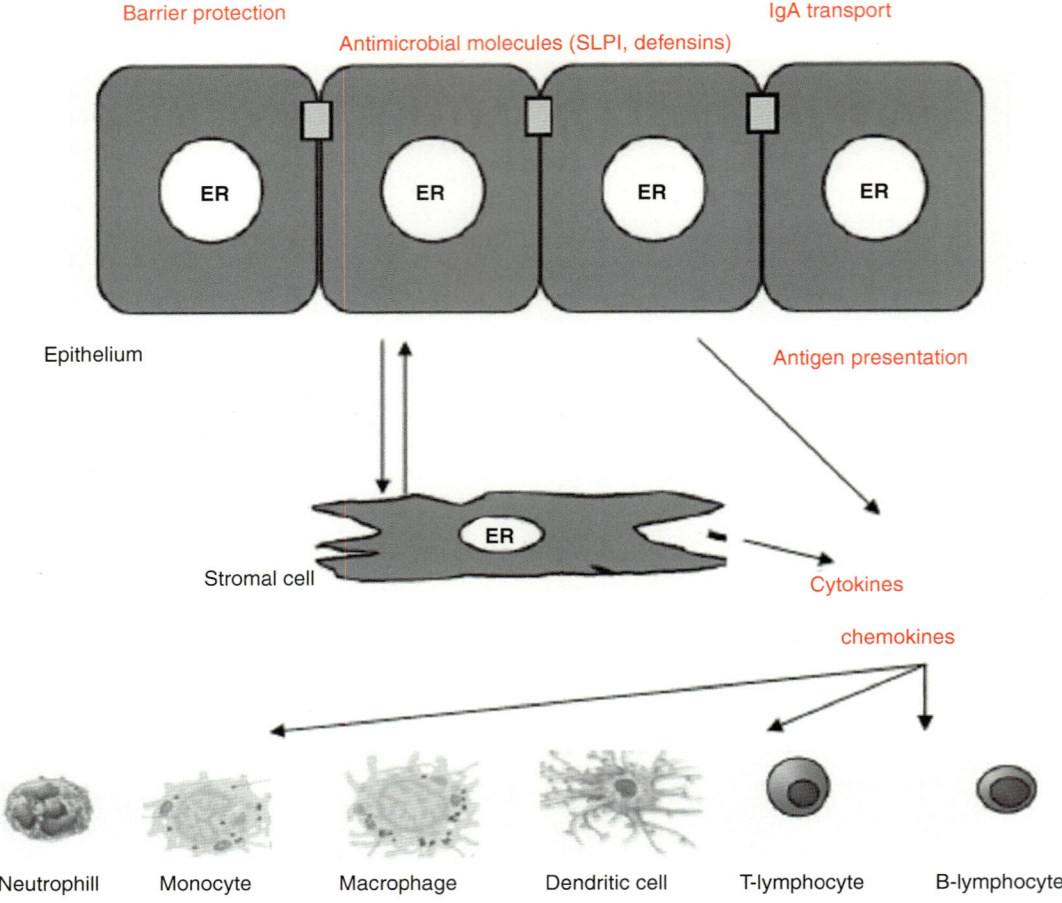

Fig. 3.1 Different immunoregulatory functions of ECs in the female reproductive tract (Adapted from Wira et al. (2005a))

IFN-β-stimulated antiviral myxovirus resistance gene 1′ and 2′, 5′-oligoadenlyate synthetase mRNA. This also suggests that ECs in the female reproductive tract are sensitive to viral infection and possess the capability to respond to RNA viruses.

To conclude, the following figure shows the multiple functions carried out by uterine ECs as sentinels of immune protection in the female reproductive tract. Acting as the first line of defense, ECs provide host protection in a number of ways that includes providing a mechanical barrier, secreting antimicrobial molecules, transporting IgA, processing and presenting antigen, and communicating with underlying immune cells by secreting cytokines and chemokines. Sex

hormone regulation of EC function is both direct via ER in ECs and indirect via ER located in the underlying stromal cells (Fig. 3.1).

3.2.2 The Role of Macrophages in the Female Genital Tract

As mentioned above, monocytes and tissue macrophages are important effector cells of innate immunity. The phenotypic characteristics of tissue macrophages reflect the unique tissue environment including cytokines, extracellular matrix, and cellular components. They are identified in tissues by their expression of cell surface receptors and can execute diverse functional activities, including phagocytosis of foreign antigens, matrix dissolution and tissue remodeling, and production of cytokines, chemokines, and growth factors.

With respect to the molecular forms of IgA, the female genital tract secretions are again unique. In contrast to plasma in which monomeric IgA constitutes 90–99 % of total IgA or to saliva and milk in which 95 % of IgA is polymeric, cervical mucus contains about 70 % polymeric IgA and vaginal secretions contain almost equal proportions of polymeric and monomeric IgA. The ratios of IgA1 and IgA2 and the predominance of polymeric IgA in cervical secretions indicate that much of the IgA originates from local production, not from plasma. However, the high representation of the serum monomeric form of IgA in the vagina clearly demonstrates that, contrary to other mucosal surfaces, this portion of the genital tract relies heavily on antibodies derived from serum and systemic immunity. Because of the intrinsic resistance of IgA2 to IgA1 proteases of many pathogenic bacteria, the increased proportions of IgA2 may provide functional advantage to certain specific antibodies.

To conclude, antigen-specific IgA, IgG, and IgM antibodies and SCs can be detected in the external secretions of the human genital tracts. IgG levels in the lower genital tract secretions seem to equal or even exceed the levels of S-IgA, whereas the dominant isotype of other mucosal secretions is S-IgA. IgG and IgA are under hormonal influence and are derived from the systemic compartment, as well as being locally produced.

3.2.2.1 Distribution and Function

Concerning distribution in the female reproductive tract, macrophages can be found throughout all tissues and represent about 10 % of the total number of leukocytes. Macrophages in mouse, rat, and human uteri are distributed throughout the endometrial stroma and myometrial connective tissue with myometrial macrophages usually larger in size than endometrial macrophages.

A large accumulation of endometrial leukocytes occurs in the periimplantation phase and during early pregnancy as well as a dramatic influx in the premenstrual phase and during menses. Pregnancy-associated leukocytes are predominantly a subpopulation of macrophages and uterine-specific NK cells, whereas in the perimenstrual period, there is a dramatic influx of inflammatory-type leukocytes: neutrophils, mast cells, and macrophages. Immediately after implantation a redistribution of uterine macrophages takes place. Macrophages are reported to flee from the implantation site and are entirely absent from the primary decidua in mice and rats. They continue to be excluded from the decidua as pregnancy progresses and are only present in small numbers in maternal blood near the placenta.

As mediators of phagocytosis of foreign pathogens and cellular debris, macrophages play an essential role in the initiation, maintenance, and resolution of host inflammatory responses in the female genital tract, for example, by secreting pro- and antiinflammatory cytokines such as TNF-α, IFN-γ, IL-1, IL-6, IL-10, and IL-12. Besides their role in the regulation of inflammation, macrophages have also been identified as important effector cells of ovarian function. The distribution of ovarian macrophages differs during the various stages of the menstrual cycle. The highest level of macrophages is in the vascular connective tissue and the theca-lutein areas of the corpus luteum during the periovulatory period. Their specific localization and variations in distribution in the ovary during different stages of the cycle as well as their presence in periovulatory human follicular fluid suggest that they play diverse roles in the folliculogenesis, tissue restructuring at ovulation, and corpus luteum formation and regression.

3.2.2.2 Regulation by Sex Hormones

Multiple studies have been examining the influence of estrogen on infectious diseases where results show that physiological levels of estrogen influence macrophage proliferation and function as well as cytokine production. It appears that the ability of estrogen to induce either pro- or antiinflammatory mediator production is concentration and cell context dependent. Human peripheral blood monocytes and human macrophages have similarly shown expression of both receptor isoforms, ERα and ERβ. Although macrophages have been shown to be affected by progesterone, nuclear progesterone receptor (PR) has rarely been detected on macrophages. This paradox between macrophage progesterone responsiveness and lack of PR expression can be explained by cross binding of progesterone to the glucocorticoid receptor. However, recent data suggest a predominantly immunosuppressive role of estrogen in modulating immune responses, mediated by nuclear ERα.

There is strong evidence that steroid hormones regulate the recruitment of uterine macrophages throughout the menstrual cycle due to regulation of cytokine and chemokine expression. The total uterine leukocyte population increased significantly on treatment with estrogen. This rise in leukocytes was due to a significant increase in both uterine macrophage populations and NK cells. Human studies have demonstrated that macrophages selectively aggregate into premenstrual endometrial stroma, concurrent with depression of estrogen and progesterone levels as the result of luteolysis. This is probably due to hormone-regulated variations in cytokine and chemokine levels as the expression of macrophage chemoattractants MCP-1, MCP-3, FKN, and MIP-1β in human endometrium is also increased perimenstrually. MCP-1 is known to play a role in controlling macrophage migration and activation, and is also produced by uterine ECs. The highest levels of MCP-1 in the endometrium were detected perimenstrually at low estrogen levels and lowest levels around the time of ovulation when estrogen levels are high. This was coincident with macrophage accumulation and depletion. Interestingly, treatment of endometrial stromal cells with estradiol significantly inhibits expression of MCP-1, which correlates with suppression of macrophage migration. This implies that fluctuations in estrogen and progesterone levels are coincident with changes in the migration of macrophages to the endometrium.

To be precise, accumulation of endometrial macrophages together with macrophage chemokines also occurs during the mid-secretory phase of the menstrual cycle with high estrogen and progesterone levels. Although these data are inconsistent with estrogen inhibition of MCP-1 expression, it is possible that regulation of MCP-1 is mediated by estrogenic modulation of another factor, such as IL-1. Estrogen has been shown to stimulate IL-1 mRNA and protein expression, and IL-1 again has been shown to induce expression of MCP-1.

Estrogen also plays an important role in the modulation of MIF expression by macrophages. MIF is produced by monocytes and macrophages as a consequence of bacterial LPS stimulation and mediates lymphocyte activation and nitric oxide synthesis as proinflammatory functions. As a counterpart of glucocorticoid-regulated antiinflammatory effects, it stimulates monocyte production of IL-6, IL-8, and IL-1β. Estrogen was demonstrated to downregulate MIF expression by LPS-activated human monocytes, directly mediated by ER.

3.2.3 Dendritic Cells

The APCs of the vaginal mucosa include the intraepithelial CD1a+, MHC class II+, fascin-bundling protein (p55)+, CD11c+, CD123-, DC-SIGN-, CD4+ Langerhans cells (LCs) and CD1a-, MHC II+, p55+, DC-SIGN+, and CD4+ DCs in the lamina propria of the mucosa. LCs are abundant in the epithelial layer of the vaginal and ectocervical mucosa, whereas DCs are predominant in the submucosal layers. These immune cells detect pathogenic invasion and/or damage of epithelial surfaces. Migration of LCs from epithelial surfaces is triggered by inflammatory cytokines induced either by pathogen invasion of mucosal surfaces or by epithelial damage.

DCs, as bone marrow-derived professional APCs, are initiators and modulators of the immune response via stimulation of B and T lymphocytes. As sentinels of immune function, DCs take up microbial antigens at sites of infection and then migrate to draining lymph nodes to stimulate antigen-specific T cell activation which is induced either by pathogen invasion of mucosal surfaces or by epithelial damage. Immature DCs reside in peripheral lymphoid tissues;

acquire antigen by phagocytosis, macropinocytosis, or adsorptive pinocytosis; and mature on pathogen stimulation, for example, through LPS. This leads to the upregulation of MHC class II and the costimulatory molecules CD80 and CD86. After migration to T cell areas of secondary lymphoid tissue, they undergo terminal maturation through ligaturing of CD40 with CD154 (CD40L) on antigen-specific T lymphocytes. Terminally mature DCs are characterized by production of IL-12 which facilitates production of IFN-γ-producing Th1 cells. DCs express mRNA for both ER isoforms at all stages in their differentiation. Nonsteroidal antiestrogens such as tamoxifen inhibit the differentiation of immature DCs and therefore the development of inflammatory Th1 responses. Antiestrogens can act as estrogen agonists or antagonists depending on the target cells and are therefore called selective estrogen receptor modulators. Human monocytes incubated with GM-CSF and IL-4 in the presence of antiestrogens failed to differentiate into immature DCs; however, this was not mediated by ER. Estradiol has been found to promote the differentiation of functional DCs from murine bone marrow precursor cells via ER. Ex vivo DC differentiation was inhibited in a steroid hormone-deficient medium and was restored by addition of physiological amounts of estradiol, but not dihydrotestosterone. This suggests a mechanism by which estradiol levels in peripheral tissues might modulate both the number and functional capabilities of DCs in vivo, thereby influencing immune responses. These contradictory results could be explained by the cell type and species-specific effects of estradiol or by the use of different hormone concentrations.

Estrogen has also been demonstrated to modulate the expression of cytokines and chemokines in human monocyte-derived DCs. Their treatment with estradiol increased production of IL-6, IL-8, and MCP-1. Moreover, mature DCs treated with estradiol had an increased ability to stimulate naïve CD4+ T cells.

Collectively, these data implicate a role for estrogen in the regulation of DC effector function and suggest that estradiol plays a key role in the induction and maintenance of inflammatory

Table 3.3 Different functions of NK cells

Cytotoxicity

NK cells can kill virally infected cells and tumor target cells regardless of their MHC expression via their cytolytic granules containing perforin

Cytokine and chemokine secretion

Besides production of IFN-γ, NK cells also secrete TNF-α, GM-CSF, IL-5, IL-13, MIP-1, and RANTES. Killing and cytokine secretion seem to be mediated by different subsets of NK cells characterized by tile intensity of expression of the CD56 marker on their surface

Contact-dependent cell costimulation

Serving as a bridge between innate and adaptive immunity, NK cells express several costimulatory ligands including CD40L which allow them to provide a costimulatory signal to T cells or B cells

Adapted from Orange JS, Ballas ZK. Natural killer cells in human health and disease. Clin Immunol. 2006;118: 1–10

responses. Nevertheless, further investigation of the influence of estrogen on DC differentiation and maturation is warranted. Considered in this context, the identification of DCs in the human reproductive tract has significant implications for the progression of inflammation and disease as well as for the maintenance of pregnancy. DCs are resident in human decidua, where they have been proposed to mediate tolerance to the conceptus as well as to mediate maternal immune responses to pathogens.

3.2.4 NK Cells

Natural killer (NK) cells are large granular lymphocytes that utilize receptors encoded in the germline DNA to become specifically activated or inhibited and are thus part of innate immunity. Similar to T cells, NK cells can utilize a variety of effector mechanisms including cytokine production and perforin-mediated cytotoxicity to help the host to eliminate pathogens and tumor cells. NK cell function can be classified into three categories (Table 3.3).

Human NK cells are found in the blood, lymphoid organs, liver, and various mucosal tissues including the lung, intestine, and uterus. They comprise about 15 % of all lymphocytes and are defined phenotypically by their expression of CD56 and lack of expression of CD3. Human blood NK cells can be divided into two major subsets based on the density of CD56 expression. CD56dim cells comprise the majority of peripheral blood NK cells (about 95 %) and express high levels of the Fc-γ receptor CD15 and killer cell Ig-like receptors (KIRs) as well as perforin. Thus, they have a high spontaneous lytic activity. CD56 NK cells express low levels of CD16, KIRs, and perforin but high levels of cytokines and are thought to be an important inflammatory subset. This is the primary NK cell subset found in lymph nodes.

3.2.4.1 Distribution and Characteristics
3.2.4.1.1 Distribution

In the female reproductive tract, NK cells can be found in all tissues. Their numbers as a percentage of leukocytes vary in different regions from 10 to 30 % in nonpregnant women. NK cells account for a substantial presence in the uterus, and altered NK cell numbers and activity have been associated with a variety of clinical conditions involving reproductive organs and reproductive failure. Reduced NK cell activity is associated with an increase in the incidence of ovarian and endometrial malignancies while higher NK cell activity has been associated with recurrent pregnancy loss. In the human endometrium, NK cells localize in large numbers especially following ovulation and account for almost 70 % of leukocytes prior to menstruation which again suggests the involvement of sex hormones in regulation of this NK cell migration.

3.2.4.1.2 Phenotype

Closer characterization of NK cells in reproductive tract tissues besides the endometrium has been performed rarely. McKenzie found CD3+, CD8+, CD16+, and CD56+ NK cells in the ectocervical epithelium which increase in number in relation to cervical intraepithelial neoplasia (CIN). In the fallopian tubes, the cervix and ectocervix there seem to be up to 20 % of all leukocytes of the CD45+, CD56+, and CD3− cell types. Endometrial NK cells also have a unique cell surface phenotype compared with peripheral

blood NK cells. They have been previously described as endometrial granulocytes, endometrial stromal cells, or decidual NK cells. Uterine NK cells express CD56 and CD94; a few also express CD16, while none express CD8 or CD57. A large amount express KIRs on their surface, but unlike blood NK cells, uterine NK cells express also CD9 and CD69 on their surface.

A large molecular study found that decidual NK cells differ in 278 genes from blood NK cells and found that the former were more similar in their gene expression profile to CD56(bright) than to CD56(dim) NK cells. The question of whether decidual NK cells are derived from blood NK cells which differentiate in the decidua or if they represent a special cell line which is produced only for the decidua is still not resolved. The hypothesis that NK cells in the decidua are derived from uterine NK cells in the endometrium at the time of implantation or from newly recruited blood NK cells has been favored. NK cells isolated from nonpregnant endometrium and decidua may not represent different phenotypes but rather a continuous process of differentiation due to alterations in hormone levels and changes in stromal cell environment. Only a few studies have been performed on NK cell phenotype in other female genital tract tissues.

3.2.4.1.3 Chemokine Receptors

Blood NK cells express a variety of chemokine receptors such as CXCR3, CXCR4, CCR5, and CCR7 and specific migration of NK cells has been induced by chemokines in vitro. Uterine NK cells demonstrated expression of CXCR3, CCR5, and CCR7. Moreover, the synthesis of CCL4, CXCL9, and CXCL10 increases during the menstrual cycle which correlates with the increasing number of NK cells in the endometrium. Additionally, estrogen and progesterone were able to induce expression of the CXC chemokine ligands 10 and 11 (CXCL10 and CXCL11), which suggests that sex hormones induce specific chemokines in nonpregnant human endometrium that can activate NK cell migration.

Several potential chemokine receptor–ligand pairs have been described in decidua that could be involved in leukocyte trafficking during pregnancy. In the maternal decidua, CD16- NK cells are found in direct contact with fetal extravillous trophoblasts. It is as yet unknown which factors contribute to the specific homing of this unique NK subset to the decidua. Hanna and colleagues reported that CXCL12, a ligand for CXCR4 which preferentially recruits CD56 NK cells, is expressed in trophoblasts. CD56 CD16- NK cells, which are the predominant type in the decidual leukocyte population, have been reported to express chemokine receptor CCR5, and its ligand CCL4 acts as a strong chemoattractant for these cells.

While the aforementioned studies show that the endometrium and decidua produce chemokines that recruit NK cells, it is not exactly clear which chemokines are involved in such NK cell recruitment. CXCL10 induced by sex hormones in the endometrium prior to implantation may recruit uterine NK cells whereas chemokines derived from trophoblasts such as CXCL12 may recruit uterine NK cells to reorganize placental arteries and facilitate trophoblast invasion of maternal tissue. NK cell attachment to uterine endometrium requires specific adhesion molecules. Leukocyte (L)-selectins and a4 integrins are important for the binding of lymphocytes. The adhesion of NK cells also involves vascular cellular adhesion molecule-1 (VCAM-1) which is expressed at the site of trophoblast invasion and might allow NK cells to migrate continuously to these sites.

3.2.4.2 Functions and Hormonal Regulation

3.2.4.2.1 Functions

Large amounts of NK cells populate the human decidua, often in close proximity to trophoblasts. These uterine NK cells have several functions in pregnancy:

- Help shield trophoblasts bearing paternal antigens from the maternal immune system
- Protect the mother from trophoblast invasion and limit their expansion
- Involved in the regulation and restructuring of maternal spiral arteries
- A component of the innate immune system, protecting against infection in the uterus

In general, NK cells as part of the innate immune system help to protect against infections. NK cells are capable of amplifying an inflammatory response and promoting macrophage activation and generation of cytotoxic T cells by producing cytokines and chemokines. Uterine NK cells have been shown to secrete IFN-γ, CSF-1, GM-CSF, TNF-α, IL-8, IL-10, and TGF-β1. Human NK cells cultured in the presence of IL-12 or IL-4 differentiate into cell populations with distinct patterns of cytokine secretion similar to Th1 and Th2 cells. NK cells grown in IL-12 produce IL-10 and IFN-γ while NK cells grown in IL-4 produce IL-5 and IL-13.

These cytokines may have significant effects on decidualization and trophoblast invasion. Uterine NK cells also produce other cytokines than blood NK cells such as angiogenic growth factors and LIF which leads to the hypothesis that uterine NK cells may play a role in endometrial angiogenesis.

In pregnancy, high numbers of decidual NK cells also seem to be involved in regulation and restructuring of maternal spiral arteries through production of angiogenic growth factors and LIF as well as in decidualization and trophoblast invasion. In the first trimester, uterine NK cells accumulate as a dense infiltrate around the trophoblast cells and spiral arteries. With further progression of pregnancy, these cells disappear from the decidua and are absent at term, which suggests that specific signals are involved in the recruitment and localization of NK cells within the uterus. Moreover, trophoblast cells can induce a subset of regulatory CD8+ T cells during the first trimester, which suggests that these cells probably regulate T cells as well as NK cell function at the maternal–fetal interface. The effects of human NK cell deficiency were investigated. These deficiencies were correlated with an increase in infections, especially herpes infections. But the role of NK cell function alone is difficult to determine as many of the NK cell deficiencies involve other immune function as well. NK cells have also been shown to actively recognize fungal infections and to play a role in the immune response against Cryptococcus.

3.2.4.2.2 Regulation Through Cytokines

NK cells can be activated by several cytokines including IL-2 and IFN-α/β as well as by prolactin and IL-15 or IL-18 in combination with IL-12. IL-15 and prolactin are both produced by the endometrium and influence NK cell differentiation. Uterine NK cells were shown to express prolactin receptors. IL-15 is present during the entire menstrual cycle with increasing levels during the mid-secretory phase and early pregnancy and is produced by endometrial and decidual stromal cells. The role of IL-15 is needed for survival, proliferation, and attachment of uterine NK cells. Perhaps expression of IL-15 by decidual endothelium is important for specific localization of NK cells close to spiral arteries. Another immunoregulatory molecule that influences NK cell is TGF-β. Inhibition of uterine NK cell cytokine production by locally produced TGF-β is a likely mechanism to regulate NK cell function in the human endometrium.

3.2.4.2.3 Regulation by Sex Hormones

There is strong evidence that uterine NK cell numbers and migration are regulated by sex hormones. NK cells are found widely within the nonpregnant endometrium and are associated with other leukocytes in small aggregates. NK cell numbers are low in the early proliferative phase and increase as the menstrual cycle progresses. In the late secretory phase prior to menstruation, NK cells account for up to 70 % of the leukocytes in the endometrium and are often seen as loose aggregates in the stratum functionalis lying next to the upper endometrial glands and the luminal epithelium. The cyclic nature of uterine NK cell appearance and the role of sex hormones in modifying changes in endometrium suggest hormonal regulation of NK recruitment and expansion in the endometrium.

Two mechanisms have been discussed as the reason for the increase of uterine NK cells: on the one hand, in situ proliferation and, on the other hand, selective recruitment from the peripheral NK cell pool. However, an active recruitment of these cells to the uterus is likely to play a major role with data indicating that uterine NK cells are derived from blood or bone marrow cells and not from NK cells within the uterus.

However, it is not exactly clear how NK cell functions are regulated by sex hormones. Various studies have yielded different and partly conflicting results. One reason may be the different kind of tissue examined, including nonpregnant endometrium as well as decidua. Estrogen has been shown to suppress human NK cell cytolysis in vivo and in vitro in a dose-dependent manner. Another study illustrated that men showed significantly higher NK cell activity in blood than women with regular menstrual cycles or women using oral contraceptives.

Uterine NK cells of decidual tissue do not express receptors for the estradiol or progesterone; therefore the activity of sex hormones on NK cell function is likely mediated via hormone action on other cells such as fibroblasts or ECs. However, NK cells do express glucocorticoid and estrogen β1 receptors, which may be mediating steroid hormonal effects on NK cells.

3.2.4.3 NK Cell Recognition and Interactions

NK cells can distinguish between healthy cells and abnormal cells by using a sophisticated repertoire of cell surface receptors that control their activation, proliferation, and effector functions. There is the hypothesis that NK cells coevolved with T cells given that they share common killing mechanism using perforin and granzymes and similar patterns of cytokine production. Both of these cells are focused on recognition of MHC molecules, and in this regard, NK cells distinguish themselves from phagocytes which rely on conserved pattern-recognition receptors such as TLRs.

NK cell recognition includes the initial binding to potential target cells, interactions between activating and inhibiting receptors with ligands available on the target, and the integration of signals transmitted by these receptors, which determines whether the NK cell responds or detaches.

Three families of cell surface receptors, KIR, Ly49, and CD94/NKG2, are expressed on NK cells which all recognize MHC I ligands and contain both activating and inhibitory isoforms.

They all share a common immunoreceptor tyrosine-based inhibitory motif (ITIM) in their cytoplasmic domains and provide protection for all cells that express normal amounts of MHC I on the cell surface. The MHC I-binding inhibitory receptors recruit tyrosine phosphatases which are believed to counteract activating receptor-stimulated tyrosine kinases. KIRs recognize epitopes on HLA-A, HLA-B, and HLA-C classes while the CD94/NKG2 receptor recognizes human HLA-E. Many of these receptors or related proteins are also found on NKT cells, memory T cells, and other immune cells.

Downregulation of MHC I due to viral infection or transformation of cells alleviates inhibition of NK cell positive signaling and results in initiation of cytotoxicity and cytokine production. It appears that there is not a single antigen receptor responsible for NK cell activation but an activity of several receptors triggering effector function. Activating receptors on NK cells include molecules with immunoreceptor tyrosine-based activation motifs (ITAM) such as NKG2D that recognizes MHC-like proteins MICA and MICB as well as 2B4 which binds to CD48. MICA and MICB are expressed by epithelial tumor cells and stressed cells; CD48 is significantly upregulated in B cell infected with Epstein–Barr virus (EBV), for example. NKG2D triggering can induce NK cell lysis of tumor cells and cytokine secretion.

Invading trophoblasts express HLA-G and can interact with the KIR receptors on uterine NK cells. Membrane-bound HLA-G has been shown to stimulate uterine NK cells and IFN-γ production and to suppress mononuclear cell effector functions. NK cell-derived IFN-γ seems to be necessary for vascular remodeling of spiral arteries and placental formation so that the recognition of HLA-G on trophoblasts by uterine NK cells may be important for placental development. Uterine NK cell-deficient mice demonstrated failure to sustain decidual integrity and loss of spiral artery modifications.

NK cell interactions with DCs are an important part of initiating the immune response. NK cells kill immature DCs. DC-derived IL-2 is essential for induction of NK cell production of

IFN-γ during bacterial infection. Moreover, IFN-α helps in activating NK cell cytotoxicity, and DCs are a good source of IFN-α in response to infection. NK cells can interact with endothelial cells through adhesion molecules and chemokine receptors. NK cells are able to recognize and kill endometrial endothelial-derived cell lines, and ECs can produce cytokines upon exposure to pathogens that can activate NK cells. However, the interactions of NK cells with these cells remain poorly understood.

3.2.4.4 Toll-Like Receptors

Like other innate immune cells, NK cells also express various TLRs. Human blood NK cells express mRNA for TLR1–TLR10. Agonists of TLR2, TLR3, and TLR9 are able to trigger IFN-γ production by NK cells, while CpG DNA, the agonist of TLR9, is not certain to activate NK cells directly or via cytokines such as IL-12, IL-8, IL-15, or TNF-α. Uterine NK cells express several TLRs such as TLR2, TLR3, and TLR4 whose agonists can trigger these cells to produce IFN-γ. The hypothesis is therefore that microorganisms may initially activate ECs which produce cytokines and these cytokines in combination with PAMPs will activate NK cell cytokine production, resulting in further activation of innate immune responses.

3.2.5 Neutrophils in the Female Genital Tract

Neutrophils comprise 40–70 % of circulating white blood cells and have always been considered as a first line of defense against pathogens. They have a relatively short lifespan of about 6 h circulating in blood before being removed by macrophages of the reticuloendothelial system (RES). When pathogenic microorganisms infect the host, neutrophils rapidly migrate to the site of infection during the first 1–4 h. Produced in the bone marrow, they enter the bloodstream by inflammatory signals originating from infection sites, adhere to the vessel wall at the sites of tissue damage, and transmigrate through endothelial cells to the infection site. When moving with the bloodstream, they roll along the vessel wall and continuously interact with the capillary walls to search for inflammation signs, a process called margination.

Tissue cell injury and infection result in increased expression of the adhesion molecules E- and P-selectins by endothelial cells as well as expression of sialomucins which interact with L-selectins on neutrophils. When rolling across the endothelial surface, the integrin molecules on the neutrophils' surface are activated, which leads to firmer adhesion. IL-8 is secreted by endothelial cells which induces shedding of integrins and L-selectin and therefore starts transmigration of neutrophils. By crossing the endothelial barrier, neutrophils unpack their granules with tissue-degrading enzymes and microbicides which facilitate this passage. Neutrophils follow both endogenous and bacterial chemoattractant signals to arrive at a site of infection. The presence of pathogens is detected by germline-encoded receptors that recognize PAMPs; human neutrophils express TLRs 2–10 except TLR3. The final elimination of pathogens is completed either by phagocytosis or production of toxic oxygen compounds by the cytoplasmic and membrane-bound nicotinamide adenine dinucleotide phosphate (NADPH) oxidase system. Other possible mechanisms are the release of microbicides such as defensins and serine proteases from intracellular granules. The neutrophils themselves produce several cytokines, for example, IL-1β, IL-8, TNF-α, and TGF-β1, that attract more neutrophils, macrophages, and other immune cells helping to initiate the adaptive immune response.

3.2.5.1 Distribution

Neutrophils can be found in all tissues of the female reproductive tract. Given the fact that the vagina is colonized by a mixture of commensal microorganisms, one would expect the highest level of neutrophils in these lower regions of the female genital tract where the most pathogens can be found. However, the highest amount of neutrophils is recovered from the fallopian tube with consistently decreasing numbers down through the lower genital tract. Patton and colleagues examined vaginal tissue of ovulating and non-ovulating women during three phases of the menstrual cycle for the number of cell layers and epithelial immune cells. The number of EC layers underwent a small reduction from menses to the postovulatory phase, and non-ovulating women had a thinner vaginal epithelium than ovulating women which suggests a hormonal influence on vaginal EC growth. However, the numbers of neutrophils as well as these of T cells and macrophages remained constant throughout the cycle.

In mice, a large number of neutrophils infiltrate into the vaginal epithelium accompanied by an increased number of neutrophils in vaginal lavage fluid after ovulation. Correspondingly, concentrations of a functional IL-8 homologue, murine MIP-2 were significantly increased. This indicates the regulation of neutrophil migration into the vagina by MIP-2 in a sexual cycle-dependent manner.

It is the consensual view that the number of neutrophils in different female genital tract tissues is dependent on IL-8; moreover, neutrophils in the female reproductive tract seem to be regulated by GM-CSF, which can potentiate induction of neutrophil chemotaxis and regulate neutrophil activation. IL-8 is a potent chemotactic and activating factor for neutrophils, and high levels of IL-8 correlate with high levels of neutrophils in the vagina. This corresponds with the findings that neutrophils cannot cross the epithelial barrier unless they are under the influence of a chemokine gradient of IL-8. The same study showed no difference between the number of neutrophils and concentration of IL-8 in healthy women compared to women with bacterial vaginosis (BV). When women were experimentally infected with *Candida albicans*, which can be either a commensal or a pathogen, there was no neutrophil infiltration in the vagina when the infection was asymptomatic or did not occur. In the case of vaginal infection, there was neutrophil infiltration and inflammation. Production of chemokines that attract neutrophils and neutrophil infiltration seems to occur only after infection of the vaginal epithelial layer. Vaginal lavage fluid from women with symptomatic infection, but not those asymptomatically colonized, promoted the chemotaxis of neutrophils. In animals, a rapid subepithelial influx of neutrophils into the vagina occurs not only due to insemination but also in response to a sterile liquid solution instilled into the vagina. Similar results were produced in women after insemination, although more in association with the cervix.

3.2.5.1.1 Cervix

Compared with other leukocytes, neutrophils represent the highest population with 83 % of all leukocytes in human cervical secretions. Both insemination with increased local production of IL-8 and infection of the cervix increase the number of neutrophils in the cervix significantly. In case of infection, cervical cells secrete IL-8 to promote neutrophil invasion in response to pathogen-associated substances such as LPS, but human cervical tissue is generally capable of producing IL-8 in vitro with decreasing activity postmenopausal.

3.2.5.1.2 Uterus

The complex cycle of the endometrium is regulated by hormonally controlled interactions between cytokines, chemokines, endometrial cells, and leukocytes. During most phases of the menstrual cycle, the numbers of neutrophils are low. However, prior to menses, a decrease in progesterone levels is responsible for a rise in IL-8 production in perivascular cells, epithelia, and glands. At this time, there is also a significant increase in endometrial neutrophils which comprise up to 15 % of all tissue cells, which serve to guard against infection at this time of lower epithelial defenses. Neutrophils may aid in endometrial breakdown as neutrophil granules release elastase and membrane-type matrix metalloproteinase (MT1-MMP) by chemotaxis, both of which are able to activate MMPs 2 and 3. The degranulation of neutrophils also releases antimicrobial components such as defensins, SLPI, or the neutrophil protease inhibitor and SLPI-related microbicide elafin, which also peaks at menses. Endometrial neutrophils are also capable of producing IFN-γ both in vitro and in vivo, especially in the endometrial stromal layer. This production

of IFN-γ also shows no variation during the menstrual cycle. By altering the local cytokine environment, neutrophils seem to be able to bias immune responses in the endometrium.

3.2.5.1.3 Fallopian Tube

The fallopian tubes represent the tissue with the highest number of neutrophils in the female reproductive tract mostly distributed in the lamina propria and a few in the epithelium. The expression of IL-8 is highest in the late proliferative phase around ovulation. This may suggest a greater influx of neutrophils at this time, but there seem to be no studies on neutrophil number variation in the fallopian tubes during the menstrual cycle. IL-8 was also present in greater amounts in the distal compared with the proximal tube. The degradative enzyme aminopeptidase N is found in tubal stromal tissue at the epithelial stromal border and may limit the effect of epithelial IL-8 in recruiting neutrophils. However, the exact role of neutrophils in the fallopian tubes as part of the local immune system remains quite unclear.

3.2.5.1.4 Ovary

Neutrophils are also present in the ovary throughout the menstrual cycle. It has been shown that low numbers of neutrophils infiltrate ovarian stroma but high numbers are present in the wall of the developing ovarian follicle. At ovulation, there was a marked increase in the density of these cells in the follicle wall, especially in the thecal layer, where they accumulate particularly around the point of imminent rupture. This suggests an active role for neutrophils in tissue remodeling during the ovulatory process.

Following rupture of the follicle and release of the ovum, the empty follicle becomes the corpus luteum. In the corpus luteum there is a higher density of neutrophils in the theca-lutein area compared with the granulosa-lutein area. There are no significant changes in neutrophil density during early and late luteal phase. IL-8 concentrations in follicular fluid vary over the menstrual cycle and have their peak around ovulation, consistent with the peak of neutrophil influx. Exposure to follicle-stimulating hormone (FSH) and luteinizing hormone (LH) but not to estradiol or progesterone increased IL-8 secretion from granulosa cells.

Through the release of and activation of MMPs and collagenase, ovarian neutrophils seem to be effector cells in the process of ovulation whereby the oocyte is expelled from the interior of the follicle. In addition, the corpus luteum that remains after a rupture or tearing of the ovarian wall represents an injured tissue in need of protection from infection, which may also be an explanation for the presence of neutrophils in this region.

3.2.5.2 Characteristics and Functions

The different numbers and distribution of neutrophils in the female reproductive tract explains the need for investigating the distribution of neutrophil chemoattractants in the different regions of the genital tract. It was found that cervical tissue expressed the highest amount of RNA for Gro-γ (CXCL3), ENA-78 (CXCL5), GCP-2 (CXCL6), and IL-8 (CXCL8). Fallopian tube expressed the second highest amount of IL-8, but ectocervix was the second to highest in expression of ENA-78 and NAP-2. Endometrium expressed the least amounts of RNA for Gro-γ, GCP-2, NAP-2, and IL-8. These findings do not correlate with neutrophil recovery from tissues by enzyme digestion. The cervix should contain the greatest number of neutrophils if CXC chemokine expression were proportional to recruitment of neutrophils. Moreover, one would expect a higher amount of microorganisms at the cervix than in higher regions of the reproductive tract, resulting in a greater need for innate immune protection by neutrophils.

In studies with EC cultures of the reproductive tract, the high neutrophil chemoattractant activity of these cells was the result of a synergistic action between IL-8 and GM-CSF secreted by ECs.

This suggests that relatively low concentrations of GM-CSF can potentiate the activity of CXC chemokines in induction of neutrophil chemotaxis. Moreover, one of the many actions of GM-CSF on neutrophils could also be to downregulate responses when they are no longer necessary. If neutrophils have entered the lumen of the genital tract after encountering high GM-CSF levels in the epithelium, a response to IL-8 which might attract the cells back into the tissue would be counterproductive.

Concerning neutrophil crossing of the epithelial barrier, it is known that they prefer to cross monolayers of cultured ECs from the basal to the apical side provided that an IL-8 gradient exists from apical to basal. Wira and colleagues presumed that unstimulated ECs in the female genital tract secrete chemokines basally to attract neutrophils to the epithelium. In addition, they produce a higher amount of chemoattractant on the luminal side that might serve to induce neutrophils to cross the epithelium and enter the lumen. Shen and colleagues have investigated neutrophils in the fallopian tubes as this tissue has the highest numbers of neutrophils per gram of tissue. Compared with blood neutrophils, fallopian tube neutrophils express higher levels of the adhesion molecules CD31 (PECAM-1) and CD15. CD31 is expressed on leukocytes and endothelial cells and is increased on transmigrated neutrophils, which suggests that fallopian tube neutrophils have crossed the endothelial barrier and are not only part of the marginated pool associated with the luminal surface of blood vessels. CD15 is a carbohydrate antigen involved in the binding of neutrophils to endothelial lectins, E-selectin and P-selectin. When stimulated with chemotactic peptides during neutrophil migration, for example, CD15 is brought to the surface from intracellular pools. Another point is that CD15 ligation is reported to induce a release of granule content; the high CD15 expression may be important for innate immune responses in the fallopian tube. Fallopian neutrophils have also been shown to possess lower amounts of specific granule-associated molecules, which suggests that they have undergone some kind of degranulation. Furthermore, they also demonstrate high levels of intracellular VEGF and IFN-γ. As VGEF plays an important role in vasodilatation and vascular permeability, it would make a leukocyte infiltration of tissues possible. In summary, neutrophils in the reproductive tract seem to be regulated by the hormonal cycle as well as by chemokines and cytokines.

3.3   Functions and Regulation of Adaptive Humoral and Cell-Mediated Immunity

3.3.1   Immunoglobulins in the Female Genital Tract

3.3.1.1   Distribution of Immunoglobulin Classes and Subtypes

Highly variable information has been reported about the presence of different Ig classes in human female genital secretions. Such discrepancies seem to reflect both the differences in the applied sampling method and individual variability such as age and stage of menstrual cycle. The dominance of IgA in the majority of external secretions, such as intestinal and nasal fluids, saliva, tears, and milk, has for decades been considered a cardinal characteristic of the humoral arm of the mucosal immune compartment. Back in 1971 it was demonstrated that S-IgA was the predominant Ig class (45 %) in CVS, the remainder consisting of monomeric IgA (20 %) and IgG (30 %). In the same study, IgA levels were found to decrease with age in contrast to IgG which increased. More recent study results partly differ from those findings. Human urine, seminal plasma, and cervical or vaginal washings collected at various stages of the menstrual cycle contain a higher proportion of IgG than IgA. Some studies showed a predominance of IgG in cervical secretions but a higher proportion of specific IgA antibodies in secretions from women colonized with group B streptococci in their cervix or rectum. Additionally, IgG is also predominant in vaginal fluid while IgA can be detected in mucus mostly from the endocervix. However, there is a predominance of IgG in cervical mucus with a peak before the time of ovulation together with smaller preovulatory peaks of IgA and IgM. Interestingly, IgG appeared to be the predominant Ig in CVS, but the ratios of IgG to IgA varied from 2:1 to 10:1. Measurements of Ig in human uterine fluid also indicated the predominance of IgG; nevertheless, the uterus may be the primary source of IgA in vaginal fluid since the concentration of IgA in vaginal fluid from hysterectomized women was only about 10 % of normal.

IgG occurring in genital secretions was deemed to be mainly serum derived, but a significant enrichment of the IgG1 subclass suggested some local influence. However, the mechanisms involved in the appearance of IgG in cervical secretions remain unclear. There are strong suggestions that the specific activity of IgG antibodies in genital tract secretions often correlates with that present in serum which is consistent with the origin of the genital tract IgG. Others discuss that a portion of the IgG is secreted by plasma cells residing in genital tissues. Whether IgG reaches the lumen by active transport or passive diffusion remains unknown. Very little is known so far concerning IgM antibodies in the genital tract. A short-lived localized IgM response has been found during herpes simplex infection.

Concerning the IgA subclasses, female genital tract secretions resemble secretions of the lower intestinal tract rather than the upper intestinal or respiratory tract where IgA antibodies mostly belong to the IgA1 subclass. Both IgA1 and IgA2 are found in equal proportions in the female genital tract as well as in the rectum and the large intestine (Fig. 3.2).

A local hypersensitivity IgE-mediated immune response can also be induced in the vagina following exposure of susceptible women to seasonal allergens, *Candida albicans*, or components of seminal fluid. The seminal fluid-derived allergens may be intrinsic components of genital secretions or compounds ranging from foods to medications that were ingested by the male sexual partner and secreted in his ejaculate.

With respect to the molecular forms of IgA, the female genital tract secretions are again unique. In contrast to plasma, in which monomeric IgA constitutes 90–99 % of total IgA, or to saliva and milk, in which 95 % of IgA is polymeric, cervical mucus contains about 70 % polymeric IgA and vaginal secretions contain almost equal proportions of polymeric and monomeric IgA. The ratios of IgA1 and IgA2 and the predominance of polymeric IgA in cervical secretions indicate that much of the IgA originates from local production, not from plasma. However, the high representation of the serum monomeric form of IgA in the vagina clearly demonstrates

Fig. 3.2 Distribution of IgA1- and IgA2-producing cells in systemic and mucosal tissues in humans (Mestecky J, Russell MW. Immunoglobulins and mechanisms of mucosal immunity. Biochem Soc Trans. 1997;25:457–62)

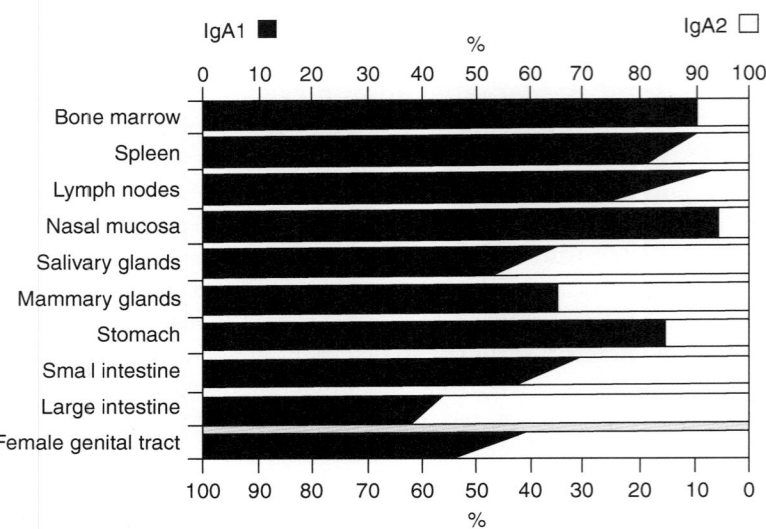

that, contrary to other mucosal surfaces, this portion of the genital tract relies heavily on antibodies derived from serum and systemic immunity. Because of the intrinsic resistance of IgA2 to IgA1 proteases of many pathogenic bacteria, the increased proportions of IgA2 may provide functional advantage to certain specific antibodies.

To conclude, antigen-specific IgA, IgG, and IgM antibodies and SCs can be detected in the external secretions of the human genital tracts. IgG levels in the lower genital tract secretions seem to equal or even exceed the levels of S-IgA whereas the dominant isotype of other mucosal secretions is S-IgA. IgG and IgA are under hormonal influence and are derived from the systemic compartment, as well as being locally produced.

3.3.1.2 Production of Immuno-globulins in Female Genital Tract Tissue

3.3.1.2.1 Cervix, Fallopian Tubes, and Vagina

IgA and IgG antibodies in the genital tract can be transported from peripheral blood and can also be produced by resident Ig-secreting cells. Studies show that the presence of antibody-containing and antibody-secreting cells is higher in the uterine endocervix than in the ectocervix, fallopian tubes, and the vagina. IgG- and IgA-secreting plasma cells are abundant in the lamina propria

Table 3.4 Distribution (percentages) of Ig-producing cells in different tissues of the female genital tract

Tissue	IgA	IgA1	IgA2	IgM	IgG
Fallopian tube	67	55	45	22	11
Endocervix	73	57	43	12	15
Ectocervix	79	59	41	10	11
Vagina	79	45	55	14	7

Adapted from Kutteh WH, Hatch D, Blackwell RE, Mestecky J. Secretory immune system of the female reproductive tract: I. Immunoglobulin and secretory-component-containing cells. Obstet Gynecol. 1988;71:56–60

of the endocervix and almost all IgA-producing cells contain J chain, a marker of synthesis of polymeric IgA. The immunocyte class proportions were similar to those reported for small intestine mucosa, with a striking predominance of IgA-producing cells. Immunohistochemical examinations by Mestecky and Kutteh found that the number of cells producing IgA, IgG, and IgM is different at various regimes in the female genital tract (Table 3.4). The endocervix and the ectocervix displayed the highest accumulation of Ig-forming cells and that such cells predominantly produced antibodies of the IgA subtype, almost equal proportions of IgA1 and IgA2 subtypes.

However, by using ELISPOT on cervical cells, at least four times more IgG- than IgA-producing cells were detected (89 % versus 17 %). Therefore, immunohistochemical studies have underestimated the IgG class because of interstitial staining. Moreover, the quantification of Ig-producing cells is difficult to perform due to their uneven distribution. The actual quantities of Ig-producing cells have been measured as density by number of cells/10 low-power fields without any accurate definition of the evaluated tissue compartment. The endocervix was found to have the largest number of cells followed by the ectocervix, fallopian tubes, and vagina. While the expression of both CD19 and CD20 is lost in terminal differentiation of B cells, CD38 is strongly expressed by plasma cells. Interestingly, CD19- or CD20-expressing cells in the cervix and vagina could not be observed. CD38 plasma cells were abundant and scattered in subepithelial stroma, reinforcing that the genital tract contains antibody-producing cells.

Cells in the single-layered epithelium of the fallopian tubes, uterus, endocervix, and ectocervix express the pIgR, the extracellular part of which is called SC. Thus, all components required for active transepithelial transport of polymeric IgA are present in a manner similar to that in other mucosal tracts. As the pIgR is not distributed equally throughout the genital tract, secretion of S-IgA takes place primarily in the cervix and to a lesser extent in the fallopian tubes and uterus. Uterine expression of polymeric IgA is under the control of hormones. Estradiol elevates expression and progesterone partly reverses this effect. Moreover, in cases of infection or inflammation, expression is also increased by the appearance of cytokines such as IFN-γ, TNF-α, and IL-4. Table 3.5 shows an overview of the presence and frequency of IgA, IgG, J chain, and SC in different female genital tract mucosae. The endocervix shows not only the highest number of Ig-producing cells but also the highest percentage of J chain, SC, and S-IgA, suggesting that the endocervix is likely to be the focal point for mucosal immunity in the genital tract.

3.3.1.2.2 Endometrium
Studies have reported that only rare and scattered Ig-producing cells are present in the normal human endometrium. Others reported the

Table 3.5 Summary of results from different studies concerning the relative distribution of IgA, IgG, SC, and J chain in the tissues of the female reproductive tract (conflicting results exist for IgG production in cervical mucosa)

	IgA	J chain	SC/sIgA	IgG
Myometrium	–	–	–	–
Fallopian tube	+	+	+	+
Ovary	–	–	–	–
Endometrium	+/–	+/–	+	+
Endocervix	+++	+++	++	+/+++
Ectocervix	++	+	+/–	+
Vagina	+	+	+/–	++

Adapted from Brandtzaeg P. Mucosal immunity in the female genital tract. J Reprod Immunol. 1997;36:23–50

predominance of IgG-containing cells in the human endometrium regardless of the stage in the menstrual cycle, followed by IgM and IgA-containing cells. When evaluated without a prefixation washing procedure, the endometrial stroma contained scattered IgG and less IgA, but there was an accumulation of IgA within the glandular lumina and apically in the epithelium without the presence of IgA immunocytes. This strongly suggested selective external transport of serum-derived polymeric IgA, which was supported by staining for J chain. Monomeric IgA without co-localization of J chain was detected in the vessel lumina, which supports this hypothesis. Also the preferential epithelial localization of IgM compared with IgG supported the idea that polymeric Igs derived from serum can actively be transported externally through endometrial glands. This was underlined by the general appearance of SC throughout the endometrial epithelium, particularly in the glands. Glandular uptake of antibody molecules from the interstitial fluid therefore seems to be dependent on SC acting as pIgR with additional paracellular diffusion of IgG. SC expression and IgA uptake in the endometrium are dependent on the phase of the menstrual cycle, showing a rise from the proliferative to the mid- and late secretory phase. The same study showed that the endometrial glands contained significantly more of all components of the secretory immune system in the mid- and late luteal phase than in the early half of the menstrual cycle (Fig. 3.3).

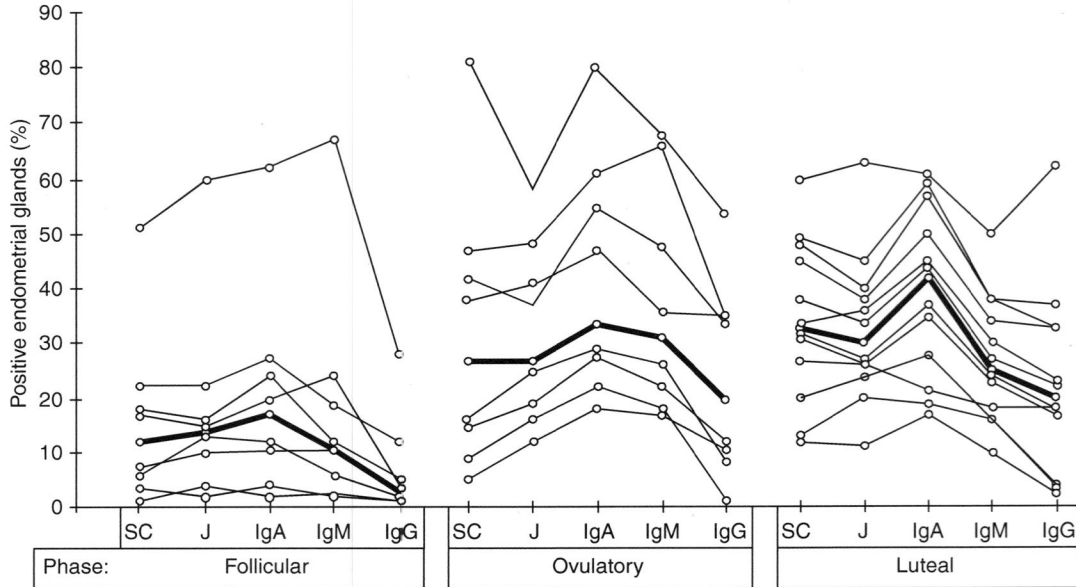

Fig. 3.3   Scatter diagram displaying the percentage distribution of human endometrial glands containing different humoral immune components throughout the menstrual cycle; each *thin line* represents one specimen, and *thick* *lines* connect medians (Bjercke S, Brandtzaeg P. Glandular distribution of immunoglobulins, J chain, secretory component, and HLA-DR in the human endometrium throughout the menstrual cycle. Hum Reprod. 1993;8:1420–5)

This again confirms the hypothesis that steroid hormones also have a significant influence on the adaptive immune system in the female reproductive tract.

3.3.1.3   Regulation of Ig Levels by Sex Hormones

Sex steroid hormones may be important in regulating both the systemic and secretory immune system. Estrogens, progesterone, and androgens directly and indirectly modify numerous immunological functions. Estrogens drive the differentiation of CD4+ helper T cells toward the Th2 subtype, increase production of Igs, and downregulate cell-mediated immunological processes. In contrast, androgens, such as dehydroepiandrosterone (DHEA), drive differentiation of CD4+ helper cells toward Th1-regulated functions and antagonize estrogen-mediated immunological effects. Progesterone increases the activity of suppressor T cells. There is clear sexual dimorphism in the immune responses of males and females which is shown by higher Ig levels in females as compared to males. Together

with more vigorous antibody responses to exogenous antigens in females, this indicates a higher level of humoral immunity in females. In addition, females seem to have a reduced incidence of tumors, a better resistance against viral and parasitic infections, and reject allografts more rapidly as compared with males, which also suggests a higher level of cellular immunity in females.

From an endocrine point of view, each organ in the female genital tract acts like a discrete reproductive organ whose contribution to reproductive success is controlled by the ovarian release of estradiol and progesterone. IgA and IgG levels in rat uterine secretions were shown to change markedly during the reproductive cycle, with the highest levels at ovulation. When ovariectomized rats were treated with estradiol, IgA and IgG levels in uterine secretions were elevated compared to saline controls. In CVS, however, levels of IgG, IgA, and SC were lowered in response to hormones. This suggests that the influence of hormone levels on immune responses may vary in different regions of the female reproductive tract.

Estradiol also upregulates the expression of pIgR in uterine ECs and thereby increases the transcytosis of polymeric IgA into the uterine lumen of intact and ovariectomized rats. Interestingly, levels of IgA, IgG, and IgM in cervical mucus are dependent on the stage of the menstrual cycle, reaching a peak before the time of ovulation. Previous experiments on IgA concentrations in cervical mucus and cervicovaginal secretions also showed a decrease at ovulation from preovulatory peaks. This relationship between the estrous cycle and specific antibody levels likely reflects the changes that occur in the female reproductive tract during the course of the estrous cycle. From the preovulatory period until the time of ovulation, or at the time of mating, the female genital tract is subjected to numerous pathogens. In fact, sperm has been shown to be a vector for bacteria, whereby the bacteria attach to the tails of sperm as they move up the reproductive tract. The need for protection of the female reproductive tract against pathogens is therefore especially high during ovulation.

Estrogen has been reported to increase total IgG and IgM production by human peripheral blood mononuclear cells (PBMCs) from normal individuals, owing to inhibition of CD8+ suppressor cells, though another study proposed secretion of IL-10 to be responsible for the increased Ig production. In the former study, the Ig-enhancing effects of estradiol were due to inhibition of CD8+ suppressor cells, while in the latter study, the effect of estradiol was neutralized by anti-IL-10 antibody and the authors suggested that the increased IgG production was mediated by secretion of IL-10 by monocytes in the PBMC cultures. It is tempting to speculate that the effects of estradiol and progesterone on Ig levels and secretion are mediated indirectly by hormonal effects on CD8+ (and possibly CD4+) T cells or accessory cells such as macrophages. In this regard it is interesting that the lymphoid aggregates found in human uterus have a central core of B lymphocytes surrounded by large numbers of CD8+ T lymphocytes which, in response to hormonal changes, would be in exactly the right anatomical location to regulate local antibody secretion.

3.3.2   Prevalence of T Lymphocytes

Leukocytes represent 6–20 % of the total number of cells in the fallopian tubes, endometrium, cervix, and vaginal mucosa with greater cell numbers in the upper tract. B lymphocytes were present in low but measurable numbers but T cells accounted for about 50 % of all leukocytes, with CD8+ T cells predominating over CD4+ T cells. This was confirmed some years later in a study by Johansson and colleagues who also showed a characteristic distribution of immune cells. They found that both CD4+ and CD8+ T cells were concentrated in a band beneath the epithelium and dispersed in the epithelium and lamina propria. They also found several lymphoid aggregates consisting of T cells and B cells in one cervical sample. Another study detected aggregates consisting of an inner core of B cells surrounded by mainly CD8+ T cells and an outer halo of macrophages in the human endometrium. Their size was found to vary with the stage of the menstrual cycle, with a larger size observed during the secretory stage than at the proliferative stage. The absence of these aggregates in uteri of postmenopausal women provided further evidence that these aggregates were under hormonal control. These aggregates had multiple features of inductive lymphoid tissue, for example, aggregated lymphocytes in follicle-like structures, lymphocyte invasion of overlying epithelium, and the presence of HEV. This suggests that these structures represent an organization of immune cells that are not dependent on the presence of infection or malignancy. Using hysterectomy specimens cocultured with IL-2 that contained CD3+ CD8+ T cells demonstrated cytolytic activity in the genital tract. Cytolysis by CD3+ CD8+ T cells was found throughout the reproductive tract and appeared to be hormonally regulated, since in the uterine endometrium, the capacity for CD3+ T cell cytolytic activity was present during the proliferative phase of the menstrual cycle and absent during the subsequent secretory phase. In contrast, in postmenopausal women the entire reproductive tract, including the uterus, retains the capacity for strong CD3+ T cell cytolytic activity. In women without inflammation, T cells

Table 3.6 Components of humoral and cellular immunity at different sites of the female reproductive tract

	Humoral immunity			Cellular immunity					
	Ig- producing cells	J chain	pIgR	T cells CD4–CD8		NK cells	MA	DC	N
Myometrium	–	–	–	–	–	–	–	–	–
Fallopian tube	+	+	+	++	++	+	+	+	+++
Ovary	–	–	–	+	+	–	+/–	+/–	+
Endometrium	+/–	+/–	++	++	++	+	+	–	++
Endocervix	+++	++	+++	++	++	+	+	++	++
Ectocervix	++	+	+	+++	+++	+	+	++	++
Vagina	+	+	–	+++	+++	+	+	++	++

Kutteh et al. (2005a)
MA macrophages, *N* neutrophils

and APCs were most prevalent in the cervical transformation zone and surrounding tissue. Intraepithelial lymphocytes were predominantly CD8+ T cells; most CD8+ cells in the transformation zone and endocervix, and a proportion of cells in the ectocervix, expressed T cell internal antigen-1, a marker of cytotoxic potential. In contrast, the normal vaginal mucosa contained few T lymphocytes and APCs. Cervicitis and vaginitis cases had increased numbers of intraepithelial CD8+ and CD4+ lymphocytes and APCs. The menstrual cycle and menopause have no apparent effect on cellular localization or abundance in any of the lower genital tract tissues. These data indicated that the cervix, especially the transformation zone, is the major inductive and effector site for cell-mediated immunity in the lower female genital tract.

Other data demonstrated that changes in circulating levels of estrogen can regulate the recruitment of bone marrow-derived cells to the uterine endometrium. The total uterine leukocyte population increased significantly when the women received oral estrogen, which resulted in higher serum estrogen levels. This rise in leukocytes was due to a significant increase in both the uterine NK cells and the macrophage populations whereas T cell numbers did not change relative to circulating estrogen levels. While further studies will be required to determine the effects of sex hormones on T cell function, receptors for estradiol have been demonstrated on both CD8+ and CD4– T cell populations whereas the presence of progesterone receptors on T lymphocytes remains controversial.

To conclude, the human systemic and mucosal compartments of the immune system, especially the female genital tract, display a remarkable degree of independence. In contrast to other mucosal systems, the genital tract mucosal system is characterized by a significant contribution of the systemic compartment with respect to Ig isotype distribution, unique distribution and phenotypes of B and T cells, strong hormonal dependency, and lack of typical lymphoepithelial inductive sites (Table 3.6). Further studies are needed to investigate the effect of sex hormones on T cell function, especially in the genital tract.

3.4   Immunization Studies

Based on the concept of a common mucosal immune system through which a fraction of lymphocytes activated at one mucosal site can disseminate immunity not only at this specific site but also to other mucosal tissues, there has been much interest in the possibility of developing vaccines against mucosal infections in the genital tract. Although the concept of a common mucosal immune system has been the dominant paradigm in mucosal immunology for more than two decades, it has become increasingly clear that there is a substantial degree of subcompartmentalization with the human reproductive tract, representing a component of this system with unique features. Indirect evidence suggests that female genital tract tissues may be preferentially supplied by cells from inductive sites located in the intestine, rectum, and nasal cavity. Remote inductive site immunizations, especially by the intranasal route or combinations of systemic and various mucosal routes, result in induction of sustained IgG- and IgA-mediated humoral immune responses.

It has been well established that the dissemination of cells from the inductive to the effector site is regulated by characteristic homing receptor–ligand interactions operational in mucosal tissue. In order to recruit leukocytes to mucosal tissue, the endothelium of the vessels expresses adhesion molecules, or addressins, that serve as ligands for homing receptors on the cells. The expression of intercellular adhesion molecule-1 (ICAM-1), VCAM-1, vascular adhesion protein-1 (VAP-1), and P-/E-selectins in cervical and vaginal tissue has also been demonstrated. However, none of the samples expressed mucosal addressin cell adhesion molecule-1 (MAdCAM-1). MAdCAM-1 has been shown in the gut-associated lymphoid tissue and is the only known vascular adhesion molecule that specifically directs lymphocytes to mucosal tissue via binding to the lymphocyte integrin $\alpha 4\beta 7$; the absence of expression of MAdCAM-1 indicates that the lymphocytes which are destined for the genital tract do not use the MAdCAM-1–integrin $\alpha 4\beta 7$ interaction used by intestinal lymphocytes, at least in non-inflamed tissue.

Immunization that produces secretory immunity in the female reproductive tract against STDs could have important practical applications. Investigators have attempted to elicit secretory immunity in the genital tract by using different routes of immunization. These local, remote, and parenteral routes are briefly outlined here.

3.4.1 Vaginal Immunization

Numerous experiments have shown that the local instillation of non-replicating antigens into the vagina of experimental animals or human female volunteers can result in the development of specific antibodies in local secretions. Studies have used a variety of antigens including those known

to have potent immunogenic and adjuvant properties following other mucosal routes of administration.

Earlier studies of immunization in the human uterine lumen with sperm, for example, failed to detect immune responses in the reproductive tract. Comparative studies have demonstrated that antibody titers in luminal fluids of the mouse female tract after intravaginal immunization were low in comparison to titers produced by systemic immunization. Adjuvants increased local immune responses to intravaginal immunization in mice as they likely damaged the uterine epithelium, thus allowing antigen to reach lymphoid cells and vessels in stroma. However, in 1973, Ogra and Ogra observed that immunization with inactivated poliovirus placed in the uterine lumen resulted in IgG antibodies in uterine secretions but not in serum. More recent studies with the potent mucosal immunogen cholera toxin (CT) B yielded analogous results. In a clinical trial women were immunized three times either orally, rectally, or vaginally with a cholera vaccine containing the recombinant CTB subunit with or without killed *Vibrio cholerae* cells. All three immunization routes increased levels of specific IgG in serum and specific IgA in saliva to similar extents. Only vaginal immunization significantly increased both specific IgA and specific IgG in both the cervix and the vagina but did not generate antibodies in the rectum. As the quality of the humoral immune response is significantly influenced by the time of immunization during the menstrual cycle, it may be necessary to administer vaccine during the follicular phase of the menstrual cycle in cases of vaginal immunization. Generally, the levels of these responses are quite modest; moreover, the responses are not disseminated either to remote mucosal sites or to the systemic compartment represented by serum antibodies. Local intravaginal immunization requires large and repeated doses of antigen; also the influence of the menstrual cycle should be taken into consideration. Furthermore, local immunization of the male tract is unlikely to be practicable. These considerations and findings support the notion that the genital tracts represent effector sites of the central mucosal immune system, but as inductive sites, they serve only for the generation of local responses.

3.4.2　Rectal Immunization

Follicular structures analogous to Peyer's patches are also found in the appendix and the large intestine, with especially pronounced accumulations in the rectum. The fact that the distribution of plasma cells produces almost equal amounts of IgA1 and IgA2 subclasses in the large intestine and female genital tract suggests that rectal lymphoid tissue may be an important source of IgA precursor cells destined for the genital tract. The potential importance of rectal lymphoid tissues as an inductive site for stimulation of humoral immune responses in the human female genital tract has been subject of several studies.

In general, the rectal immunization route generated variable results, depending on the type of antigen, frequency of vaccine administration, and stage of the menstrual cycle. Interestingly, rectal immunization was superior to other routes for inducing high levels of specific IgA and IgG in rectal secretions but was least effective for generating antibodies in female genital tract secretions. In another trial with influenza virus, rectal immunization induced significant increases in the concentration of flu-specific IgA but not IgG in cervical secretions within 28 days after vaccination. Rectal administration did not induce significant IgA responses, and only small flu-specific IgG increases in serum. Six months after administration, IgA and IgG flu-specific antibody concentrations were significantly higher than baseline levels in vaginal/cervical secretions. To generate long-lasting humoral immune responses, the combination of several mucosal immunization routes was more effective, for example, oral and rectal immunization.

3.4.3　Nasal Immunization

Animal studies also emphasized the importance of the inductive sites in the nasal cavity for the generation of mucosal, including genital, and systemic immune responses that may exceed in magnitude those induced by oral immunization. Experiments convincingly demonstrated that viral or bacterial antigens in combination with CTB instilled into the nasal cavity induced superior immune responses in local secretions as well as in saliva and female genital tract secretions. Furthermore, the complicating factor of hormonal influences could be avoided by using the nasal route, which offers the additional advantage of potentially inducing high levels of specific IgG antibodies in the circulation, and requiring lower antigen doses. Limited studies on nasal immunization performed in women suggested that intranasal immunization with CTB or CTB-*Vibrio cholerae* vaccines induced respectable titers of anti-CTB IgA and IgG antibodies in vaginal washings and cervical fluid. The results of another study comparing nasal and vaginal immunization with CTB showed that both resulted in significant IgA and IgG anti-CTB responses in serum. Only vaginal vaccination given on days 10 and 24 in the cycle induced strong specific IgG and IgA antibody responses in the cervix whereas modest responses were seen after nasal vaccination. Nasal vaccination was superior in inducing a specific IgA response in vaginal secretions, giving a 35-fold increase, while vaginal vaccination only induced a fivefold IgA increase. It was concluded that a combination of nasal and vaginal vaccination might be the best vaccination strategy for inducing protective antibody responses in both cervical and vaginal secretions, provided that the vaginal vaccination is given at optimal time points in the cycle.

When mice were immunized intravaginally with a bacterial protein antigen coupled to CTB subunit plus CT as adjuvant, weak specific antibody responses in both IgA and IgG isotypes were detected in vaginal wash fluids 7 days after the last of three immunizations. No antibodies were detected in saliva and only low levels of IgG antibodies were found in the serum. In contrast, when the same immunogen was administered without adjuvant intranasally, mice developed substantially greater levels of IgA and

IgG antibodies in vaginal fluids, and also IgA antibodies in saliva as well as IgG and IgA antibodies in serum. Analysis of the molecular forms of IgA antibodies in murine vaginal washes indicated that these were predominantly polymeric and similar to those found in saliva, consistent with S-IgA, although smaller amounts of possibly monomeric IgA were also present.

It may be concluded that the nasal immunization route deserves further testing with vaccines and potential adjuvants for prevention of STDs.

3.4.4 Systemic Immunization

Systemic immunization is of unique relevance to the induction of humoral immunity in the female genital tract. The significant contribution of IgG from the circulation to the pool of antibodies in the genital tract secretions clearly indicates that parenteral immunization may be of considerable value. Indeed, systemic vaccination with inactivated influenza virus TT elicited specific IgG antibodies in vaginal and cervical secretions. Recently, female mice were immunized at two parenteral sites in the pelvis which generated significant IgG and IgA titers in vaginal fluid. However, further studies on systemic immunization are warranted.

3.5 Immunology of Menstruation: Menstruation as an Inflammatory Process

In order to be prepared for implantation, the endometrium undergoes predictable, sequential phases of proliferation and secretory changes. Menstruation results from partial breakdown of the superficial or functionalis layer of the endometrium and ends in almost complete loss of the functionalis due to a fall in estrogen and progesterone. Re-epithelialization occurs simultaneously with tissue destruction and is followed by regeneration of the stromal components. This also occurs by withdrawal of exogenous hormones as in the case of contraceptive use or by administration of progesterone receptor antagonists such as mifepristone at the appropriate stage of cycle. However, although levels of these hormones fall significantly with corpus luteum degeneration in all mammals with an estrous cycle, only women and some primates menstruate. The molecular mechanisms by which steroids induce these changes involve interactions between the endocrine and immune system.

3.5.1 Classic Concepts of Menstruation

Markee, in 1940, examined the morphological changes in autologous endometrium transplanted to the eye of the rhesus monkey. Prior to menstruation there was vasoconstriction of the spiral arterioles followed by vasodilatation. His thesis was that the tissue destruction occurred by necrosis coming from anoxia. Already in 1961 it was observed that menstruation still occurred in primate atrophic endometrium without such coiled arteries. Overall endometrial blood flow was not reduced just prior to menstruation and the thesis of the presence of anoxia has not been demonstrated in human endometrium.

Later on it has been demonstrated that the onset of bleeding is clearly not the first significant event in the process. Prior to bleeding as the first outward sign of menstruation, one can see degeneration in the basal lamina supporting the decidualized endometrial cells and the endothelium of blood vessels in the late luteal phase of the cycle. Small lesions in the luminal epithelium have been observed on day 28 of the cycle followed by degeneration of the functionalis layer. The first event in menstruation seems to be degradation of the extracellular matrix which leads to a loss of blood vessel integrity resulting in bleeding. Disruption of the luminal epithelium then allows the escape of blood into the uterine lumen.

Since the 1980s, the concept of menstruation as the result of an inflammatory event has been proposed. Several features during the late secretory phase involving the presence of tissue edema and decidual cells and the influx of migratory cells have been observed, as well as leukocyte invasion and subsequent production of inflammatory mediators. The more recent identification of a variety of types of inflammatory cells using specific markers and also of chemokines and MMPs in premenstrual and menstrual tissue strongly supports this hypothesis. Current views of the mechanism of menstruation fall into two different categories: those supporting a key role for vasoactive substances and those proposing a central role for tissue destruction. Both theories fit the concept that menstruation is initiated at the stage when cells bearing proinflammatory molecules dramatically increase in number in the tissue. During the immediate premenstrual phase, progesterone withdrawal induces expression of uterine cytokines that attract leukocytes into the uterine environment and expression of MMPs by both endometrial and leukocytic cells. However, knowledge of the exact local mechanisms involved is still incomplete.

3.5.2 Distinct Features of the Endometrium During Menstruation

During the secretory phase one of the characteristic features is a progressive rise in the number of apoptotic cells within the endometrial glands. Withdrawal of factors such as interleukins as well as of steroid hormones leads to apoptosis in steroid-sensitive tissues. Estrogen regulates proliferation and apoptosis in endometrium as shown by studies in animals; its withdrawal induced apoptosis. The secretory epithelium loses its integrity during the menstrual phase. The loss of key proteins in cell–cell adhesion may be responsible for the loss of integrity of the epithelial lining in endometrium during menstruation. Menstruation is also associated with a compromise in vascular integrity. Progesterone withdrawal also involves a severe constriction of the spiral arteries with consequent hypoxia in the regions closest to the uterine lumen. There have been other proposed endometrial vasoconstrictors besides prostaglandins such as endothelins and angiotensin II whose activity was increased in perivascular stromal cells around spiral arterioles in the secretory phase.

Kelly has proposed two different phases of menstruation. Vasoconstriction and cytokine changes at the onset of menstruation are initiated by progesterone withdrawal and are probably reversible. Subsequent activation of lytic mechanisms due to hypoxia is then inevitable. This latter phase seems to be progesterone independent and involves cells that may not express progesterone receptor such as uterine leukocytes. Hypoxia stimulates local mediators such as the angiogenic vascular endothelial growth factor (VEGF) in endometrial stromal cells. VEGF, a heparin-binding glycoprotein, is a very potent mitogen for endothelial cells and induces vascular permeability and acts as a chemoattractant for monocytes. It is also one of the most potent angiogenic factors and is produced by monocytes, macrophages, and smooth muscle cells. It has been shown that VEGF protein is localized predominantly in endometrial glands. Estradiol increases the expression of VEGF gene in normal human endometrium. Hypoxia, IL-1, PDGF and TGF-β, EGF, and prostaglandin E2 are other factors known to upregulate VEGF expression. VEGF also induces expression of certain MMPs in the endometrium. Endometrium repair starts as early as 36 h after the beginning of menstrual bleeding while tissue breakdown is still in progress. Macrophages are partly responsible for the removal of detritus. Cytokines and growth factors produced by inflammatory cells induce the process of wound healing. Macrophages, for example, express TGF-α, TGF-β, fibroblast growth factors, PDGF, VEGF, and activin βB.

3.5.2.1 Nonresident Cellular Components of Human Endometrium

Both the extracellular matrix composition and the cellular components of the human endometrium change in parallel with hormonal changes during the normal menstrual cycle. Recently, the contribution of infiltrating cells of lymphomyeloid origin has been recognized. The population of various lymphomyeloid cells varies with the different phases of the cycle and has highest levels during the premenstrual and menstrual phases (Table 3.7).

Table 3.7 Relative distribution of specific inflammatory cells in the functional endometrium at three stages of the normal menstrual cycle, with the percentage of total endometrial cells at menses

	Proliferative phase (days 10–12)	Secretory phase (days 22–23)	Menses (days 26–28)
Macrophages	+	++	+++ (6–15 %)
Eosinophils	–	–	++ (3–5 %)
Neutrophils	–	–	+++ (6–15 %)
Mast cells	++	++	++ (3–5 %)
T lymphocytes	+	+	+ (1–2 %)
B lymphocytes	+/–	+/–	+
NK cells	–	+/++	+++ (5–6 %)

Adapted from Salamonsen LA, Woolley DE. Menstruation: Induction by matrix metalloproteinases and inflammatory cells. J Reprod Immunol. 1999;44:1–27

Evidence has emerged that at any time subsets of these cell types, represented by different phenotypes, are present in the endometrium and that apparently similar cells in the endometrium can be functionally different from those in the blood of the same individual. Thus, at least some of the cells which traffic into the endometrium must change in phenotype in response to the new environment. However, there is no doubt that during the perimenstrual and menstrual phase, there is a significant influx of inflammatory cells into the endometrium, comprising up to 40 % of the total cell number within the functional endometrium.

The leukocyte population in the endometrium is dynamic. Fluctuations in the number of cells are probably a consequence of migration from the blood, cellular proliferation within the tissue, apoptosis, and cell loss during the shedding of the functionalis. Eosinophils and neutrophils become apparent in the endometrium during the premenstrual phase only whereas increased numbers of macrophages and NK cells can be found earlier in the cycle (Table 3.7).

3.5.2.1.1 Neutrophils

Neutrophils, the most abundant leukocytes in humans, are closely related to tissue damage in inflammatory disorders. During most of the cycle, neutrophils are barely detectable in the normal endometrium but the amount raises perimenstrually, comprising about 6–15 % of the total cell number at this time. Densities compared to those seen during menses are also reached in areas of endometrial breakdown in patients treated with progestins. Neutrophils may aid in endometrial breakdown as neutrophil granules release elastase and membrane-bound MT1-MMP by chemotaxis which activate MMPs 2 and 3. The degranulation of neutrophils also releases antimicrobial contents such as defensins, SLPI, and the neutrophil protease inhibitor and microbicide related to SLPI, elafin, which also peaks at menses. However, not all neutrophils have been observed to be immunopositive for MMP-9, activin βA which is responsible for cellular differentiation, and MT11-MMP. This suggests that there is more than one neutrophil phenotype. Endometrial neutrophils are also capable of producing IFN-γ both in vitro and in vivo, especially in the endometrial stromal layer. This production of IFN-γ also shows no variation during the menstrual cycle.

3.5.2.1.2 Eosinophils

Eosinophils have been detected in the human endometrium by immunolocalization of eosinophil cationic proteins (ECP) 1 and 2. They are absent from normal endometrium during most of the cycle but immediately prior to menstruation increase dramatically in their numbers. Most of them are found in aggregates and the extracellular localization of the ECP suggests activation of the cells. Also some eosinophils are positive for MMP-9, and also the eosinophil chemoattractant, the chemokine eotaxin, and its receptor CCR3 were localized in endometrial cells.

3.5.2.1.3 Macrophages

Macrophages (CD68+) are present throughout the cycle with an increase in the early secretory phase and a further increase in the late secretory phase. On days 27–28, their numbers are similar to those of neutrophils comprising approximately 6–15 % of all cells in the functionalis. These cells are distributed throughout the tissue with some aggregates and some concentration around endometrial glands. Increased numbers of macrophages are found in progestin-exposed endometrium, particularly in association with abnormal uterine bleeding. Macrophages also show phenotypic differences concerning the expression of MMP-9, activin βB, and MT1-MMP.

3.5.2.1.4 Mast Cells

Mast cells secrete many vasoactive and proinflammatory molecules and participate in inflammation through vasodilatation and enhancing leukocyte infiltration as well as causing direct tissue damage through their proteases. Mast cells are found in endometrial tissue throughout the cycle without any changes in their number or distribution. However, by detecting the mast cell-specific proteases tryptase and chymase, one can tell that there are defined phases of mast cell activation. Activated mast cells are seen in the mid-proliferative (days 10–12) and mid-secretory (days 20–23) phases and immediately prior to and during menstruation, coinciding with the stages of tissue edema. Mid-secretory activation occurs at a time when implantation would be initiated in a fertile cycle. Two different phenotypes have been detected in the endometrium: those in the functionalis are positive for tryptase and negative for chymase while those in the basalis contain both mast cell-specific proteinases. Thus, tryptase, more than chymase, seems to have an important function in the process of shedding of the functionalis. It can activate proMMP-3, a key enzyme in the activation cascade of MMPs, and could be an important factor in degradation of the interstitial matrix through its actions on collagen type VI. Endometrial interstitial stroma contains a matrix composed of collagen types I, III, V, and VI and fibronectin, whereas basement membrane structures are composed of laminin and collagen type IV. As compositional changes during menstruation include the depletion of collagen VI during periimplantation period and at times of edema, tryptase seems to be of immediate relevance to the stromal disruption and edematous changes that apparently coincide with endometrial mast cell degranulation. Mast cell products, histamine and heparin, mediate changes in endometrial vasopermeability, bleeding, and angiogenesis. Mast cell activation also has the potential to stimulate the production of matrix-degrading metalloproteinases through their expression of interleukins and TNF-α.

3.5.2.1.5 NK Cells

NK cells are among the most numerous hematopoietic cells in perimenstrual endometrium. Only a few can be detected during the proliferative phase, but numbers increase during the secretory phase and their numbers rise up to 15 % of the total number of cells in the stroma perimenstrually. They are found distributed throughout the stroma and in intraepithelial locations. They are present during the decidual changes, and the very large number of these cells found in the decidua of pregnancy suggests an important role in the decidualization process. In contrast, the death of uterine NK cells could be an early event in the onset of endometrial breakdown at menstruation. In premenstrual endometrium, NK cells undergo morphological changes with their nuclei becoming pyknotic and fragmented. Probably they influence the critical decision that the mid- to late secretory endometrium has to make either to decidualize or to undergo menstruation. Due to their expression of CD56, they seem to be relatives of the CD56 CD16+ NK cells in peripheral blood. Compared to peripheral NK cells, endometrial granulated lymphocytes (eGLs) have cytotoxic activity beginning in the late proliferative phase. At this phase the proportion of eGLs expressing the activation antigens CD69 and HLA-DR is highest and decreased during the menstrual phase suggesting anti-infectious abilities. eGLs contain perforin, granzyme A, T cell intracytoplasmic antigen-1 granules, and MT1-MMP, which all can contribute to cell and tissue degradation.

3.5.2.1.6 Lymphocytes

CD3+ T lymphocytes are present in the endometrium throughout the menstrual cycle and their numbers increase prior to menstruation. Their total numbers are much less than those of other leukocytes, comprising only 1–2 % of the total number of cells. Concerning their distribution they are found as basal lymphoid aggregates, in intraepithelial sites, and scattered throughout the stroma. The CD4+ to CD8+ ratio in endometrium is inverted when compared with peripheral blood T cells (66 % CD8+ to 33 % CD4+ in endometrium). The cells are cytolytically active during the proliferative phase but not in the same manner in the secretory phase which could mean that progesterone may downregulate its activity. T cell activity may be related also to local secretion of cytokines such as IFN-γ, which is apparent in lymphoid aggregates in the stratum basalis but less consistently in functionalis throughout the cycle. Other T cell activation markers, CD69 and DR, are similar in both proliferative and secretory phases and suggest that T cells are in a state of persistent activation. At the time when cytolytic activity is low in these cells in the endometrium, it is high in these cells within the blood, indicating that endometrial CD3+ cells are functionally different. Subsets of endometrial T cells also express MMP-9.

CD45RA + B lymphocytes can also be detected in low numbers during the entire cycle and are present in perimenstrual tissue in clusters among stromal cells. So far, Ig synthesis or its specificity at this site remains unknown.

3.5.2.2 Regulation of Leukocytes in the Endometrium
3.5.2.2.1 Steroid Hormones

Although there is also the possibility of leukocyte regulation by estrogen, the greatest changes in leukocyte numbers and activation occur during alterations in progesterone levels. Leukocyte numbers are negatively regulated by progesterone in ovine endometrium while the influx is coincident with the fall in progesterone. It seems to be the PR-expressing cells such as stromal, epithelial, and endothelial cells that regulate the influx and activation of leukocytes. These act as effector cells that mediate the destruction and remodeling of the endometrial tissue together with factors produced by resident endometrial cells. The question arises as to how inflammatory cells differentiate to unique phenotypic subsets in the endometrium and how are they activated to release their mediators at the appropriate time

and place for menstruation. Besides entering the endometrium from the blood, some leukocytes, especially granulocytes, have been observed to proliferate in the endometrium, mostly during the secretory phase. CD45+ T cells, macrophages, and CD56+ NK cells express the proliferation markers Ki67 and BrdU within the endometrium throughout the menstrual cycle with a marked increase in the secretory phase.

Endometrial receptors of both hormones are upregulated during the follicular phase by ovarian estrogen and subsequently downregulated in the luteal phase by progesterone. The predominant form of the ER in all cell types in the uterus is ERα with only weak expression of ERβ. ERα expression in the functionalis increases in both glandular and stromal cells in the proliferative phase and declines in the secretory phase due to progesterone suppression. ERβ, however, has also been detected in vascular endothelial cells, which suggests a direct influence of estrogen on endometrial blood vessels. Such direct effects may be involved in endometrial angiogenesis and vascular permeability changes during the cycle. The PR isoform PRA is present in human glandular and stromal cells during the proliferative phase but is present only in stromal cells by the end of the secretory phase. The other isoform, PRB, is also detected in both cellular compartments in the proliferative phase and absent in the late secretory phase.

In rodents, however, steroid hormone receptors have been identified on several immune cell types with low-binding affinities but numerous steroidal effects which would support direct actions. Studies in sheep suggest that endometrial leukocytes are negatively regulated by progesterone, either directly or indirectly. The finding of PR on leukocytes would confirm this hypothesis, but most studies show a lack of evidence for PR or ER expression on endometrial leukocytes which suggests that effects of steroid hormones on human leukocytes may only be indirect. Except for the study of Paldi and colleagues, there has also been no evidence for PR-encoding mRNA in peripheral blood lymphocytes. However, there are PR-independent effects of progesterone which still have to be investigated in the case of endometrial leukocytes.

Table 3.8 Distribution of different chemokines and adhesion molecules in endometrium during the menstrual cycle

	Localization in endometrium	Cyclic expression
Chemokines		
IL-8 (47,639)	Surface epithelium, glands, perivascular	Increase in late secretory phase
MCP-1 (501)	Epithelial > stromal > vascular	Proliferative and secretory phase
MCP-2 (501)	Epithelial	Proliferative and secretory phase
RANTES (567)	Stromal	
Eotaxin (1580)	Epithelial > decidualized stromal cells/perivascular/eosinophils	Proliferative and secretory phase
MIP-1α (17)	Epithelial	Proliferative and secretory phase
Adhesion molecules		
ICAM-1 (1413)	Epithelial, vascular, stromal	Entire cycle, peak at menses
ICAM-2 (1413)	Vascular endothelium	Entire cycle
PECAM (1397)	Vascular endothelium, stromal	Peak at menses
VCAM/E-selectin (1380)	Glands	Entire cycle
	Vascular endometrium	Secretory phase
	Stromal	Secretory phase

M. Wirth 2006, Personal communication

3.5.2.2.2 Cytokines and Adhesion Molecules

Leukocyte migration into the endometrium is likely to be mediated by chemokines, which bind a large family of G-protein-coupled receptors on their target cells. In addition to their role in cell migration, they also stimulate degranulation and promote angiogenesis. Most of these intercellular mediators are multifunctional and synergistic as well as antagonistic properties exist for specific cytokine combinations. Different chemokine receptors expressed on the same cell can induce specific signals, giving weight to the theory that the receptors couple to distinct pathways. Steroid hormones could modulate the influx of inflammatory cells via actions on chemokines. Most chemokines are stimulated by IL-1 and inhibited by glucocorticoids. Glucocorticoid receptors are similar to PRs; both belong to a superfamily of homologous transcription factors. Therefore it is highly likely that progesterone could act in progesterone-dependent tissues in a similar manner to glucocorticoids in other tissues. Each of the nonresident cells in the endometrium is able to synthesize and release a variety of cytokines and growth factors. The distribution pattern of chemokines in the normal endometrium (Table 3.8) supports their role in the influx of inflammatory cells prior to menstruation although data are partly inconsistent.

IL-8 was detected in the surface epithelium and glands but not in stromal cells whereas others demonstrated the presence of IL-8 in perivascular cells of blood vessels increasing in the late secretory phase. MCP-1 was also detected in perivascular cells of blood vessels and was increased in both the late secretory and proliferative phases while other studies localized MCP-1 in ECs. Kelly and colleagues demonstrated that progesterone inhibited the synthesis of MCP-1 from cell lines and the synthesis of IL-8 from endometrial explants. Progesterone withdrawal thus can stimulate the premenstrual rise in these chemokines. RANTES production from endometrial stromal or ECs was stimulated by IL-1 and TNF-α in vitro, but not by sexual hormones. Eotaxin, a chemoattractant for eosinophils which is only detectable in the late secretory phase, was found in eosinophils and perivascular and decidualized stromal cells at this stage. The highest concentrations were seen in luminal and glandular ECs throughout the proliferative and secretory phases of the cycle. Its CCR3 receptor was expressed not only by eosinophils but also by endometrial ECs. Therefore the role of eotaxin and its receptor is not limited to recruitment of eosinophils premenstrually, but they may also have additional functions due to their overall expression by ECs. These results may give the conclusion that chemokines modulate the recruitment of leukocytes into the endometrium and their expression is stimulated by the withdrawal of progesterone at the end of the cycle.

Adhesion molecules are necessary for the attachment of leukocytes to the endothelium and for their extravasation and trafficking through tissues. ICAM-1 has been demonstrated in the stroma of the functionalis during the menstrual phase of the cycle. This molecule was also expressed by CD3+ cells in the lymphoid aggregates in the basalis layer and was present on vascular endothelium throughout the cycle with an overall peak in expression at menstruation. ICAM-2 expression has been detected in vascular endothelium without changes during the menstrual cycle. Platelet endothelial cell adhesion molecule (PECAM) was also stained in the stroma during menstruation and in endothelial cells of all vessel types. VCAM-1 and E-selectin appeared in stromal cells in the upper functionalis in the secretory phase. It seems likely that unique cell and site-specific expression of adhesion molecules in the endometrium may account partly for the distinct distribution of leukocytes.

3.5.2.3 Matrix Metalloproteinases

The integrity of endometrial tissues is maintained by cell–cell and cell–matrix interactions and binding as well as an intact fibrovascular meshwork. Shedding of the endometrium seems to require participation of factors that display the ability to cause the breakdown of these cell–cell and cell–matrix adhesions and compromise the integrity of the fibrovascular stroma.

MMPs are a family of highly homologous endopeptidases that degrade components of both interstitial and basement membrane extracellular matrix. The MMPs can be divided into major subfamilies: collagenases, gelatinases, stromelysins, and MT-MMPs. Most of them are secreted as zymogens that can be activated in vitro by a number of natural proteases and can be inhibited by specific inhibitors of metalloproteinases (TIMPs) by the formation of 1:1 complexes. The localization of various MMPs and TIMPs in the human endometrium is shown in Table 3.9.

Most of the MMPs such as MMP-1, MMP-2, and MMP-3 are produced by endometrial

Table 3.9 Distribution of MMPs and TIMPs mRNA or protein in human endometrium during the menstrual cycle

MMP	Localization in human endometrium	Cyclic expression
Collagenases		
MMP-1 (1209)	Stroma, connective tissue cells	Increase prior and during menses
MMP-8	Neutrophils	
Gelatinases		
MMP-2 (1209)	Stroma, most cells	Entire cycle
MMP-7 (1209)	Glandular epithelium	Increase prior and during menses
MMP-9 (1209)	Neutrophils, macrophages	Increase prior and during menses
Stromelysins		
MMP-3 (1209)	Stroma	Increase prior and during menses
MMP-10 (1209)	Stroma	
MMP-11	Stroma, epithelium	
Others		
MT1-MMP (1579)	Epithelium, most cells	Increase prior and during menses
MT2-MMP (1579)	Most cells	Increase prior and during menses
TIMPs		
TIMP-1 (1582)	Epithelium, stroma, vascular smooth muscle	Entire cycle
TIMP-2 (1582)	Epithelium, stroma, vascular smooth muscle	Entire cycle
TIMP-3 (1582)	Epithelium, stroma, vascular smooth muscle	Entire cycle

M. Wirth 2006, Personal communication

stromal/decidual cells except MMP-7 which is an EC product and MMP-9 which is mainly produced by leukocytes including eosinophils, neutrophils, and macrophages. MMP-2 and MT1-MMP are distributed more widely and are found in almost all cells in the endometrium.

MMPs are regulated at the transcriptional level by a variety of cytokines, growth factors, and steroid hormones by tissue- and cell-specific mechanisms. The patterns of expression of MMPs during the menstrual cycles are different in the normal human endometrium. MMP-1, MMP-3, MMP-7, MMP-9, and MT1-MMP mRNA and protein are all substantially increased immediately prior to and during menstruation, which has led them to be regarded as the mediators of tissue breakdown at menstruation. TIMPs have been demonstrated to be present throughout the cycle and can be localized in most cell types.

Leukocytes can produce MMPs and other enzymes with the potential to degrade components of the extracellular matrix (Table 3.10). These factors produced by leukocytes have the potential to stimulate the production of latent MMP generated by adjacent cells or participate in MMP activation.

For example, when MMP-3 is present, a cascade of MMP activation can be initiated. Besides production of plasminogen activator and chymotrypsin, mast cells produce tryptase which can activate proMMP-3 and chymase which can activate proMMP-1 and proMMP-3. Neutrophil elastase acts directly on substrates elastin, proteoglycan, and collagen, but they also produce MMP-8, MMP-9, and MT1-MMP themselves. Eosinophils can produce MMP-1 and MMP-9 while macrophages can generate MMP-9 and MT1-MMP. Thus, activation of leukocytes at any site can result in substrate-degrading enzyme or activators of such enzymes being released into the surrounding tissue. Studies have examined the regulation of MMP production and activation by endometrial cells in vitro. Endometrial stromal cells were put in culture with the human mast cell line (HMC)-1 or with peripheral blood neutrophils. HMC-1 produced the mast cell products tryptase, IL-1, and TNF-α. The HMC-1 cells stimulated stromal cell proMMP-1 and proMMP-3 and to a lesser extent also proMMP-2, with an increasing stimulation as mast cell numbers increased. When cultured with peripheral blood neutrophils, proMMP-2, proMMP-3, and proMMP-9 were activated while TIMP-1 and TIMP-2 produced by stromal cells were degraded. Withdrawal of progesterone may contribute to the recruitment and activation of leukocytes by

Table 3.10 Production of proteases relevant to menstruation

Leukocyte	Protease	Potential substrate
Mast cell	Tryptase	proMMP-3
	Chymase	proMMP-1, pro-MMP-3
	Chymotrypsin	Broad spectrum
	Plasminogen activator	Plasminogen
Neutrophil	Elastase	Elastin, proteoglycans, collagens
	MMP-8	Collagens
	MMP-9	Collagens, elastin
	MT1-MMP	ProMMP-2, proMMP-13
	Heparanase	Proteoglycans
	Cathepsin G	Elastin, proteoglycans, collagens
Eosinophil	MMP-1	Collagens
	MMP-9	Collagens
	β-Glucorunidase	Proteoglycans
	Arylsulphatase	Proteoglycans
Macrophage	MMP-9	Proteoglycans
	Metalloelastase	Elastase, collagens
	MT1-MMP	Elastase, collagens
	Plasminogen activator	Elastase, collagens
T lymphocyte	MMP-2	Elastase, collagens
	MMP-9	Elastase, collagens
NK cells	MT1-MMP	Elastase, collagens

Adapted from Salamonsen LA, Lathbury LJ. Endometrial leukocytes and menstruation. Hum Reprod Update. 2000; 6:16–27

inducing the production of cytokines and chemokines by endometrial and ECs of the endometrium. Furthermore, withdrawal of progesterone may directly promote MMP production by resident endometrial cells. Several in vitro studies demonstrate that progesterone is a potentially important player in regulation of MMPs in the endometrium. Physiological concentrations of progesterone cocultured with endometrial explants almost completely inhibited the release of both latent and active MMPs. Salamonsen

Fig. 3.4 Summary of menstruation hypothesis (Adapted from Critchley et al. 2001a)

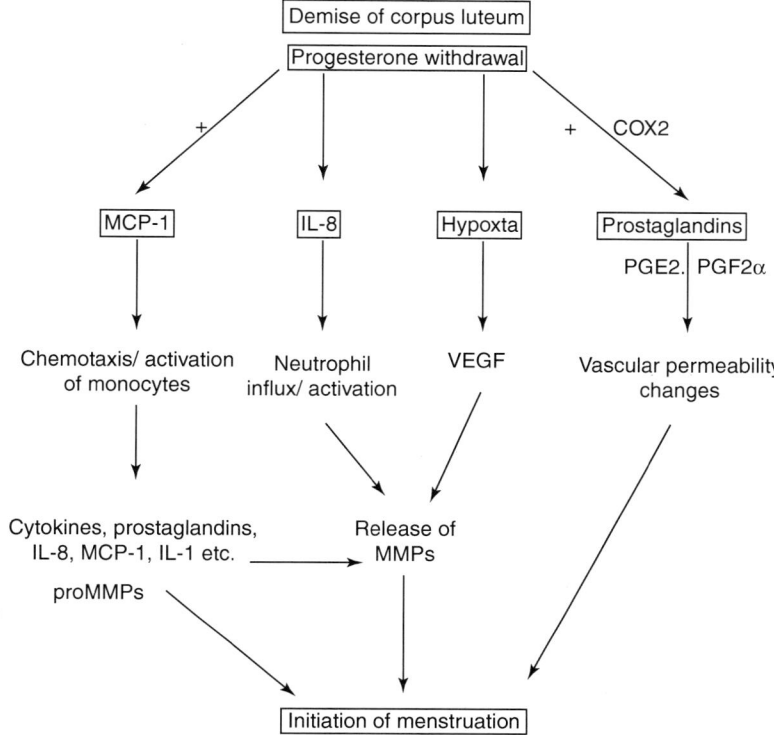

demonstrated the upregulation of MMP-1, MMP-2, and MMP-3 productions by withdrawal of progesterone in a cell culture model. There are several arguments for indirect actions of progesterone withdrawal accounting for the upregulation of MMPs at menstruation. Menstruation exclusively happens in women and some primates while all mammals undergo demise of the corpus luteum in a nonfertile cycle. Furthermore, withdrawal of progesterone is an endocrine mechanism and would result in systemic actions whereas MMP production is focal. There are also many local mediators in endometrial cells that modulate MMP production which are maximally produced during the late secretory and menstrual phase. These include TGF-β, TNF-α, IL-1, LIF, GM-CSF, and prostaglandins. In vitro studies support their potential for MMP regulation in the endometrium. For example, TNF-α and IL-1 are both products of epithelial and stromal cells and increase MMP-1 and MMP-3 production by stromal cells. Prostaglandins are present in high concentrations in endometrium where the synthesis

and metabolism of prostaglandin is regulated via estrogen and progesterone. Increased production of prostaglandin F2α induces myometrial contractions and vasoconstriction whereas other prostaglandins are vasodilatators that work together with bradykinin to increase pain and edema. Cyclooxygenase 2 (COX2) is the inducible form of prostaglandin synthetase and is present in human endometrium, particularly in the menstrual phase. A summary of the latest hypotheses of menstruation is given in Fig. 3.4.

Further Reading

Distinct Features of the Genital Mucosal Tissue

Crowley-Norwick PA, Bell MC, Edwards RP, McCallister D, Gore H, Kanbour-Shakir A, Mestecky J, Partridge EE. Normal uterine cervix: characterization of isolated lymphocyte phenotypes and immunoglobulin secretion. Am J Reprod Immunol. 1995;34:241–7.

Janeway Jr CA, Medzhitov R. Innate immune recognition. Annu Rev Immunol. 2002;20:197–216.

Johansson M, Lycke NJ. Immunology of the human genital tract. Curr Opin Infect Dis. 2003;16:43–9.

Kozlowski PA, Williams SB, Lynch RM, Flanigan TP, Patterson RR, Cu-Uvin S, Neutra MR. Differential induction of mucosal and systemic antibody responses in women after nasal, rectal, or vaginal immunization: influence of the menstrual cycle. J Immunol. 2002; 169:566–74.

Kutteh WH, Mestecky J. The concept of mucosal immunology. In: Bronson RA, Alexander NJ, Anderson D, Branch DW, Kutteh WH, editors. Reproductive immunology. Ann Arbor: Blackwell Science; 1996. p. 28–51.

Kutteh WH, Prince SJ, Hammonds KR, Kutteh CC, Mestecky J. Variations in immunoglobulins and IgA subclasses of human uterine cervical secretions around the time of ovulation. Clin Exp Immunol. 1996;104:538–42.

Kutteh WH, Mestecky J, Wira CR. Mucosal immunity in the human female reproductive tract. In: Mestecky J, Lamm ME, Strober W, Bienenstock J, McGhee JR, Mayer L, editors. Handbook of mucosal immunology. Oxford: Elsevier Academic Press; 2005a. p. 1631–46.

Lamm ME, Mestecky J. Immunology and immunopathology of the genitourinary tract: an overview. In: Mestecky J, Lamm ME, Strober W, Bienenstock J, McGhee JR, Mayer L, editors. Handbook of mucosal immunology. Oxford: Elsevier Academic Press; 2005. p. 1575–7.

Mestecky J, Moldoveanu Z, Russell MW. Immunologic uniqueness of the genital tract: challenge for vaccine development. Am J Reprod Immunol. 2005;53:208–14.

Neurath MF, Finotto S, Glimcher LH. The role of Th1/ Th2 polarization in mucosal immunity. Nat Med. 2002;8:567–73.

Pudney J, Quayle AJ, Anderson DJ. Immunological microenvironments in the human vagina and cervix: mediators of cellular immunity are concentrated in the cervical transformation zone. Biol Reprod. 2005;73: 1253–63.

Quayle AJ. The innate and early immune response to pathogen challenge in the female genital tract and the pivotal role of ECs. J Reprod Immunol. 2002;57 61–79.

Quayle AJ, Porter EM, Nussbaum AA, Wang YM, Brabec C, Yip KP, Mok SC. Gene expression, immunolocalization, and secretion of human defensin-5 in human female reproductive tract. Am J Pathol. 1998;152: 1247–58.

Schöllmann C, Stauder G, Schäffer A, Schwarz G, Rusch K, Peters U. Grundlagen der immunologie. Ein repetitorium. Germering: Forum Medizin; 2004.

Tomasi TB. The immune system of secretions. Englewood cliffs. New York: Prentice-Hall; 1976.

Wira CR, Fahey JV, Sentman CL, Pioli PA, Shen L. Innate and adaptive immunity in female genital tract: cellular responses and interactions. Immunol Rev. 2005a;206: 306–35.

Wira CR, Grant-Tschudy KS, Crane-Godreau MA. ECs in the female reproductive tract: a central role as sentinels of immune protection. Am J Reprod Immunol. 2005;53:65–76.

Functions and Regulations of Innate Immune Responses in the Human Reproductive Tract

Akira S, Takeda K. Toll-like receptor signaling. Nat Rev Immunol. 2004;4:499–511.

Arici A, Senturk LM, Seli E, Bahtiyar MO, Kim G. Regulation of monocyte chemotactic protein-1 expression in human endometrial stromal cells by estrogen and progesterone. Biol Reprod. 1999;61:85–90.

Beagley KW, Gockel CM. Regulation of innate and adaptive immunity by the female sex hormones estradiol and progesterone. FEMS Immunol Med Microbiol. 2003;38:13–22.

Chen D, Xu X, Cheon YP, Bagchi MK, Bagchi IC. Estrogen induces expression of secretory leukocyte protease inhibitor in rat uterus. Biol Reprod. 2004;71:508–14.

Cook DG, Fantini J, Spitalnik SL, Gonzalez-Scarano F. Binding of human immunodeficiency virus I (HIV-1) gp120 to galactosylceramide (GalCer): relationship to the V3 loop. Virology. 1994;201:206–14.

Crane-Godreau MA, Wira CR. Effect of Escherichia coli on rat uterine EC transepithelial resistance and basolateral release of TGFβ and TNFα. Infect Immun. 2004;72:1866–73.

Critchley HOD, Brenner RM, Drudy TA, Williams K, Nayak NR, Slayden OD, Millar MR, Saunders PTK. Estrogen receptor beta, but not estrogen receptor alpha, is present in vascular endothelium of the human and nonhuman primate endometrium. J Clin Endocrinol Metab. 2001a;86:1370–8.

Cunha GR, Chung L, Shannon J, Taguchi O, Fujii H. Hormone-induced morphogenesis and growth: role of mesenchymal-epithelial interactions. Recent Prog Horm Res. 1983;39:559–98.

Cunha GR, Cooke PS, Kurita T. Role of stromal-epithelial interactions in hormonal responses. Arch Histol Cytol. 2004;67:417–34.

Denison FC, Kelly RW, Calder AA, Riley SC. Secretory leukocyte protease inhibitor concentration increases in amniotic fluid with the onset of labor in women: characterization of sites of release within the uterus. J Endocrinol. 1999;161:299–306.

Fahey JV, Wira CR. Effect of menstrual status an antibacterial activity and secretory leukocyte protease inhibitor production by human uterine ECs in culture. J Infect Dis. 2002;185:1606–13.

Fahey JV, Kaushic C, Wira CR. Human uterine ECs: influence of culture conditions and stromal cells on EC transEC resistance. In: Gupta SK, editor. Reproductive immunology. New Delhi: Narosa Publishing House; 1999a. p. 366–78.

Fahey JV, Prabhala RH, Guyre PM, Wira CR. Antigen-presenting cells in the human female reproductive tract: analysis of antigen presentation in pre- and postmenopausal women. Am J Reprod Immunol. 1999b;42:49–57.

Fahey JV, Schaefer TM, Channon JY, Wira CR. Secretion of cytokines and chemokines by polarized human ECs from the female reproductive tract. Hum Reprod. 2005;20:1439–46.

Fleming DC, King AE, Williams AR, Critchley HO, Kelly RW. Hormonal contraception can suppress natural antimicrobial gene transcription in human endometrium. Fertil Steril. 2003;79:856–63.

Franklin RD, Kutteh WH. Characterization of immunoglobulins and cytokines in human cervical mucus: influence of exogenous and endogenous hormones. J Reprod Immunol. 1999;42:93–106.

Ganz T. Defensins: antimicrobial peptides of innate immunity. Nat Rev Immunol. 2003;3:710–20.

Grant KS, Wira CR. Effect of mouse uterine stromal cells on EC transepithelial resistance (TER) and TNF-α and TGF-β release in culture. Biol Reprod. 2003;69: 1091–8.

Grant-Tschudy KS, Wira CR. Effect of estradiol on mouse uterine EC transepithelial resistance (TER). Am J Reprod Immunol. 2004;52:252–62.

Grant-Tschudy KS, Wira CR. Hepatocyte growth factor regulation of uterine EC transepithelial resistance (TER) and TNF alpha release in culture. Biol Reprod. 2005a;72:814–21.

Grant-Tschudy KS, Wira CR. Paracrine mediators of mouse uterine EC transepithelial resistance in culture. J Reprod Immunol. 2005b;67:1–12.

Hashimoto C, Hudson KL, Anderson KV. The Toll gene of Drosophila, required for dorsal- ventral embryonic polarity, appears to encode a transmembrane protein. Cell. 1988;52:269–79.

Hocini H, Becquart P, Bouhlal H, Adle-Biassette H, Kazatchkine M, Belec L. Secretory leukocyte protease inhibitor inhibits infection of monocytes and lymphocytes with human immunodeficiency virus type 1 but does not interfere with transcytosis of cell-associated virus across tight epithelial barriers. Clin Diagn Lab Immunol. 2000;7:515–8.

Hoover DM, Boulegue C, Yang D, Oppenheim JJ, Tucker K, Lu W, Lubkowski J. The structure of human macrophage inflammatory protein-3alpha/CCL20. Linking antimicrobial and CC chemokine receptor-6 binding activities with human beta-defensins. J Biol Chem. 2002;277:37647–54.

Hunt JS, Miller L, Roby KF, Huang J, Platt JS, DeBrot BL. Female steroid hormones regulate production of pro-inflammatory molecules in uterine leukocytes. J Reprod Immunol. 1997;35:87–99.

Inaba T, Wiest WG, Strickler RC, Mori J. Augmentation of the response of mouse uterine ECs to estradiol by uterine stroma. Endocrinology. 1988;123:1253–8.

Jacobsson B, Holst RM, Wennerholm UB, Andersson B, Lilja H, Hagberg H. Monocyte chemotactic protein-1 in cervical and amniotic fluid: relationship to microbial invasion of the amniotic cavity, intra-amniotic inflammation, and preterm delivery. Am J Obstet Gynecol. 2003;189:1161–7.

Kaushic C, Grant K, Crane M, Wira CR. Infection of polarized primary ECs from rat uterus with Chlamydia trachomatis: cell-cell interaction and cytokine secretion. Am J Reprod Immunol. 2000;44:73–9.

Kayisli UA, Mahutte NG, Arici A. Uterine chemokines in reproductive physiology and pathology. Am J Reprod Immunol. 2002;47:213–21.

King AE, Critchley HOD, Kelly RW. Presence of secretory leukocyte protease inhibitor in human endometrium and first trimester decidua suggests an antibacterial protective role. Mol Hum Reprod. 2000;8:191–6.

King AE, Fleming DC, Critchley HOD, Kelly RW. Differential expression of the natural antimicrobials, beta-defensins 3 and 4, in human endometrium. J Reprod Immunol. 2003a;59:1–16.

King AE, Morgan K, Sallenave JM, Kelly RW. Differential regulation of secretory leukocyte protease inhibitor and elafin by progesterone. Biochem Biophys Res Commun. 2003b;310:594–9.

Leth-Larsen R, Floridon C, Nielsen O, Holmskov U. Surfactant protein D in the female genital tract. Mol Hum Reprod. 2004;10:149–54.

LeVine AM, Whitsett JA. Pulmonary collectins and innate host defense of the lungs. Microbes Infect. 2001;3: 161–6.

MacNeill C, Umstead TM, Phelps DS, Lin Z, Floros J, Shearer DA, Weisz J. Surfactant protein A, an innate immune factor, is expressed in the vaginal mucosa and is present in the vaginal lavage fluid. Immunology. 2004;111:99–107.

MasCasullo V, Fam E, Keller MJ, Herold BC. Role of mucosal immunity in preventing genital herpes infection. Viral Immunol. 2005;18:595–606.

Medzhitov R, Preston-Hurlburt P, Janeway C. A human homologue of the Drosophila Toll protein signals activation of adaptive immunity. Nature. 1997;388: 394–7.

Menge AC, Mestecky J. Surface expression of secretory component and HLA class II DR antigen on glandular ECs from human endometrium and two endometrial adenocarcinoma cell lines. J Clin Immunol. 1993; 13:259–64.

Niyonsaba F, Ogawa H, Nagaoka I. Human β-defensin-2 functions as a chemotactic agent for tumor necrosis factor-α-treated human neutrophils. Immunology. 2004;111:273–81.

Nusrat A, Turner JR, Madara JL. Molecular physiology and pathophysiology of tight junctions IV. Regulation of tight junctions by extracellular stimuli: nutrients, cytokines, and immune cells. Am J Physiol Gastrointest Liver Physiol. 2000;279:G851–7.

Parsons AK, Cone RA, Moench TR. Uterine uptake of vaginal fluids; implications for microbicides. Microbicides. Antwerp. 2002.

Pierro E, Mincini F, Alesiani O, Miceli F, Proto C, Screpanti I, Mancuso S, Lanzone A. Stromal- epithelial interactions modulate estrogen responsiveness in normal human endometrium. Biol Reprod. 2001;64:831–8.

Pioli PA, Amiel E, Schaefer TM, Connolly JE, Wira CR, Guyre PM. Differential expression of toll-like receptors 2 and 4 in tissues of the human female reproductive tract. Infect Immun. 2004;72:5799–806.

Pudney J, Quayle AJ, Anderson DJ. Immunological microenvironments in the human vagina and cervix: mediators of cellular immunity are concentrated in the cervical transformation zone. Biol Reprod. 2005;73: 1253–63.

Quayle AJ, Porter EM, Nussbaum AA, Wang YM, Brabec C, Yip KP, Mok SC. Gene expression, immunolocalization, and secretion of human defensin-5 in human female reproductive tract. Am J Pathol. 1998;152:1247–58.

Robertson SA, Mayrhofer G, Seamark RF. Uterine ECs synthesize granulocyte-macrophage colony-stimulating factor and interleukin-6 in pregnant and nonpregnant mice. Biol Reprod. 1992;46:1069–79.

Robertson SA, Mayrhofer G, Seamark RF. Ovarian steroid hormones regulate granulocyte- macrophage colony-stimulating factor synthesis by uterine ECs in the mouse. Biol Reprod. 1996;54:183–96.

Salamonsen LA, Woolley DE. Menstruation: induction by matrix metalloproteinases and inflammatory cells. J Reprod Immunol. 1999;44:1–27.

Schaefer TM, Desouza K, Fahey JV, Beagley KW, Wira CR. Toll-like receptor (TLR) expression and TLR-mediated cytokine/chemokine production by human uterine ECs. Immunology. 2004;112:428–36.

Schaefer TM, Fahey JV, Wright JA, Wira CR. Migration inhibitory factor secretion by polarized uterine ECs is enhanced in response to the TLR3 agonist poly (I:C). Am J Reprod Immunol. 2005;54:193–202.

Schieferdecker HL, Ullrich R, Hirseland H, Zeitz M. T cell differentiation antigens on lymphocytes in human intestinal lamina propria. J Immunol. 1994;149:2816–22.

Selsted ME, Ouellette AJ. Mammalian defensins in the antimicrobial immune response. Nat Immunol. 2005;6:551–7.

Shen L, Fahey JV, Hussey SB, Asin SN, Wira CR, Fanger MW. Synergy between IL-8 and GM- CSF in reproductive tract EC secretions promotes enhanced neutrophil chemotaxis. Cell Immunol. 2004;230:23–32.

Tabizadeh S, Santhanam U, Sehgal PB, May LT. Cytokine-induced production of IFN-beta 2/IL-6 by freshly explanted human endometrial stromal cells: modulation by estradiol-17 beta. J Immunol. 1989;142:3134–9.

Valore EV, Park CH, Quayle AJ, Wiles KR, McCray PB, Ganz T. Human β-defensin-1: an antimicrobial peptide of urogenital tissue. J Clin Invest. 1998;101:1633–42.

Wallace PK, Yeaman GR, Johnson K, Collis JE, Guyre PM, Wira CR. MHC class II expression and antigen presentation by human endometrial cells. J Steroid Biochem Mol Biol. 2001;76:203–11.

Wira CR, Rossoll RM. Antigen-presenting cells in the female reproductive tract: influence of sex hormones on antigen presentation in the vagina. Immunology. 1995;84:505–8.

Wira CR, Rossoll RM. Estradiol regulation of antigen presentation by uterine stromal cells: role of TGF-β production by ECs in mediating antigen presenting cell function. Immunology. 2003;109:398–406.

Wira CR, Sandoe CP. Hormone regulation of immunoglobulins: influence of estradiol on IgA and IgG in the rat uterus. Endocrinology. 1980;106:1020–6.

Wira CR, Sullivan DA. Estradiol and progesterone regulation of IgA, IgG and secretory component in cervico-vaginal secretions of rat. Biol Reprod. 1985;32:90–5.

Wira CR, Fahey JV, White HD, Yeaman GR, Givan AL, Howell AL. The mucosal immune system in the human female reproductive tract: influence of stage of the menstrual cycle and menopause on mucosal immunity in the uterus. In: Glasser S, Aplin J, Giudice L, Tabizadeh S, editors. The endometrium. New York: Taylor & Francis; 2002. p. 371–404.

Wira CR, Fahey JV, Sentman CL, Pioli PA, Shen L. Innate and adaptive immunity in female genital tract: cellular responses and interactions. Immunol Rev. 2005;206:306–35

Wira CR, Grant-Tschudy KS, Crane-Godreau MA. ECs in the female reproductive tract: a central role as sentinels of immune protection. Am J Reprod Immunol. 2005;53:65–76.

Yang D, Chertov O, Bykovskaia SN, Chen Q, Buffo MJ, Shogan J, Anderson M, Schröder JM, Wang JM, Howard OMZ, Oppenheim JJ. β-defensins: linking innate and adaptive immunity through dendritic and T cell CCR6. Science. 1999;286:525–8.

Yeaman GR, Guyre PM, Fanger MW, Collins JE, White HD, Rathbun W, Orndorff KA, Gonzalez J, Stern JE, Wira CR. Unique CD8+ T cell-rich lymphoid aggregates in human uterine endometrium. J Leukoc Biol. 1997;61:427–35.

Yoshimura T, Inaba M, Sugiura K, Nakajima T, Ito T, Nakamura K, Kanzaki H, Ikehara S. Analyses of dendritic cell subsets in pregnancy. Am J Reprod Immunol. 2003;50:137–45.

Young A, Thomson AJ, Ledingham MA, Jordan F, Greer IA, Norman JE. Immunolocalization of proinflammatory cytokines in myometrium, cervix, and fetal membranes during human parturition at term. Biol Reprod. 2002;66:445–9.

Young SL, Lyddon TD, Jorgensson RL, Misfeldt ML. Expression of Toll-like receptors in human endometrial ECs and cell lines. Am J Reprod Immunol. 2004;52:67–73.

Zarmakoupis PN, Rier SE, Maroulis GB, Becker JL. Inhibition of human endometrial stromal cell proliferation by interleukin 6. Hum Reprod. 1995;10:2395–9.

The Role of Macrophages in the Female Genital Tract

Akoum A, Jolicoeur C, Boucher A. Estradiol amplifies interleukin-1-induced monocyte chemotactic protein-1 expression by ectopic endometrial cells of women with endometriosis. J Clin Endocrinol Metab. 2000;85:896–904.

Arici A, Senturk LM, Seli E, Bahtiyar MO, Kim G. Regulation of monocyte chemotactic protein- 1 expression in human endometrial stromal cells by estrogen and progesterone. Biol Reprod. 1999;61:85–90.

Ashcroft GS, Mills SJ, Lei K, Gibbons L, Jeong MJ, Taniguchi M, Burow M, Horan MA, Wahl SM, Nakayama T. Estrogen modulates cutaneous wound healing by downregulating macrophage migration inhibitory factor. J Clin Invest. 2003;111:1309–18.

DeLoia JA, Stewart-Akers AM, Brekosky J, Kubik CJK. Effects of exogenous estrogen on uterine leukocyte recruitment. Fertil Steril. 2002;77:548–54.

Hunt JS. Immunologically relevant cells in the uterus. Biol Reprod. 1994;50:461–6.

Jones RL, Kelly RW, Critchley HO. Chemokine and cyclooxygenase-2 expression in human endometrium coincides with leukocyte accumulation. Hum Reprod. 1997;12:1300–6.

Jones RL, Hannan NJ, Kaitúu TJ, Zhang J, Salamonsen LA. Identification of chemokines important for leukocyte recruitment to the human endometrium at the times of embryo implantation and menstruation. J Clin Endocrinol Metab. 2004;89:6155–67.

Kamat BR, Isaacson PG. The immunocytochemical distribution of leukocytic subpopulations in human endometrium. Am J Pathol. 1987;127:66–73.

Kutteh WH, Prince SJ, Hammonds KR, Kutteh CC, Mestecky J. Variations in immunoglobulins and IgA subclasses of human uterine cervical secretions around the time of ovulation. Clin Exp Immunol. 1996;104: 538–42.

Kutteh WH, Mestecky J, Wira CR. Mucosal immunity in the human female reproductive tract. In: Mestecky J, Lamm ME, Strober W, Bienenstock J, McGhee JR, Mayer L, editors. Handbook of mucosal immunology. Oxford: Elsevier Academic Press; 2005. p. 1631–46.

Lambert KC, Curran EM, Judy BM, Lubahn DB, Estes DM. Estrogen receptor-α deficiency promotes increased TNF-α secretion and bacterial killing by murine macrophages in response to microbial stimuli in vitro. J Leukoc Biol. 2004;75:1166–72.

Merogi AJ, Marrogi AJ, Ramesh R, Robinson WR, Fermin CD, Freeman SM. Tumor-host interaction: analysis of cytokines, growth factors, and tumor-infiltrating lymphocytes in ovarian carcinomas. Hum Pathol. 1997;28:321–31.

Meter RA, Wira CR, Fahey JV. Secretion of monocyte chemotactic protein-1 by human uterine epithelium directs monocyte migration in culture. Fertil Steril. 2005;84:191–201.

Mor G, Sapi E, Abrahams VM, Rutherford T, Song J, Hao XY, Muzaffar S, Kohen F. Interaction of the estrogen receptors with the Fas ligand promoter in human monocytes. J Immunol. 2003;170:114–22.

Phiel KL, Henderson RA, Adelman SJ, Elloso MM. Differential estrogen receptor gene expression in human peripheral blood mononuclear cell populations. Immunol Lett. 2005;97:107–13.

Roger T, Glauser MP, Calandra T. Macrophage migration inhibitory factor (MIF) modulates innate immune responses induced by endotoxin and gram-negative bacteria. J Endotoxin Res. 2001;7:456–60.

Wira CR, Fahey JV, Sentman CL, Pioli PA, Shen L. Innate and adaptive immunity in female genital tract: cellular responses and interactions. Immunol Rev. 2005;206: 306–35.

Wu R, Van der Hoek KH, Ryan NK, Norman RJ, Robker RL. Macrophage contribution to ovarian function. Hum Reprod Update. 2004;10:119–33.

Dendritic Cells

Abbas AK, Lichtman AH, Pober JS. Immunologie. Verlag Hans Huber: Bern Göttingen Toronto Seattle; 1996.

Akira S. Mammalian Toll-like receptors. Curr Opin Immunol. 2003;15:5–11.

Balu RB, Savitz DA, Ananth CV, Hartmann KE, Miller WC, Thorp JM, Heine RP. Bacterial vaginosis and vaginal fluid defensins during pregnancy. Am J Obstet Gynecol. 2002;187:1267–71.

Bengtsson AK, Ryan EJ, Giordano D, Magaletti DM, Clark EA. 17beta-estradiol (E2) modulates cytokine and chemokine expression in human monocyte-derived dendritic cells. Blood. 2004;104:1404–10.

Bjercke S, Scott H, Braathen LR, Thorsby E. HLA-DR-expressing Langerhans'-like cells in vaginal and cervical epithelium. Acta Obstet Gynecol Scand. 1983; 62:585–9.

Cella M, Scheidegger D, Palmer-Lehmann K, Lane P, Lanzavecchia A, Alber G. Ligation of CD40 on dendritic cells triggers production of high levels of interleukin-12 and enhances T cell stimulatory capacity: T-T help via APC activation. J Exp Med. 1996;184:747–52.

Dawson RD. Modern concepts of humoral and cellular immunity. In: Bronson RA, Alexander NJ, Anderson D, Branch DW, Kutteh WH, editors. Reproductive immunology. Ann Arbor: Blackwell Science; 1996. p. 3–27.

Finlay BB, Cossart P. Exploitation of mammalian host cell functions by bacterial pathogens. Science. 1997;276:718–25.

Gardner L, Moffett A. Dendritic cells in the human decidua. Biol Reprod. 2003;69:1438–46.

Heine H, Lien E. Toll-like receptors and their function in innate and adaptive immunity. Int Arch Allergy Immunol. 2003;130:180–92.

Hughes A. Evolution of the host defense system. In: Kaufmann SHE, Sher A, Ahmed R, editors. Immunology of infectious diseases. Washington: ASM Press; 2002. p. 67–78.

Jablonowska B, Selbing A, Palfi M, Ernerudh J, Kjellberg S, Lindton B. Prevention of recurrent spontaneous abortion by intravenous immunoglobulin: a double blind, placebo-controlled study. Hum Reprod. 1999; 14:838–41.

Janeway Jr CA, Medzhitov R. Innate immune recognition. Annu Rev Immunol. 2002;20:197–216.

Kaufmann SHE, Kabelitz D. The immune response to infectious agents. In: Kaufmann SHE, Kabelitz D, editors. Immunology of infection. Methods in microbiology volume 32. 2nd ed. London: Academic; 2002. p. 1–20.

Komi J, Lassila O. Nonsteroidal anti-estrogens inhibit the functional differentiation of human monocyte-derived dendritic cells. Blood. 2000;95:2875–82.

Lieu PT, Heiskala M, Peterson PA, Yang Y. The roles of iron in health and disease. Mol Aspects Med. 2001;22: 1–87.

Medzhitov R, Biron CA. Innate immunity. Curr Opin Immunol. 2003;15:2–4.

Neutra MR, Kraehenbuhl JP. Regional immune response to microbial pathogens. In: Kaufmann SHE, Sher A, Ahmed R, editors. Immunology of infectious diseases. Washington: ASM Press; 2002. p. 191–206.

Paharkova-Vatchkova V, Maldonado R, Kovats S. Estrogen preferentially promotes the differentiation of CD11c+CD11b dendritic cells from bone marrow precursors. J Immunol. 2004;172:1426–36.

Roitt I. Essential immunology. 8th ed. Oxford: Blackwell Science; 1994.

Schöllmann C, Stauder G, Schäffer A, Schwarz G, Rusch K, Peters U. Grundlagen der immunologie. Ein repetitorium. Germering: Forum Medizin; 2004.

NK Cells

Bulmer JN, Morrison L, Longfellow M, Ritson A, Pace D. Granulated lymphocytes in human endometrium: histochemical and immunohistochemical studies. Hum Reprod. 1991;6:791–8.

Cassatella MA. The production of cytokines by polymorphonuclear neutrophils. Immunol Today. 1995;16:21–6.

Cella M, Scheidegger D, Palmer-Lehmann K, Lane P, Lanzavecchia A, Alber G. Ligation of CD40 on dendritic cells triggers production of high levels of interleukin-12 and enhances T cell stimulatory capacity: T-T help via APC activation. J Exp Med. 1996;184:747–52.

Chegini N, Ma C, Roberts M, Williams RS, Ripps BA. Differential expression of interleukin (IL) IL-13 and IL-15 throughout the menstrual cycle in endometrium of normal fertile women and women with recurrent spontaneous abortion. J Reprod Immunol. 2002;56:93–110.

Cooper MA, Fehniger TA, Caligiuri MA. The biology of human natural killer-cell subsets. Trends Immunol. 2001;22:633–40. 253.

Degli-Esposti MA, Smyth MJ. Close encounters of different kinds: dendritic cells and NK cells take centre stage. Nat Rev Immunol. 2005;5:112–24.

Dosiou C, Giudice LC. Natural killer cells in pregnancy and recurrent pregnancy loss: endocrine immunologic perspectives. Endocr Rev. 2004;26:44–62.

Dunn CL, Critchley HO, Kelly RW. IL-15 regulation in human endometrial stromal cells. J Clin Endocrinol Metab. 2002;87:1898–901.

Eriksson M, Meadows SK, Wira CR, Sentman CL. Unique phenotype of human uterine NK cells and their regulation by endogenous TGF-β. Leukocyte Biol. 2004;76:667–75.

Fausch SC, Da Silva DM, Rudolf MP, Kast WM. Human papillomavirus virus-like particles do not activate Langerhans cells: a possible immune escape mechanism used by human papillomaviruses. J Immunol. 2002;169:3242–9.

Givan AL, White HD, Stern JE, Colby E, Gosselin EJ, Guyre PM, Wira CR. Flow cytometric analysis of leukocytes in the human female reproductive tract: a comparison of fallopian tube, uterus, cervix, and vagina. Am J Reprod Immunol. 1997;38:350–9.

Greenwood JD, Minhas K, di Santo JP, Makta M, Kiso Y, Croy BA. Ultrastructural studies of implantation sites from mice deficient in uterine natural killer cells. Placenta. 2000;21:693–702.

Hanna J, Wald O, Goldman-Wohl D, Prus D, Markel G, Gazit R, Katz G, Haimov-Kochman R, Fuji N, Yagel S, Peled A, Mandelboim O. CXCL12 expression by invasive trophoblasts induces the specific migration of CD16- human natural killer cells. Blood. 2003;102:1569–77.

Hayashi F, Means TK, Luster AD. Toll-like receptors stimulate human neutrophil function. Blood. 2003; 102:2660–9.

Hedges SR, Sibley D, Mayo MS, Hook 3rd EW, Russell MW. Cytokine and antibody responses in women infected with Neisseria gonorrhoeae: effects of concomitant infections. J Infect Dis. 1998;178:742–51.

Hornung V, Rothenfusser S, Britsch S, Krug A, Jahrsdörfer B, Giese T, Endres S, Hartmann G. Quantitative expression of toll-like receptor 1-10 mRNA in cellular subsets of human peripheral blood mononuclear cells and sensitivity to CpG oligodeoxynucleotides. J Immunol. 2002;168:4531–7.

Hunt JS. Immunologically relevant cells in the uterus. Biol Reprod. 1994;50:461–6.

Ishikawa F, Miyazaki S. New biodefense strategies by neutrophils. Arch Immunol Ther Exp. 2005;53:226–33.

Jokhi PP, King A, Sharkey AM, Smith SK, Loke YW. Screening for cytokine messenger ribonucleic acids in purified human decidual lymphocyte populations by the reverse- transcriptase polymerase chain reaction. J Immunol. 1994;153:4427–35.

Kalish RB, Vardhana S, Gupta M, Perni SC, Chasen ST, Witkin SS. Polymorphisms in the tumor necrosis factor-a gene at position -308 and the inducible 70 kDa heat shock protein gene at position +1267 in multifetal pregnancies and preterm premature rupture of fetal membranes. Am J Obstet Gynecol. 2004;191:1368–74.

Kitaya K, Yasuda J, Yagi I, Tada Y, Fushiki S, Honjo H. IL-15 expression at human endometrium and decidua. Biol Reprod. 2000;63:683–7.

Kitaya K, Nakayama T, Daikoku N, Fushiki S, Honjo H. Spatial and temporal expression of ligands for CXCR3 and CXCR4 in human endometrium. J Clin Endocrinol Metab. 2004;89:2470–6.

Koopman LA, Kocow HD, Rybalov B, Boyson JE, Orange JS, Schatz F, Masch R, Lockwood CJ, Schachter AD, Park PJ, Strominger JL. Human decidual natural killer cells are a unique NK cell subset with immunomodulatory potential. J Exp Med. 2003;198:1201–12.

Krieg AM. Now I, know my CpGs. Trends Microbiol. 2001;9:249–52.

Lanier LL. NK cell recognition. Annu Rev Immunol. 2005;23:225–74.

Ley K. Integration of inflammatory signals by rolling neutrophils. Immunol Rev. 2002;186:8–18.

Li XF, Charnock-Jones S, Zhang E, Hiby S, Malik S, Day K, Licence D, Bowen JM, Gardner L, King A, Loke YW, Smith SK. Angiogenic growth factor messenger ribonucleic acids in uterine natural killer cells. J Clin Endocrinol Metab. 2001;86:1823–34.

Ma D, Gu MJ, Liu BQ. A preliminary study on natural killer activity in patients with gynecologic malignancies. J Tongji Med Univ. 1990;10:159–63.

McKenzie J, King A, Hare J, Fulford T, Wilson B, Stanley M. Immunocytochemical characterization of large granular lymphocytes in normal cervix and HPV-associated disease. J Pathol. 1991;165:75–80.

McMahon CW, Raulet DH. Expression and function of NK cell receptors in CD8+ T cells. Curr Opin Immunol. 2001;13:465–70.

Orange JS. Human natural killer cell deficiencies and susceptibility to infection. Microbes Infect. 2002;4:1545–58.

Orange JS, Ballas ZK. Natural killer cells in human health and disease. Clin Immunol. 2006;118:1–10.

Patton D, Thwin SS, Meier A, Hooton TM, Stapleton AE, Eschenbach DA. EC layer thickness and immune cell populations in the normal human vagina at different stages of the menstrual cycle. Am J Obstet Gynecol. 2000;183:967–73.

Peritt D, Robertson S, Gri G, Showe L, Aste-Amezaga M, Trinchieri G. Cutting edge: differentiation of human NK cells into NK1 and NK2 subsets. J Immunol. 1998;161:5821–4.

Ravetch JV, Lanier LL. Immune inhibitory receptors. Science. 2000;290:84–9.

Schöllmann C, Stauder G, Schäffer A, Schwarz G, Rusch K, Peters U. Grundlagen der immunologie. Ein repetitorium. Germering: Forum Medizin; 2004.

Sentman CL, Meadows SK, Wira CR, Eriksson M. Recruitment of uterine NK cells: induction of CXC chemokine ligands 10 and 11 in human endometrium by estradiol and progesterone. J Immunol. 2004;173:6760–6.

Shao L, Jacobs AR, Johnson VV, Mayer L. Activation of CD8+ regulatory T cells by human placental trophoblasts. J Immunol. 2005;174:7539–47.

Stricker RB, Steinleitner A, Bookoff CN, Weckstein LN, Winger EE. Successful treatment of immunologic abortion with low-dose intravenous immunoglobulin. Fertil Steril. 2000;73:536–40.

Sun R, Li AL, Wei HM, Tan ZG. Expression of prolactin receptor and response to prolactin stimulation of human NK cell lines. Cell Res. 2004;14:67–73.

Todd HM, Dundoo VL, Gerber WR, Cwiak CA, Baldassare JJ, Hertelendy F. Effect of cytokines on prostaglandin E2 and prostacyclin production in primary cultures of human myometrial cells. J Matern Fetal Med. 1996;5:161–7.

Watari M, Watari H, Fujimoto T, Yamada H, Nishihira J, Strauss JF, Fujimoto S. Lipopolysaccharide induces interleukin-8 production by human cervical smooth muscle cells. J Soc Gynecol Investig. 2003;10:110–7.

Wells M, Bennett J, Bulmer JN, Jackson P, Holgate CS. Complement component deposition in uteroplacental (spiral) arteries in normal human pregnancy. J Reprod Immunol. 1987;12:125–35.

Wira CR, Fahey JV, Sentman CL, Pioli PA, Shen L. Innate and adaptive immunity in female genital tract: cellular responses and interactions. Immunol Rev. 2005;206:306–35.

Xu P, Alfaidy N, Challis JR. Expression of matrix metalloproteinase (MMP)-2 and MMP-9 in human placenta and fetal membranes in relation to preterm and term labor. J Clin Endocrinol Metab. 2002;87:1353–61.

Yeaman GR, Guyre PM, Fanger MW, Collins JE, White HD, Rathbun W, Orndorff KA, Gonzalez J, Stern JE, Wira CR. Unique CD8+ T cell-rich lymphoid aggregates in human uterine endometrium. J Leukoc Biol. 1997;61:427–35.

Neutrophils in the Female Genital Tract

Bates DO, Lodwick D, Williams B. Vascular endothelial growth factor and microvascular permeability. Microcirculation. 1999;6:83–96.

Bohmer JT, Schemmer G, Harrison Jr FN, Kreft W, Elliot M. Cervical wet mount as a negative predictor for gonococci- and Chlamydia trachomatis-induced cervicitis in a gravid population. Am J Obstet Gynecol. 1999;181:283–7.

Brännström M, Enskog A. Leukocyte networks and ovulation. J Reprod Immunol. 2002;57:47–60.

Brännström M, Pascoe V, Norman RJ, McClure N. Localization of leukocyte subsets in the follicle wall and in the corpus luteum throughout the human menstrual cycle. Fertil Steril. 1994;61:488–95.

Cassatella MA. The production of cytokines by polymorphonuclear neutrophils. Immunol Today. 1995;16:21–6.

Cauci S, Guaschino S, de Aloysio D, Driussi S, De Santo D, Penacchioni P, Quadrifoglio F. Interrelationships of interleukin-8 with interleukin-1β and neutrophils in vaginal fluid of healthy and bacterial vaginosis positive women. Mol Hum Reprod. 2003;9:53–8.

Critchley HOD, Jones RL, Lea RG, Drudy TA, Kelly RW, Williams ARW, Baird DT. Role of inflammatory mediators in human endometrium during progesterone withdrawal and early pregnancy. J Clin Endocrinol Metab. 1999;84:240–8.

Faurschou M, Borregard N. Neutrophil granules and secretory vesicles in inflammation. Microbes Infect. 2003;5:1317–27.

Fidel Jr PL, Barousse M, Espinosa T, Ficarra M, Sturtevant J, Martin DH, Quayle AJ, Dunlap K. An intravaginal live Candida challenge in humans leads to new hypothesis for the immunopathogenesis of vulvovaginal candidiasis. Infect Immun. 2004;72:2939–46.

Givan AL, White HD, Stern JE, Colby E, Gosselin EJ, Guyre PM, Wira CR. Flow cytometric analysis of leukocytes in the human female reproductive tract: a comparison of fallopian tube, uterus, cervix, and vagina. Am J Reprod Immunol. 1997;38:350–9.

Hayashi F, Means TK, Luster AD. Toll-like receptors stimulate human neutrophil function. Blood. 2003;102:2660–9.

Heit B, Tavener S, Raharjo E, Kubes P. An intracellular signaling hierarchy determines direction of migration in opposing chemotactic gradients. J Cell Biol. 2002; 159:91–102.

Huber AR, Kunkel SL, Todd RF, Weiss SJ. Regulation of transendothelial neutrophil migration by endogenous interleukin-8. Science. 1991;254:99–102.

Ishikawa F, Miyazaki S. New biodefense strategies by neutrophils. Arch Immunol Ther Exp. 2005;53:226–33.

Kidney JC, Proud D. Neutrophil transmigration across human airway epithelial monolayers. Mechanisms and dependence on electrical resistance. Am J Respir Cell Mol Biol. 2000;23:389–95.

King AE, Critchley HOD, Sallenave JM, Kelly RW. Elafin in human endometrium: an antiprotease and antimicrobial molecule expressed during menstruation. J Clin Endocrinol Metab. 2003;88:4426–31.

Krause W. Leitlinie immunologische Infertilität. J Dtsch Dermatol Ges. 2005;3:650–5.

Ley K. Integration of inflammatory signals by rolling neutrophils. Immunol Rev. 2002;186:8–18.

Luu NT, Rainger GE, Buckley CD, Nash GB. CD31 regulates direction and rate of neutrophil migration over and under endothelial cells. J Vasc Res. 2003;40:467–79.

Palter SF, Mulayim N, Senturk L, Arici A. Interleukin-8 in the human fallopian tube. J Clin Endocrinol Metab. 2001;86:2660–7.

Pandya IJ, Cohen J. Leukocyte reaction of the human cervix to spermatozoa. Fertil Steril. 1985;43:412–21.

Patton D, Thwin SS, Meier A, Hooton TM, Stapleton AE, Eschenbach DA. EC layer thickness and immune cell populations in the normal human vagina at different stages of the menstrual cycle. Am J Obstet Gynecol. 2000;183:967–73.

Runesson E, Ivarsson K, Janson PO, Brännström M. Gonadotropin- and cytokine-regulated expression of the chemokine interleukin-8 in the human preovulatory follicle of the menstrual cycle. J Clin Endocrinol Metab. 2000;85:4387–95.

Schöllmann C, Stauder G, Schäffer A, Schwarz G, Rusch K, Peters U. Grundlagen der immunologie. Ein repetitorium. Germering: Forum Medizin; 2004.

Shen L, Fahey JV, Hussey SB, Asin SN, Wira CR, Fanger MW. Synergy between IL-8 and GM-CSF in reproductive tract EC secretions promotes enhanced neutrophil chemotaxis. Cell Immunol. 2004;230:23–32.

Sonoda Y, Mukaida N, Wang J, Shimada-Hiratsuka M, Naito M, Kasahara T, Harada A, Inoue M, Matsushima K. Physiologic regulation of postovulatory migration into vagina in mice by a C-X-C chemokine(s). J Immunol. 1998;160:6159–65.

Thompson LA, Tomlinson MJ, Barratt CL, Bolton AE, Cooke ID. Positive immunoselection-a method of isolating leukocytes from leukocytic reacted human cervical mucus samples. Am J Reprod Immunol. 1991;26:58–61.

Wira CR, Fahey JV, Sentman CL, Pioli PA, Shen L. Innate and adaptive immunity in female genital tract: cellular responses and interactions. Immunol Rev. 2005;206: 306–35

Wollen AL, Sandvei R, Mork S, Marandon JL, Matre R. In situ characterization of leukocytes in the fallopian tube in women with or without an intrauterine contraceptive device. Acta Obstet Gynecol Scand. 1994;73:103–12.

Yeaman GR, Collins JE, Currie JK, Guyre PM, Wira CR, Fanger MW. IFN-γ is produced by polymorphonuclear neutrophils in human uterine endometrium and by cultured peripheral blood polymorphonuclear neutrophils. J Immunol. 1998;16:5145–53.

Zhang J, Hampton AL, Nie GY, Salamonsen LA. Progesterone inhibits activation of latent matrix metalloproteinase (MMP)-2 by membrane-type 1 MMP: enzymes co-ordinately expressed in human endometrium. Biol Reprod. 2000;62:85–94.

Immunoglobulins in the Female Genital Tract

Beagley KW, Gockel CM. Regulation of innate and adaptive immunity by the female sex hormones estradiol and progesterone. FEMS Immunol Med Microbiol. 2003;38:13–22.

Bjercke S, Brandtzaeg P. Glandular distribution of immunoglobulins, J chain, secretory component, and HLA-DR in the human endometrium throughout the menstrual cycle. Hum Reprod. 1993;8:1420–5.

Brandtzaeg P. Mucosal immunity in the female genital tract. J Reprod Immunol. 1997;36:23–50.

Crowley-Norwick PA, Bell MC, Edwards RP, McCallister D, Gore H, Kanbour-Shakir A, Mestecky J, Partridge EE. Normal uterine cervix: characterization of isolated lymphocyte phenotypes and immunoglobulin secretion. Am J Reprod Immunol. 1995;34:241–7.

Hocini H, Barra A, Belec L, Iscaki S, Preud'Homme JL, Pillot J, Bouvet JP. Systemic and secretory humoral immunity in the normal human vaginal tract. Scand J Immunol. 1995;42:269–74.

Hordnes K, Tynning T, Brown TA, Haneberg B, Jonsson R. Nasal immunization with group B streptococci can induce high levels of specific IgA antibodies in cervicovaginal secretions of mice. Vaccine. 1997;15:1244–51.

Jackson S, Mestecky J, Moldoveanu Z, Spearman P. Appendix I: collection and processing of human mucosal secretions. In: Mestecky J, Bienenstock J, Lamm ME, Mayer L, McGhee JR, Strober W, editors. Mucosal immunology. 3rd ed. Amsterdam: Elsevier Academic Press; 2005. p. 1829–39.

Jalanti R, Isliker H. Immunoglobulin in human cervicovaginal secretions. Int Arch Allergy Appl Immunol. 1977;53:402–8.

Johansson EL, Rudin A, Wassen L, Holmgren J. Distribution of lymphocytes and adhesion molecules in human cervix and vagina. Immunology. 1999;96: 272–7.

Kanda N, Tamaki K. Estrogen enhances immunoglobulin production by human PBMCs. J Allergy Clin Immunol. 1999;103:282–8.

Kutteh WH, Mestecky J. Secretory immunity in the female reproductive tract. Am J Reprod Immunol. 1994;31:40–6.

Kutteh WH, Hatch D, Blackwell RE, Mestecky J. Secretory immune system of the female reproductive tract: I. Immunoglobulin and secretory-component-containing cells. Obstet Gynecol. 1988;71:56–60.

Kutteh WH, Prince SJ, Hammonds KR, Kutteh CC, Mestecky J. Variations in immunoglobulins and IgA subclasses of human uterine cervical secretions around the time of ovulation. Clin Exp Immunol. 1996;104:538–42.

Kutteh WH, Mestecky J, Wira CR. Mucosal immunity in the human female reproductive tract. In: Mestecky J, Lamm ME, Strober W, Bienenstock J, McGhee JR, Mayer L, editors. Handbook of mucosal immunology. Oxford: Elsevier Academic Press; 2005. p. 1631–46.

Mestecky J, Fultz PN. Mucosal immune system of the human genital tract. J Infect Dis. 1999;179 Suppl 3:S470–4.

Mestecky J, Russell MW. Immunoglobulins and mechanisms of mucosal immunity. Biochem Soc Trans. 1997;25:457–62.

Mestecky J, Lue C, Russell MW. Selective transport of IgA. Cellular and molecular aspects. Gastroenterol Clin North Am. 1991;20:441–71.

Michaels RM, Rogers KD. A sex difference in immunologic responsiveness. Pediatrics. 1971;47:120–3.

Paavonen T, Andersson LC, Adlercreutz H. Sex hormone regulation of in vitro immune response. Estradiol enhances human B cell maturation via inhibition of suppressor T cells in pokeweed mitogen-stimulated cultures. J Exp Med. 1981;154:1935–45.

Parr MB, Parr EL. Mucosal immunity in the female and male reproductive tracts. In: Ogra PL, Mestecky J, Strober W, McGhee JR, Bienenstock J, editors. Handbook of mucosal immunology. San Diego: Academic; 1994. p. 677–89.

Profet M. Menstruation as a defense against pathogens transported by sperm. Q Rev Biol. 1993;68: 335–86.

Quesnel A, Cu-Uvin S, Murphy D, Ashley RL, Flanigan T, Neutra MR. Comparative analysis of methods for collection and measurement of immunoglobulins in cervical and vaginal secretions of women. J Immunol Methods. 1997;202:153–61.

Russell MW, Mestecky J. Humoral immune responses to microbial infections in the genital tract. Microbes Infect. 2002;4:667–77.

Thaler CJ, Samtleben W. Einfluss von Sexualsteroiden auf physiologische and pathologische Reaktionen des Immunsystems. Überlegungen zur postmenopausalen Hormonsubstitution. Gynakologe. 2000;33: 393–401.

Waldman RH, Cruz JM, Rowe DS. Immunoglobulin levels and antibody to Candida albicans in human cervicovaginal secretions. Clin Exp Immunol. 1971;9:427–34.

Wira CR, Sandoe CP. Sex steroid hormone regulation of IgG and IgA in rat uterine secretions. Nature. 1977;268:534–6.

Wira CR, Sandoe CP. Hormone regulation of immunoglobulins: influence of estradiol on IgA and IgG in the rat uterus. Endocrinology. 1980;106:1020–6.

Wira CR, Sullivan DA. Estradiol and progesterone regulation of IgA, IgG and secretory component in cervicovaginal secretions of rat. Biol Reprod. 1985;32:90–5.

Prevalence of T Lymphocytes

Beagley KW, Gockel CM. Regulation of innate and adaptive immunity by the female sex hormones estradiol and progesterone. FEMS Immunol Med Microbiol. 2003;38:13–22.

Givan AL, White HD, Stern JE, Colby E, Gosselin EJ, Guyre PM, Wira CR. Flow cytometric analysis of leukocytes in the human female reproductive tract: a comparison of fallopian tube, uterus, cervix, and vagina. Am J Reprod Immunol. 1997;38:350–9.

Johansson EL, Rudin A, Wassen L, Holmgren J. Distribution of lymphocytes and adhesion molecules in human cervix and vagina. Immunology. 1999;96:272–7.

Kutteh WH, Mestecky J, Wira CR. Mucosal immunity in the human female reproductive tract. In: Mestecky J, Lamm ME, Strober W, Bienenstock J, McGhee JR, Mayer L, editors. Handbook of mucosal immunology. Oxford: Elsevier Academic Press; 2005. p. 1631–46.

Pudney J, Quayle AJ, Anderson DJ. Immunological microenvironments in the human vagina and cervix: mediators of cellular immunity are concentrated in the cervical transformation zone. Biol Reprod. 2005;73:1253–63.

White HD, Crassi KM, Givan AL, Stern JE, Gonzalez JL, Memoli VA, Green WR, Wira CR. CD3 + CD8 + CTL activity within the human female reproductive tract. J Immunol. 1997;158:3017–27.

Yeaman GR, Guyre PM, Fanger MW, Collins JE, White HD, Rathbun W, Orndorff KA, Gonzalez J, Stern JE, Wira CR. Unique CD8+ T cell-rich lymphoid aggregates in human uterine endometrium. J Leukoc Biol. 1997;61:427–35.

Immunization Studies

Bergquist C, Johansson EL, Lagergård T, Holmgren J, Rudin A. Intranasal vaccination of humans with recombinant Cholera Toxin B subunit induces systemic and local antibody responses in the upper respiratory tract and the vagina. Infect Immun. 1997;65:2676–84.

Crowley-Norwick PA, Bell MC, Brockwell R, Edwards RP, Chen S, Partridge EE, Mestecky J. Rectal immunization for induction of specific antibody in the genital tract of women. J Clin Immunol. 1997;17:370–9.

Czerkinsky C, Anjuere F, McGhee JR, George-Chandy A, Holmgren J, Kieny MP, Fujiyashi K, Mestecky JF, Pierrefite-Carle V, Rask C, Sun JB. Mucosal immunity and tolerance: relevance to vaccine development. Immunol Rev. 1999;170:197–222.

Johansson EL, Rask C, Fredriksson M, Eriksson K, Czerkinsky C, Holmgren J. Antibodies and antibody-secreting cells in the female genital tract after vaginal or intranasal immunization with Cholera Toxin B subunit or conjugates. Infect Immun. 1998;66:514–20.

Johansson EL, Rudin A, Wassen L, Holmgren J. Distribution of lymphocytes and adhesion molecules in human cervix and vagina. Immunology. 1999;96:272–7.

Johansson EL, Wassen L, Holmgren J, Jertborn M, Rudin A. Nasal and vaginal vaccinations have differential effects on antibody responses in vaginal and cervical secretions in humans. Infect Immun. 2001;69:7481–6.

Kozlowski PA, Cu-Uvin S, Neutra MR, Flanigan TP. Comparison of the oral rectal and vaginal immunization routes for induction of antibodies in rectal and genital tract secretions. Infect Immun. 1997;65:1387–94.

Kozlowski PA, Cu-Uvin S, Neutra MR, Flanigan TP. Mucosal vaccination strategies for women. J Infect Dis. 1999;179:493–8.

Kozlowski PA, Williams SB, Lynch RM, Flanigan TP, Patterson RR, Cu-Uvin S, Neutra MR. Differential induction of mucosal and systemic antibody responses in women after nasal, rectal, or vaginal immunization: influence of the menstrual cycle. J Immunol. 2002;169:566–74.

Kutteh WH, Kantele A, Moldoveanu Z, Crowley-Nowick PA, Mestecky J. Induction of specific immune responses in the genital tract of women after oral or rectal immunization and rectal boosting with Salmonella typhi Ty 21a vaccine. J Reprod Immunol. 2001;52:61–75.

Ogra PL, Ogra SS. Local antibody response to polio vaccine in the female genital tract. J Immunol. 1973a;110:1307–11.

Rodriguez A, Tjarnlund A, Ivanji J, Singh M, Garcia I, Williams A, Marsh PD, Troye-Blomberg M, Fernandez C. Role of IgA in the defense of respiratory infections. IgA-deficient mice exhibited increased susceptibility to intranasal infection with Mycobacterium bovis BCG. Vaccine. 2005;23:2565–72.

Rudin A, Johansson E-L, Bergquist C, Holmgren J. Differential kinetics and distribution of antibodies in serum and nasal and vaginal secretions after nasal and oral vaccination of humans. Infect Immun. 1998;66:3390–6.

Russell MW, Mestecky J. Humoral immune responses to microbial infections in the genital tract. Microbes Infect. 2002;4:667–77.

Thapar M, Parr EL, Parr MB. Secretory immune responses in mouse vaginal fluid after pelvic, parenteral, or vaginal immunization. Immunology. 1990;70:121–5.

Thapar M, Parr EL, Parr MB. The effect of adjuvants on antibody titers in mouse vaginal fluid after intravaginal immunization. J Reprod Immunol. 1990;17:207–16.

Wu H-Y, Abdu S, Stinson D, Russell MW. Generation of female genital tract antibody responses by local or central (common) mucosal immunization. Infect Immun. 2000;68:5539–45.

Immunology of Menstruation: Menstruation as an Inflammatory Process

Ahmed A, Li XF, Shams M, Gregory J, Rollason T, Barnes NM, Newton JR. Localization of the angiotensin II and its receptor subtype expression in human endometrium and identification of a novel high-affinity angiotensin II binding site. J Clin Invest. 1995;96:848–57.

Ben-Baruch A, Michiel DF, Oppenheim JJ. Signals and receptors involved in recruitment of inflammatory cells. J Biol Chem. 1995;270:11703–6.

Bergquist C, Johansson EL, Lagergård T, Holmgren J, Rudin A. Intranasal vaccination of humans with recombinant Cholera Toxin B subunit induces systemic and local antibody responses in the upper respiratory tract and the vagina. Infect Immun. 1997;65:2676–84.

Birkedal-Hansen H, Moore WGI, Bodden MK, Windsor LJ, Birkedal-Hansen B, DeCarlo A, Engler JA. Matrix metalloproteinases: a review. Crit Rev Oral Biol Med. 1993;4:197–250.

Chen CK, Huang SC, Chen CL, Yen MR, Hsu HC, Ho HN. Increased expressions of CD69 and HLA-DR but not of CD25 or CD71 on endometrial T lymphocytes of non-pregnant women. Hum Immunol. 1995;42:227–32.

Critchley HOD, Brenner RM, Drudy TA, Williams K, Nayak NR, Slayden OD, Millar MR, Saunders PTK. Estrogen receptor beta, but not estrogen receptor alpha, is present in vascular endothelium of the human and nonhuman primate endometrium. J Clin Endocrinol Metab. 2001;86:1370–8.

Critchley HOD, Kelly RW, Brenner RM, Baird DT. The endocrinology of menstruation-a role for the immune system. Clin Endocrinol. 2001;55:701–10.

Crowley-Norwick PA, Bell MC, Brockwell R, Edwards RP, Chen S, Partridge EE, Mestecky J. Rectal immunization for induction of specific antibody in the genital tract of women. J Clin Immunol. 1997;17:370–9.

Czerkinsky C, Anjuere F, McGhee JR, George-Chandy A, Holmgren J, Kieny MP, Fujiyashi K, Mestecky JF, Pierrefite-Carle V, Rask C, Sun JB. Mucosal immunity and tolerance: relevance to vaccine development. Immunol Rev. 1999;170:197–222.

Finn CA. Implantation, menstruation and inflammation. Biol Rev Camb Philos Soc. 1986;61:313–28.

Gottschall SL, Hansen PJ. Regulation of leukocyte subpopulations in the sheep endometrium by progesterone. Immunology. 1992;76:636–41.

Hornung D, Ryan IP, Chao VA, Vigne JL, Schriock D, Taylor RN. Immunolocalization and regulation of the chemokine RANTES in human endometrial and endometriosis tissues and cells. J Clin Endocrinol Metab. 1997;82:1621–8.

Jeziorska M, Salamonsen LA, Woolley DE. Mast cell and eosinophil distribution and activation in human endometrium throughout the menstrual cycle. Biol Reprod. 1995;53:312–20.

Johansson EL, Rask C, Fredriksson M, Eriksson K, Czerkinsky C, Holmgren J. Antibodies and antibody-secreting cells in the female genital tract after vaginal or intranasal immunization with Cholera Toxin B subunit or conjugates. Infect Immun. 1998;66:514–20.

Johansson EL, Rudin A, Wassen L, Holmgren J. Distribution of lymphocytes and adhesion molecules in human cervix and vagina. Immunology. 1999;96:272–7.

Johansson EL, Wassen L, Holmgren J, Jertborn M, Rudin A. Nasal and vaginal vaccinations have differential effects on antibody responses in vaginal and cervical secretions in humans. Infect Immun. 2001;69:7481–6.

Jolicoeur C, Boutouil M, Drouin R, Paradis I, Lemay A, Akoum A. Increased expression of monocyte chemotactic protein-1 in the endometrium of women with endometriosis. Am J Pathol. 1998;152:125–33.

Jones RL, Kelly RW, Critchley HO. Chemokine and cyclooxygenase-2 expression in human endometrium coincides with leukocyte accumulation. Hum Reprod. 1997;12:1300–6.

Jones RK, Bulmer JN, Searle RF. Phenotypic and functional studies of leukocytes in human endometrium and endometriosis. Hum Reprod Update. 1998;4:702–9.

Jones RL, Hannan NJ, Kaitúu TJ, Zhang J, Salamonsen LA. Identification of chemokines important for leukocyte recruitment to the human endometrium at the times of embryo implantation and menstruation. J Clin Endocrinol Metab. 2004;89:6155–67.

Kelly RW, King AE, Critchley HOD. Cytokine control in human endometrium. Reproduction. 2001;121:3–19.

King A. Uterine leukocytes and decidualization. Hum Reprod Update. 2000;6:28–36.

King A, Balendran N, Wooding P, Carter NP, Loke YW. CD3 leukocytes present in the human uterus during early placentation: phenotypic and morphologic characterisation of the CD56+ population. Dev Immunol. 1991;1:169–90.

King AE, Critchley HOD, Sallenave JM, Kelly RW. Elafin in human endometrium: an antiprotease and antimicrobial molecule expressed during menstruation. J Clin Endocrinol Metab. 2003;88:4426–31.

Kodama T, Hara T, Okamoto E, Kusunoki Y, Ohama K. Characteristic changes of large granular lymphocytes that strongly express CD56 in endometrium during the menstrual cycle and early pregnancy. Hum Reprod. 1998;13:1036–43.

Kozlowski PA, Cu-Uvin S, Neutra MR, Flanigan TP. Comparison of the oral rectal and vaginal immunization routes for induction of antibodies in rectal and genital tract secretions. Infect Immun. 1997;65:1387–94.

Kozlowski PA, Cu-Uvin S, Neutra MR, Flanigan TP. Mucosal vaccination strategies for women. J Infect Dis. 1999;179:493–8.

Kozlowski PA, Williams SB, Lynch RM, Flanigan TP, Patterson RR, Cu-Uvin S, Neutra MR. Differential induction of mucosal and systemic antibody responses in women after nasal, rectal, or vaginal immunization: influence of the menstrual cycle. J Immunol. 2002;169:566–74.

Kutteh WH, Kantele A, Moldoveanu Z, Crowley-Nowick PA, Mestecky J. Induction of specific immune responses in the genital tract of women after oral or rectal immunization and rectal boosting with Salmonella typhi Ty 21a vaccine. J Reprod Immunol. 2001;52:61–75.

Ludwig H, Spornitz HM. Microarchitecture of the endometrium by scanning electron microscopy: menstrual desquamation and remodelling. Ann N Y Acad Sci. 1991;622:28–46.

Markee JE. Menstruation in intraocular endometrial transplants in the rhesus monkey. Contrib Embryol. 1940;177:220–30.

Martin P. Wound healing-aiming for perfect skin regeneration. Science. 1997;276:75–81.

Matsuzaki S, Fukaya T, Suzuki T, Murakami T, Sasano H, Yajima A. Estrogen receptor alpha and beta mRNA expression in human endometrium throughout the menstrual cycle. Mol Hum Reprod. 1999;5:559–64.

Ogra PL, Ogra SS. Local antibody response to poliovaccine in the female genital tract. J Immunol. 1973b;110:1307–11.

Paldi A, d'Auriol L, Misrahi M, Bakos AM, Chaouat G, Szerkeres-Bartho J. Expression of the gene coding for the progesterone receptor in activated human lymphocytes. Endocr J. 1994;2:317–9.

Roberts DK, Parmley TH, Walker NJ, Horbelt DV. Ultrastructure of the microvasculature in human endometrium throughout the normal menstrual cycle. Am J Obstet Gynecol. 1993;168:1393–406.

Rodgers WH, Matrisian LM, Guidice LC, Dsupin B, Cannon P, Svitek C, Gorstein F, Osteen KG. Patterns of matrix metalloproteinase expression in cycling endometrium imply different functions and regulation by steroid hormones. J Clin Invest. 1994;94:946–53.

Rodriguez A, Tjarnlund A, Ivanji J, Singh M, Garcia I, Williams A, Marsh PD, Troye-Blomberg M, Fernandez C. Role of IgA in the defense of respiratory infections. IgA-deficient mice exhibited increased susceptibility to intranasal infection with Mycobacterium bovis BCG. Vaccine. 2005;23:2565–72.

Rudin A, Johansson E-L, Bergquist C, Holmgren J. Differential kinetics and distribution of antibodies in serum and nasal and vaginal secretions after nasal and oral vaccination of humans. Infect Immun. 1998;66:3390–6.

Russell MW, Mestecky J. Humoral immune responses to microbial infections in the genital tract. Microbes Infect. 2002;4:667–77.

Salamonsen LA, Lathbury LJ. Endometrial leukocytes and menstruation. Hum Reprod Update. 2000;6:16–27.

Salamonsen LA, Woolley DE. Menstruation: induction by matrix metalloproteinases and inflammatory cells. J Reprod Immunol. 1999;44:1–27.

Salamonsen LA, Zhang J, Brasted M. Leukocyte networks and human endometrial remodelling. J Reprod Immunol. 2002;57:95–108.

Shifren JL, Tseng JF, Zaloudek CJ, Ryan IP, Meng YG, Ferrara N, Jaffe RB, Taylor RN. Ovarian steroid regulation of vascular endothelial growth factor in the human endometrium: implications for angiogenesis during the menstrual cycle and in the pathogenesis of endometriosis. J Clin Endocrinol Metab. 1996;81:3112–8.

Song JY, Russell P, Markham R, Manconi F, Fraser IS. Effects of high dose progestogens on white cells and necrosis in human endometrium. Hum Reprod. 1996;11:1713–8.

Stewart JA, Bulmer JD, Murdoch AP. Endometrial leukocytes: expression of steroid hormone receptors. J Clin Pathol. 1998;51:121–6.

Tabibzadeh S. Proliferative activity of lymphoid cells in human endometrium throughout the menstrual cycle. J Clin Endocrinol Metab. 1990;70:437–43.

Tabibzadeh S, Kong QF, Babaknia A. Expression of adhesion molecules in human endometrial vasculature throughout the menstrual cycle. J Clin Endocrinol Metab. 1994a;79:1024–32.

Tabibzadeh S, Kong QF, Satyaswaroop PG. Distinct regional and menstrual cycle dependent distribution of apoptosis in human endometrium. Potential regulatory role of T cells and TNF- α. Endocr J. 1994b;2:87–95.

Tawia SA, Beaton LA, Rogers PA. Immunolocalization of the cellular adhesion molecules, intercellular adhesion molecule-1 (ICAM-1) and platelet endothelial cell adhesion molecule (PECAM), in human endometrium throughout the menstrual cycle. Hum Reprod. 1993;8:175–81.

Thapar M, Parr EL, Parr MB. Secretory immune responses in mouse vaginal fluid after pelvic, parenteral, or vaginal immunization. Immunology. 1990;70:121–5.

Thapar M, Parr EL, Parr MB. The effect of adjuvants on antibody titers in mouse vaginal fluid after intravaginal immunization. J Reprod Immunol. 1990;17:207–16.

Thelen M. Dancing to the tune of chemokines. Nat Immunol. 2001;2:129–34.

Thompson AJ, Greer MR, Young A, Boswell F, Telfer JF, Cameron IT, Norman JE, Campbell S. Expression of intercellular adhesion molecules ICAM-1 and ICAM-2 in human endometrium: regulation by interferon-gamma. Mol Hum Reprod. 1999;5:64–70.

Wang H, Critchley HOD, Kelly RW, Shen D, Baird DT. Progesterone receptor subtype B is differentially regulated in human endometrial stroma. Mol Hum Reprod. 1998;4:407–12.

White HD, Crassi KM, Givan AL, Stern JE, Gonzalez JL, Memoli VA, Green WR, Wira CR. CD3 + CD8 + CTL activity within the human female reproductive tract. J Immunol. 1997;158:3017–27.

Wu H-Y, Abdu S, Stinson D, Russell MW. Generation of female genital tract antibody responses by local or central (common) mucosal immunization. Infect Immun. 2000;68:5539–45.

Yeaman GR, Collins JE, Currie JK, Guyre PM, Wira CR, Fanger MW. IFN-γ is produced by polymorphonuclear neutrophils in human uterine endometrium and by cultured peripheral blood polymorphonuclear neutrophils. J Immunol. 1998;16:5145–53.

Zhang J, Nie GY, Wang J, Woolley DE, Salamonsen LA. Mast cell regulation of endometrial stromal cell matrix metalloproteinases: a mechanism underlying menstruation. Biol Reprod. 1998;59:693–703.

Zhang J, Hampton AL, Nie GY, Salamonsen LA. Progesterone inhibits activation of latent matrix metalloproteinase (MMP)-2 by membrane-type 1 MMP: enzymes co-ordinately expressed in human endometrium. Biol Reprod. 2000;62:85–94.

Zhang J, Lathbury LJ, Salamonsen LA. Expression of the chemokine eotaxin and its receptor, CCR3, in human endometrium. Biol Reprod. 2000;62:404–11.

Immunology of Genital Tract Infections

4

Contents

4.1   Introduction

The understanding of the immune system in the genital tract is of critical importance when considering the increasing prevalence of STDs. The World Health Organization (WHO) estimated a global incidence of 340 million curable STDs in 1999 compared to 250 million cases in 1990. Especially in the developing world, limited access to diagnosis and treatment causes STDs to be the second leading cause of healthy years of life lost by women of reproductive age. In the United States, it is estimated that approximately 18.9 million new cases of STD infections occurred in the year 2000, of which 9.1 million (48 %) were among young persons aged between 15 and 24. Among them, three STDs, HPV, trichomoniasis, and *Chlamydia*, accounted for 88 % of all new STI cases. The epidemiology of each STD is different and dependent on many factors including individual behavior, social conditions, pathogen characteristics, and access to treatment. In the following sections, the latest developments and current studies on the most essential STDs will be discussed with an emphasis on immune responses and chances for vaccination.

4.2   Viral Infections of the Genital Tract

4.2.1   Herpes Simplex Virus

The family of human herpesviridae includes the herpes simplex virus types 1 and 2 (HSV-1 and HSV-2) which are of essential clinical importance in gynecology and obstetrics (Table 4.1).

HSV is an enveloped, linear, double-stranded DNA virus whose only known hosts are humans. HSV-1 and HSV-2 are distinguished by antigenic differences in their envelope proteins. There are 11 glycoproteins in HSV, which are inserted into the envelope of the virus and perform different biological functions (Fig. 4.1).

Typically, HSV infects ECs at mucosal surfaces or abraded skin. HSV-1 normally is associated with oral infections and HSV-2 with genital

Table 4.1 Overview of human herpesviridae

Alpha-herpesviridae	Herpes simplex virus 1
	Herpes simplex virus 2
	Varicella zoster virus
Beta-herpesviridae	Cytomegalovirus
	Human herpes virus 6
	Human herpes virus 7
Gamma-herpesviridae	Epstein–Barr virus
	Human herpes virus 6

M. Wirth 2006, Personal communication

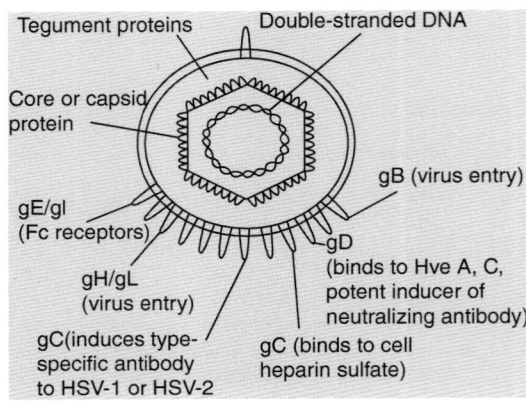

Fig. 4.1 Structural elements of an HSV virion and their biological functions (Cunningham AL, Mikloska Z. The Holy Grail: immune control of human herpes simplex virus infection and disease. Herpes. 2001;8 Suppl 1:6A–10)

infections, but either type can infect a person anywhere on the skin. HSV-2 is usually sexually transmitted and is clinically manifested in the genital or adjacent area as primary or recurrent infection. HSV-1 is becoming an increasingly common cause of primary genital infection but is less commonly a cause of recurrent infection.

The natural history of HSV infection includes an acute or subclinical first-episode mucocutaneous infection, establishment of viral latency in the dorsal root ganglion, and subsequent reactivation. With reactivation, the virus travels back down the nerve root to create a mucocutaneous outbreak, or it may produce no detectable symptoms. Genital herpes infection caused by HSV-2 is one of the most prevalent STDs worldwide and is the most common cause of genital ulcers. The percentage of HSV-2 infections varies between

6 % and 50 % among different populations and its prevalence is increasing. An estimated 20–35 % of pregnant women are HSV-2 seropositive. Genital herpes is more common in women than in men, with approximately one in four women versus one in five men having specific antibodies to HSV-2; this gender difference suggests that the female genital tract provides a more permissive environment for HSV-2 infection and the establishment of latency. Subclinical viral shedding has been documented in more than 80 % of HSV-2-seropositive persons who report no lesions. Only 10–25 % of persons who are HSV-2 seropositive report a history of genital herpes, which suggests that most infected persons have unrecognized symptomatic or completely asymptomatic infections. However, once patients are told of their positive antibody status, more than 50 % identify clinically symptomatic recurrences that previously were ascribed to other conditions. It is thought that viral shedding in persons who are unaware of their infection is responsible for at least 70 % of HSV transmission. There is a concerning relationship between HIV and genital HSV infection because the interaction of HSV-2 and HIV-1 may result in more efficient transmission of HIV-1 and an increased rate of HIV replication during HSV reactivation.

Although oral treatment with acyclovir can reduce the severity of infections, development of a vaccine to prevent or control HSV-2 infections in the genital tract would greatly contribute to preventive health care. To achieve this goal, it is important to understand the host defense mechanisms that are available at genital mucosal sites to protect against this STD.

4.2.1.1 Innate Immune Responses in Genital Herpes Infections

The role of immune factors in the control of HSV infection, especially recurrent lesions after viral reactivation, appears complex. There is a general difference between immune responses to primary and recurrent disease, which is clinically demonstrated in the much longer median duration of lesions and viral shedding in initial infection. There is a mean of 21 days for lesions and 10 days for viral shedding in primary infection

compared to 10 days for lesions and 4 days for viral shedding in recurrent infections.

Basic innate immune responses have been implicated in the protection against genital HSV infection, and extensive studies have identified responses that are important in limiting viral replication and spread to uninfected cells. The first line of defense against genital HSV infection consists of cervical mucus, the endogenous bacterial flora, acidic pH, and secreted proteins such as complement, defensins, and SLPI. The second line of defense is composed of early viral-induced responses by ECs and resident DCs, which are characterized predominantly by IFN production. The third is the recruitment of cellular effectors. IFN type 1 responses are produced within hours after infection, and neutrophils are found within 24 h after vaginal infection. Moreover, macrophages, NK cells, and submucosal DCs have been shown to capture HSV-2 antigen and stimulate T-cell activation in regional lymph nodes.

4.2.1.1.1 pH

The acidic environment of the human vagina in healthy premenopausal women with a pH of 4.0–4.5 contributes to the first line of innate immune defenses in the genital tract. Therefore, early studies developed acid-buffering compounds as candidate microbicides and tested anti-HSV activity provided by the acidic pH. Interestingly, acidic buffers with a pH ≤ 4.5 irreversibly inactivated HSV-1 or HSV-2 and reduced viral yield at least 1,000-fold in vitro, whereas exposure to pH of 5.0 had only a minor effect. The significance of these in vitro findings was confirmed in a murine model in which a vaginal acid-buffering formulation with pH 3.5 named AmpHora was tested. AmpHora significantly protected mice from genital herpes when challenged with the virus delivered in human seminal fluid compared to mice that received a placebo gel.

4.2.1.1.2 Antimicrobial Peptides

Antimicrobial peptides, with their subgroups α- and β-defensins and cathelicidins, have a broad spectrum of activity against different microorganisms and are also presumed to contribute to antiviral activity in the genital tract. HNP1-4 demonstrated to protect human cells with respect to HSV infection in vitro. Further studies indicated that synthetic HNP-4 is less active than HNP1-3 in protecting against HSV and that the EC defensins HD-5 and HD-6 also inhibit HSV-2 infection. Cervicovaginal secretions (CVS) obtained from healthy women by cervicovaginal lavage (CVL) were shown to inhibit HSV infection. There was a reduction of HSV-2 infection by at least 90 % if cells were cultured with CVL from healthy women. The anti-HSV activity of CVL was independent of age, vaginal pH, and the presence of HSV antibodies in serum. The same study indicated that this anti-HSV activity correlated with the concentration of HNP1-3 in the fluid. Both CVL samples and HNP1-3 interacted with virus and prevented virus entry after binding. Preliminary work failed to demonstrate any in vitro anti-HSV activity for synthetic HBD-1 and HBD-2, but further studies are needed to assess whether HBD in cervical secretions contribute to intrinsic anti-HSV activity. The only known human cathelicidin, LL-37, has also not been tested for its anti-HSV activity.

These findings suggest that CVS contributes to innate resistance to HSV-2 infection and identify defensins as participants in this activity (Table 4.2). CVS defensins may provide a prototype for future topical microbicides.

Various other genital tract proteins, such as secretory leukocyte protease inhibitor (SLPI), lactoferrin, and surfactant protein D (SP-D), may also play a role in innate immunity against HSV. Although SLPI is known to protect human macrophages and CD4+ T cells from HIV-1 infection, not much has been found out about the influence of SLPI in protection against HSV. Preliminary studies showed that SLPI inhibits HSV-2 infection in vitro, but HSV-2 significantly decreases SLPI concentrations in cervical cell culture supernatants, implying that the virus may downregulate this antiviral protein. Lactoferrin was shown to inhibit HSV-1 infection in vitro by interfering with the binding of glycoprotein C to cell surface heparin sulfate receptors. This may only partially explain the anti-HSV-2 activity of lactoferrin as binding of HSV-2 to cells is

Table 4.2 Antiviral activity of antimicrobial peptides against HSV-2

	Antiviral activity against HSV-2
α-*Defensins*	
HNP1-3	Yes
HNP-4	Less
HD-5	Yes
HD-6	Yes
β-*Defensins*	
HBD1-2	No; further studies needed
Cathelicidins	
LL-37	Not tested

M. Wirth 2006, Personal communication

primarily mediated by glycoprotein B. SP-D was lately demonstrated in the genital tract mucosa and may play a role in inhibiting HIV transmission as well as in protecting against other STDs.

4.2.1.1.3 Complement

As another factor of innate immunity, complement recognizes infectious agents using three different molecules. These are C1q, mannose-binding lectin (MBL), and C3, which trigger the classical, lectin, and alternative pathways of complement activation, respectively. All three of these molecules are detected in vaginal secretions from healthy women. Notably, HSV has evolved several strategies to evade immune attack by the classical and alternative complement pathways, which include inhibiting activities mediated by C3, C5, and properdin. Specifically, glycoprotein C binds C3 and its activation products, C3b, iC3b, and C3c, and accelerates the decay of the alternative complement pathway C3 convertase. In a murine genital tract model, viruses deleted of HSV-1 glycoprotein C are less virulent. Less is known about the role played by MBL and the lectin pathway as a host defense against genital herpes infection. Recent studies indicate that MBL binds to HSV-2 in vitro. Interestingly, MBL deficiency increases the generalized susceptibility of an individual to infectious diseases, and increased susceptibility to HIV infection in MBL-deficient individuals has been described.

4.2.1.1.4 Dendritic Cells

The precise role played by the different DC populations in the immune response to HSV in the female genital tract is not clear. HSV-1 has been shown to productively infect immature DCs with progressive loss of DCs. Infection is associated with downregulation of CD1a, CD40, CD54 (ICAM-1), CD80, and CD86, which may lead to delayed activation of T cells and allows more time for replication of HSV type 1 in epidermal cells. This may be yet another novel strategy of immune evasion, and these findings support the notion that immature DCs respond to HSV challenge by impaired maturation. Further results indicate that HSV-1-infected mature DCs have a limited capacity to migrate to lymph nodes, thus inhibiting an antiviral immune response. In a study on rhesus macaques, HSV-2 was found to induce apoptotic death, decreased expression of costimulatory molecules, and increased release of cytokines by monocyte-derived DCs. This coincided with HSV-2-infected DCs stimulating weak T-cell responses. Similar effects were observed in HSV-2-exposed human DCs.

In contrast, results from other studies suggest a previously unanticipated role for submucosal DCs in the generation of protective Th1 immune responses to HSV-2 in the vaginal mucosa. In a murine model, HSV-2 infection of the epithelium induces activation of neighboring uninfected submucosal DCs. Intravaginal inoculation of mice with HSV-2 led to a rapid recruitment of submucosal DCs to the infected epithelium. Subsequently, DCs harboring viral peptides emerged in the draining lymph nodes and were found to be responsible for the stimulation of IFN-γ secretion from HSV-specific CD4+ T cells.

These results demonstrate a role for submucosal DCs in the generation of protective Th1 immune responses to HSV-2 in the vaginal mucosa and indicate that DCs are the primary cells responsible for T-cell priming in the draining lymph nodes. The inference that DCs, but not Langerhans cells (LCs), have such a role is supported by the fact that LCs from the vaginal epithelium did not migrate to the draining iliac

lymph nodes after intravaginal HSV-2 infection. LCs may be inhibited from performing antigen-presenting functions as a result of the lytic destruction of the epithelial layer. This notion is supported by the progressive reduction of the number of LCs in draining lymph nodes after HSV-2 infection. Similar results have been obtained by using immature human monocyte-derived CD11c+DCs, which showed limited productive viral replication and increased expression of CD86, CD83, and HLA DR as well as release of proinflammatory cytokines and chemokines after exposure to HSV-2.

Blood DCs infected with HSV-2 activated CD8+ T cells, which again blocked CD4+ T-cell proliferation. These DC could transform CD25-CD8+ T cells into Treg cells that blocked both antigen-specific and allogeneic CD4+ T-cell activation in vitro.

Further studies are ongoing to better define the role that DCs play in mucosal response to HSV infection in the genital tract.

4.2.1.1.5 NK Cells

Several studies have also shown a role for NK cells, NK T cells, and IL-15 as regulatory factors in an innate immune response to HSV. Mice lacking IL-15 or NK/NK T cells were significantly more susceptible to intravaginal HSV-2 infection than control mice. The lack of NK and NK T cells in these mice and, as a result, lack of early IFN-γ response impaired the innate immune response against HSV-2. A follow-up study by the same group indicated that IL-15 also has direct antiviral activity independent of NK/NK T cells in mediating innate defense against HSV-2 infection.

A role of NK cells in innate immune responses against HSV-2 in humans also seems essential, and a number of examples of NK cell deficiencies in humans have been reported and are associated with an increase in herpes virus infections. However, because NK cell deficiencies involve other immune functions, it is difficult to determine the precise role played by NK cells in these cases.

Studies on lymphocyte-deficient mice suggest that their impaired innate resistance to HSV-1 is not dependent on NK cells, but owing to differences in these study models one probably cannot transfer these results to human HSV infection.

4.2.1.1.6 Neutrophils

The role played by neutrophils in the innate immune response to genital herpes in human beings is not exactly known.

In a murine model, depletion of neutrophils before HSV-2 intravaginal inoculation did not increase the incidence of infection, suggesting that the small population of resident neutrophils was ineffective in preventing infection by a viral pathogen. However, neutrophils did help in virus clearance from the genital mucosa after primary infection. The mechanisms by which neutrophils mediate antiviral activity are not well understood. They bind HSV virions or HSV-infected cells in vitro and kill them by oxygen-dependent or oxygen-independent systems. Furthermore, neutrophils may mediate antiviral activity through release of antiviral cytokines such as

TNF-α, IFN-α, and IFN-γ or oxygen and nitrogen metabolites.

4.2.1.1.7 Toll-Like Receptors

As mentioned earlier, the recognition of infectious pathogens like HSV-2 by the innate immune system relies on TLRs. TLR2 and TLR9 seem to be involved in cell signaling in response to HSV. TLR9 mediates HSV-2 induced IFN-α secretion from DCs, and HSV-1 also elicits inflammatory cytokine secretion through TLR2. A summary of the innate immune responses of the female genital tract against HSV is shown in Fig. 4.2.

4.2.1.2 Specific Immune Responses in Genital Herpes Infection

Despite the recognition that innate immunity provides the first line of defense during both primary and recurrent HSV infection and plays a critical role in preventing infection and in limiting viral replication, the specific factors such as antimicrobials and TLRs that contribute to the mucosal response in the female genital tract have only recently begun to receive attention. Further studies are needed to provide a better understanding of

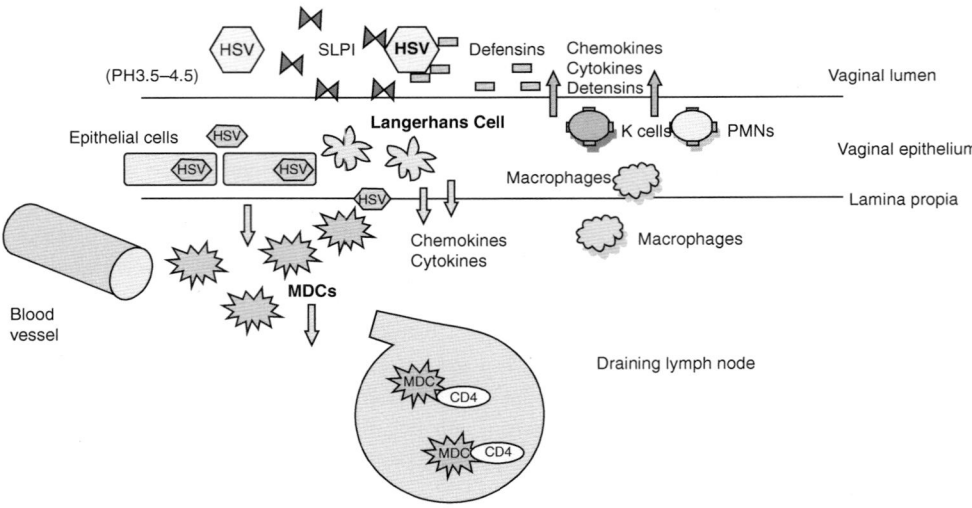

Fig. 4.2 Mucosal innate immune response to HSV in the female genital tract. Viral particles may be inactivated by acidic pH and substances secreted into the vaginal lumen, including defensins, SLPI, and complement. Resident immune cells, including ECs, DCs, NK cells, and PMNs, respond to viral exposure by killing virus or virally infected cells directly or by releasing cytokines and chemokines. These initial responses trigger the recruitment

of additional immune cells, notably monocyte-derived CD11c + DCs, which endocytose viral antigens, mature, and then migrate to the draining lymph node to stimulate CD4+ T cells and initiate the adaptive immune response (MasCasullo V, Fam E, Keller MJ, Herold BC. Role of mucosal immunity in preventing genital herpes infection. Viral Immunol. 2005;18:595–606) the contribution of specific components of mucosal immunity and the mechanisms by which the virus may evade these immune strategies. Defining this activity is crucial, as these factors might be exploited in the development of microbicides.

4.2.1.2.1 T Lymphocytes

For decades, the questions about T-cell subtypes and the specific role of neutralizing antibodies in HSV infection have been dominating issues. The longer prevalence of herpetic lesions in AIDS patients as well as the high frequency in patients after organ transplantation indicates the dominant influence of T-cell responses rather than the persistence of neutralizing antibodies in recurrent infections. Moreover, only very high levels of neutralizing antibodies could prevent the axonal spread of HSV-1 to epidermal cells in vitro contributing to control of HSV spread and shedding. Mice depleted of CD4+ and CD8+ T cells prior to genital HSV-2 infection shed virus for a prolonged period, confirming a role for T cells in virus clearance.

Early murine studies of the immunology of HSV infection suggested that IFNs and macrophages were an important part of the initial immune response and that the most important protective specific T-lymphocyte response was mediated by CD8+ lymphocytes. However, immunohistology of biopsies of human recurrent herpetic lesions revealed a sequence of immune cell infiltration beginning with CD4+ lymphocytes and macrophages in the first 2 days around the infected epidermal cells, which also develop strong HLA-DR expression. This was followed by an influx of CD8+ lymphocytes, which normalized the balance between CD4+ and CD8+ lymphocytes. The CD4/CD8 ratio is not restored to that of the blood until after 2 days, indicating an early CD4+ and a later CD8+ lymphocyte influx.

Several studies have demonstrated that Th1 CD4+ T cells are necessary and sufficient to provide protective immunity to HSV-2. A murine model of genital HSV infection was utilized to examine the local T-cell response in the genital mucosa and the draining genital lymph nodes. HSV-specific T cells with a higher rate of CD4+ and Th1-like T cells were first detected 4 days after vaginal HSV inoculation in the genital lymph nodes, followed by their appearance in the genital

tract 1 day later. Additionally, experiments with T-cell subtype knockout animals and depletion with T-cell subset-specific monoclonal antibody indicated that immunity following vaginal HSV challenge was principally dependent on the function of CD4+ T cells. Furthermore, it has been shown that the CD4+ T-cell-mediated protection is linked to the cells' ability to secrete IFN-γ.

The mechanism of the Th1-mediated protective immunity to HSV-2 likely involves several pathways. It is possible that CD4+ T cells are involved in the direct killing of HSV-infected ECs, as these effector cells are rapidly recruited to the sites of secondary infection. IFN-γ has also been shown to act on vaginal ECs to restore MHC class I expression and upregulate MHC class II expression, which may contribute to the recognition by CD4+ effector T cells. Alternatively, IFN-γ could exert protection by activating macrophages and neutrophils for enhanced phagocytosis of infected cells, resulting in the secretion of TNF-α and the release of NO. Finally, IFN-γ secreted during the secondary viral challenge may also be important in the recruitment of memory and effector lymphocytes to the infected vaginal epithelium. Antigen-specific T cells have been detected in the uterine cervix of women with genital HSV-2 infection where CTL activity was associated with both CD4+ and CD8+ T-cell populations. This is consistent with the finding that clearance of HSV-2 skin lesions correlated with the infiltration of CTLs of both CD4+ and CD8+ phenotypes. Addressing the specificity of CTLs, it has been reported that CD8+ T cells from genital herpes lesions recognize viral tegument and immediate-early proteins as their targets.

An immune evasion mechanism that allows the infected cell to escape scrutiny by cytotoxic CD8+ lymphocytes is the ability of HSV to downregulate MHC class I on the surface when infecting epidermal keratinocytes. The immediate-early viral protein of HSV, infected cell protein 47 (ICP 47), complexes with and inhibits the human transporter associated with antigen presentation (TAP) on the surface of the endoplasmic reticulum in humans but not in mice. TAP is responsible for transporting small antigenic viral peptides into the lumen of the endoplasmic reticulum, where it assembles into the MHC class I peptide complex before transport to the cell surface. Inhibition of TAP inhibits the assembly of MHC class I peptide and recognition by CD8+ cytotoxic T lymphocytes. However, as mentioned above, IFN-γ, which is produced by CD4+ lymphocytes in the lesion, partly restores MHC class I expression on the surface of infected cells by the cellular production of TAP and also stimulates MHC class II expression. Specific activated CD4+ lymphocytes are able to recognize infected epidermal cells and probably uninfected cells expressing MHC class II. This may result in the production of more IFN-γ or destruction of infected cells by CD4 T lymphocytes, which is normally mediated by CD8 lymphocytes. The restoration of MHC class I expression on infected epidermal cells allows recognition by CD8 cytotoxic T lymphocytes, which are then apparently able to destroy the remaining infected epidermal cells. HSV-specific CD8+ demonstrated precursor CTL in HSV-1 and HSV-2 seropositive persons with recurrent genital herpes.

A summary of the adaptive immune mechanisms with T-cell priming in genital herpes infection is provided in Fig. 4.3.

4.2.1.2.2 B Lymphocytes

Studies among B-cell-deficient mice have been used to further illustrate the contributions of humoral and cellular immunity in protection against vaginal infection in the HSV-2 mouse model. In this model, progesterone-treated adult mice are inoculated intravaginally with a thymidine kinase (TK)-deficient, attenuated strain of HSV-2. The deletion in the TK gene, which is required for the reactivation of the latent HSV-2, renders the virus only infectious during the primary mucosal infection without the neurovirulence associated with the wild-type (WT) virus. Although B cell-deficient mice in these studies developed an early transient genital inflammation upon primary infection with TK-deficient HSV-2, during secondary challenge of immune mice with the WT-HSV-2, all of the mice cleared the infection completely. Further, mice immunized with TK-HSV-2 were completely protected from subsequent WT-HSV-2 challenge. These results also indicate that B cells are not critical APCs

required to activate T cells following TK-HSV-2 infection.

4.2.1.2.3 Immunoglobulins

Women with symptomatic genital herpes have antibodies to HSV-2 of both IgA and IgG isotypes, as well as IgM in CVS and in serum. External secretions including cervical mucus contain both IgG and IgA antibodies, but these differ in their specificity for various HSV-2 antigens. Moreover, cervical anti-HSV IgA antibodies either free or with SC as S-IgA also differ with respect to their levels and specificities for various HSV-2 antigens, suggesting their origin from the circulation as well as by local production.

Despite the fact that S-IgA was the predominant Ig in progestin-treated mouse vaginal mucus, nearly all specific viral antibodies in HSV-immune mice were of the IgG isotype. However, these observations did not eliminate the possibility of a contribution of vaginal IgA in immune protection against HSV-2, since ELISA titers of specific antibodies do not necessarily predict functional virus neutralization.

The role of antibodies in protection of the female genital tract against HSV-2 remains controversial. Anti-HSV mAb failed to protect against vaginal challenge infection, and specific antibody was not detected in vaginal secretions after parenteral immunization that produced high antibody titres in serum. Immunity against vaginal HSV-2 infection was comparable in intact and IgA-deficient mice, and only little vaginal-specific S-IgA was detected after local immunization in the vagina. Intranasal immunization of mice with recombinant vaccinia virus produced high titers of specific IgG and IgA in the vagina but failed to prevent epithelial infection. These results would suggest a protective immunity in vaginal mucosa that is mainly based on T cells, which was underlined by other experiments as well. Passive transfer of serum IgG from immune mice diminished a vaginal challenge infection even though mean antibody titer in vaginal secretions of mice was only 8 % of that measured in actively immunized mice. Purified IgG from vaginal secretions of immunized mice

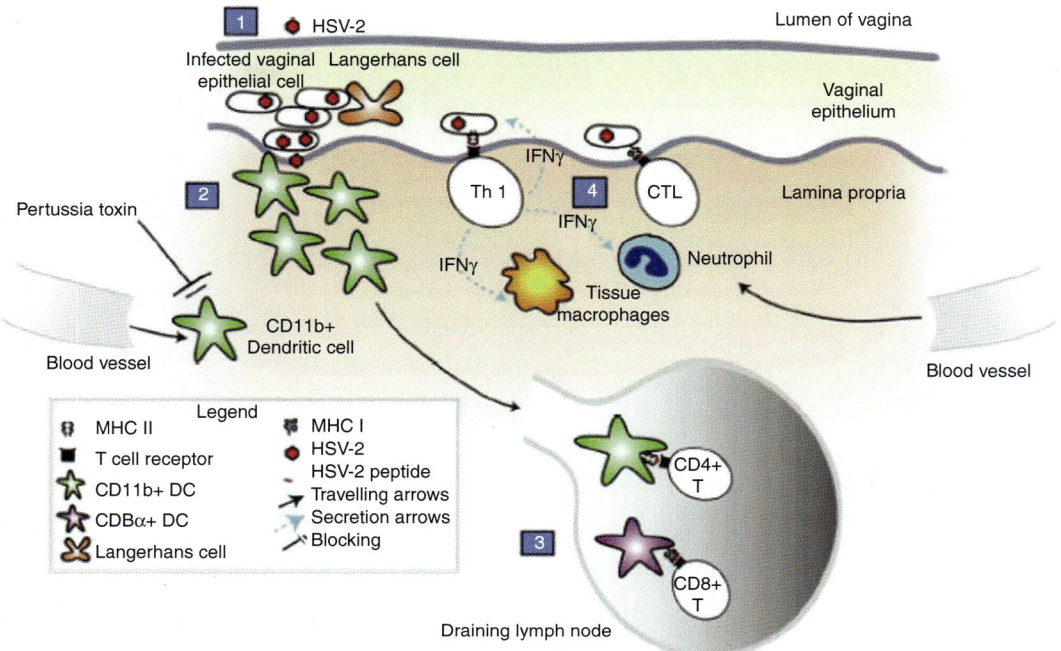

Fig. 4.3 T-cell priming in genital herpes infection. The virus replicates within the infected keratinocytes, resulting in the induction of signals necessary for the recruitment of the CD11b+DCs to the submucosa beneath the infected ECs. This signal likely involves chemokines, since pertussis toxin treatment of mice at the time of infection prevents DC accumulation at the infected sites. Once recruited, submucosal DCs can take up virus antigens from the infected keratinocytes and migrate to the draining lymph nodes. By the time the CD11b+DCs enter the lymph nodes, they assume an activated phenotype, expressing higher levels of costimulatory molecules such as CD80 and CD86. Within the lymph nodes, the virus antigen-loaded CD11b+DCs can stimulate CD4+ T cells, which undergo differentiation to Th1 cells. It is possible that CD8+ T cells are also stimulated within the lymph nodes, by a separate group of DCs expressing CD8a. Once activated, the effector Th1 and CTLs exit the lymph nodes and migrate back to the vaginal mucosa, where they mediate clearance of infected keratinocytes. The IFN-γ secreted from the Th1 cells has multiple effector functions, including upregulation of MHC class II molecules on the infected keratinocytes, making these cells susceptible to recognition by CD4+ effector cells. Some of these CD4+ T cells may act as CTLs and eliminate infected cells. The IFN-γ secreted from the effector Th1 cells may also activate phagocytes such as tissue macrophages and neutrophils directly or via chemokines, resulting in the clearance of infected cells (Iwasaki A. The role of dendritic cells in immune responses against vaginal infection by herpes simplex virus type 2. Microbes Infect. 2003;5:1221–30)

neutralized HSV-2 in vitro. The protective effect of HSV-2-specific antibodies has also been demonstrated by passive intravaginal immunization shortly before HSV-2 challenge given by the same route.

The protective role of antibodies in vaginal secretions of mice that were immune to vaginal challenge with HSV-2 was further investigated by neutralization and passive transfer. These neutralization studies were carried out by incubation of WT-HSV-2 in antibody preparations in vitro, followed by inoculation into vaginae of nonimmune mice. The results showed that HSV-2 was effectively neutralized both by unfractionated antibody and by purified IgG from immune vaginal secretions, but not by purified S-IgA from immune secretions or by unfractionated antibody from nonimmune mice. The protective effect of IgG in vivo was further investigated by passively transferring purified serum IgG from immune and nonimmune donors to nonimmune recipients before vaginal challenge infection. Immune IgG significantly reduced the percentage of vaginal epithelium infected, shed virus protein concentrations in the vaginal lumen, and illness scores, even though the viral antibody titers in the serum and vaginal secretions of recipient mice at the time of challenge were only 29 and 8 %, respectively, of those in actively immunized mice. Although Igs do not play a critical role during secondary challenge with HSV-2 in mice immunized with TK-HSV-2, passive transfer of immune IgG can significantly reduce local virus replication. Further, neutralizing antibodies may be important in the prevention of viral shedding from neuronal axons to the epidermis during reactivation. The importance of IgG in HSV immunity is evidenced by the immune evasion mechanism employed by the virus. The HSV genome encodes glycoprotein E and I, which together comprise a high-affinity Fc receptor expressed by infected cells for the purpose of absorbing and inactivating anti-HSV IgG. Data indicate that IgG antibody in vaginal secretions of immune mice provides early protection against vaginal HSV challenge infection, whereas S-IgA contributed very little to protection.

Concerning the origin of IgG, observations suggest that the titer of viral IgG in vaginal secretions of mice that were intravaginally immunized with HSV-2 may be higher than can be accounted for by passive transudation from serum. The relative contributions of humoral and cell-mediated adaptive immunity against HSV-2 infection in the mouse model have recently been studied. Antibody is supposed to mainly act early during immune resistance to challenge infection, whereas cell-mediated immunity primarily acts later. An early role for antibody is consistent with the presence of neutralizing IgG in vaginal secretions of immunized mice, whereas memory T cells, on the other hand, require several hours to secrete substantial amounts of IFN-γ in the vagina in response to the challenge antigen and may require even longer developing cytolytic activity.

Women with symptomatic genital herpes have antibodies to HSV-2 of both IgA and IgG isotypes, as well as IgM antibodies in CVS and in serum. Another study aimed at detecting HSV antibodies and neutralizing activity in CVS of women seropositive for both HSV-1 and HSV-2

and to stratify the HSV-2-specific antibody activity according to their HSV-2 DNA genital shedding status. HSV-specific binding antibodies were detected at rates of nearly 70 % (IgG) and 51 % (IgA), with similar proportions of Igs to HSV-1 and HSV-2. The presence of detectable HSV-specific antibodies was inversely associated with HSV-2 DNA genital asymptomatic shedding and a subset of these women (17 %) had functional neutralizing activity against HSV-2 in their CVS.

4.2.1.3 Sex Hormones and the Immune Response to Genital Herpes Infection

Susceptibility and immune responses to STDs, including genital HSV-2 infection, are profoundly affected by sex hormones. Studies have indicated that intake of oral contraceptives influences susceptibility to candidiasis, HSV-2, HIV-1, and chlamydial infections in women.

Interestingly, previous studies have shown that mice are susceptible to intravaginal HSV-2 infection primarily during the diestrous phase of the estrous cycle. Thus, treatment of mice with progesterone, which maintains the mice at a diestrus-like stage, is often required for consistent intravaginal infection with HSV-2. However, the precise mechanism by which progesterone treatment increases the susceptibility to intravaginal HSV-2 infection is unknown. It is suggested that this effect is due to diminishing thickness and increased permeability of the vaginal epithelial layer during diestrus coinciding with high progesterone levels. Progesterone treatment of mice led to a 100-fold increase in susceptibility to genital HSV-2 compared with untreated mice at the diestrous phase. Further, long-term effects of this depot progesterone treatment included reduction in protective immunity to HSV-2. Therefore, progesterone might have an immunosuppressive role with the thickness and gross morphology of the vaginal epithelium alone might not account for the susceptibility to HSV-2 infection.

As another possible mechanism for the increased susceptibility to HSV-2 in the diestrous phase, it can be hypothesized that APCs are less abundant in the vagina during the susceptible diestrous phase and more abundant during the resistant estrous stage. However, analysis of the distribution of DCs during the estrous cycle revealed that these cells are abundantly present in the epithelium of mice at diestrus, whereas they are only sparsely present in the basal layer of the vaginal epithelium in estrus, which suggests that the distribution of the APCs per se does not account for the susceptibility to virus infection at different stages of the estrous cycle.

Finally, it is possible that the virus entry receptors are expressed differently during the hormonal cycle and that the relevant receptors are expressed only during the susceptible stages. Interestingly, nectin-1, the major coreceptor for HSV entry in the genital tract, is expressed in the epithelium of the mouse vagina only during stages of the estrous cycle in which mice are susceptible to vaginal HSV. Limited clinical studies suggest that asymptomatic HSV viral shedding is not related to contraceptive use or menstrual cycle. Moreover, nectin-1 is expressed throughout the menstrual cycle in human beings. Further studies are needed to elucidate the relationship between mucosal immunity, the hormonal environment, and response to HSV challenge.

4.2.1.4 The Role of Cytokines

Both HSV-specific CD4+ and CD8+ T-cell cytotoxicity have been demonstrated in vitro and in lymphocytes cloned from recurrent herpetic lesions ex vivo. In vivo, CD8+ lymphocyte cytotoxicity is presumably dependent upon upregulation of MHC class I by IFN-γ secreted from earlier infiltrating CD4+ lymphocytes. Furthermore, the mechanism for the enhancement of CD8+ T-cell cytotoxicity by adjuvants in this system appears to be via increased levels of IL-12. The specific infiltration of monocytes and CD4+ and CD8+ lymphocytes in sequence associated with only a few B lymphocytes suggests a leukocyte-specific chemotactic stimulus rather of β-chemokines than of α-chemokines that are chemoattractant for neutrophils but not for monocytes and lymphocytes.

In the mouse model that after HSV-2 inoculation, a rapid synthesis of IFN-γ by lymphocytes and macrophages was observed which occurred only in immune/challenged but not in nonimmune/non-challenged mice indicating that it required memory T cells. Virus-specific memory T cells in the vagina of immune mice encountered challenge virus antigen, rapidly secreted IFN-γ, leading to T- and B-cell recruitment into the vagina. Thus, IFN-γ seems to be an early and important mediator of T-cell immunity in HSV-2 infection.

The high concentration of IFN-γ in herpetic lesion fluid also suggests a Th1 pattern of cytokine response. The Th2 pattern leads to predominantly neutralizing antibody secretion by B cells, whereas a Th1 pattern leads to production of the antiviral cytokines, IFN-γ and TNF-α, and the activation of cytotoxic CD8+ lymphocytes, through IL-12 and IFN-γ. A Th1 pattern of cytokine induction is important in the control of persistent virus infections since only CTLs are able to eradicate infected cells, and IFN-γ and TNF-α can purge infected cells of viral proteins. A Th2 pattern leading to neutralizing antibody production may prevent cell-to-cell transmission of the virus.

Concerning the presence of cytokines, on the first day of the lesion, high concentrations of IL-1β and IL-6, moderate concentrations of IL-1α and IL-10, and low concentrations of IL-12 and β chemokines were found; levels of MIP-1β were significantly higher than levels of MIP-1α and RANTES. At day 3, the concentrations of IL-1β, IL-6, and MIP-1β were lower, whereas the levels of IL-10, IL-12, and MIP-1α remained similar, and the level of TNF-α was now detectable. These cytokines may play a role in early recruitment, activation, and IFN-γ production of CD4+ cells in herpetic lesions. β-chemokines attract monocytes and T lymphocytes into the lesions, in particular, MIP-1β for CD4+ lymphocytes, and IL-12 entrains CD4+ lymphocyte secretion to a Th1 pattern. Macrophages probably also secrete IL-12, IFNs, and other cytokines within the lesion. Immune processes in a recurrent herpetic lesion are shown in Fig. 4.4.

Fig. 4.4 Immune processes and in vivo secretions of cytokines and chemokines in herpetic lesions. *M*, macrophage; *K*, keratinocyte (Cunningham AL, Mikloska Z. The Holy Grail: immune control of human herpes simplex virus infection and disease. Herpes. 2001;8 Suppl 1:6A–10)

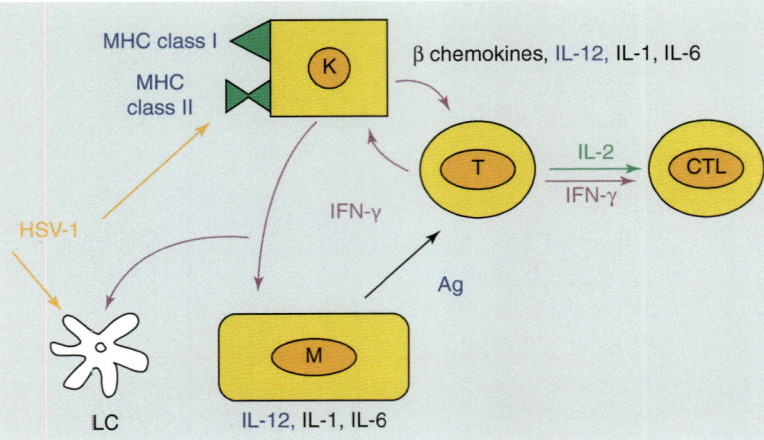

4.2.1.5 New Immunological Therapeutic Approaches

4.2.1.5.1 Resiquimod

Current treatment of genital herpes focuses on the direct inhibition of viral replication. The nucleoside analogs, in particular acyclovir, dominate the treatment recommendations for genital herpes. Most antiviral therapy is aimed at the treatment or suppression of recurrent episodes. Both episodic and long-term suppressive therapies are prescribed, but nucleoside analogs have no long-term effect on the disease; genital herpes episodes recur at the pretreatment rate if therapy is stopped. Given the limitations of current therapy directed against viral replication, a regimen utilizing an immune modulator may be more acceptable to patients. Therefore, the development of the immune response modifiers (IRMs) as a potential new treatment option for genital herpes is briefly presented. IRMs, as, for example, imiquimod and resiquimod, are synthesized ring-structured nucleoside structures. They induce immune cells to produce cytokines and, thus, initiate the immune response, which can result in antiviral or antitumor effects. Especially resiquimod was shown to stimulate the development of Th1 immune responses in guinea pig models of genital herpes. Resiquimod stimulated the secretion of IFN-α, TNF-α, IL-6, IL-8, and IL-12 from various cells including DCs, monocytes, and macrophages. Resiquimod induces the functional maturation of DC, LC, and B lymphocytes into effective APCs, and it promotes the

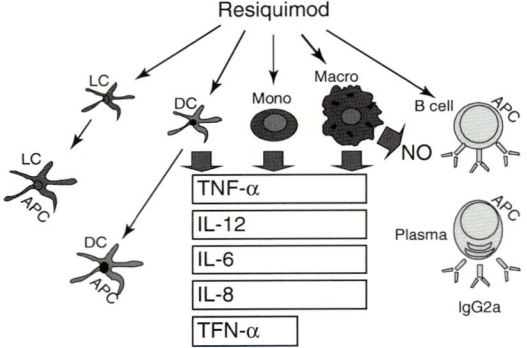

Fig. 4.5 Stimulation of immune responses by the IRM resiquimod. Resiquimod stimulates the secretion of IFN-α, TNF-α, IL-6, IL-8, and IL-12 from various cells, including DCs, monocytes (*mono*), and macrophages (*macro*). Resiquimod induces the functional maturation of DCs, LCs, and B lymphocytes into effective APCs and promotes the development of B lymphocytes into plasma cells and the subsequent secretion of IgG2a. Resiquimod also stimulates nitric oxide (NO) production from macrophages (Miller RL, Tomai MA, Harrison CJ, Bernstein DI. Immunomodulation as a treatment strategy for genital herpes: review of the evidence. Int Immunopharmacol. 2002;2:443-451)

development of B lymphocytes into plasma cells (Fig. 4.5).

Resiquimod was shown to inhibit herpetic lesions and delay genital herpes recurrence in the guinea pig model. The decrease in recurrence was correlated with an increase of the in vitro IL-2 produced by peripheral mononuclear cells in response to HSV antigen but not with levels of IFN or circulating anti-HSV-2 antibodies. The rationale for the use of resiquimod as a treatment for genital herpes is to stimulate the secretion of key cytokines, e.g., IFN-α, IL-12, and TNF-α, by the innate immune system in order to induce an HSV-specific Th1-acquired immune response. In a randomized vehicle-controlled phase II clinical study on 52 patients with a history of six or more recurrences per year, topical application of resiquimod reduced recurrences of genital herpes even after cessation of dosing. The median time to the next recurrence was 169 days in the resiquimod-treated group in comparison to 57 days in the vehicle-treated group. The percentage of patients without a recurrence during the 6-month observation period after dosing was 6 % in the vehicle-treated group compared to 32 % in the resiquimod-treated group.

This apparent continued posttreatment benefit of resiquimod could be an important improvement to current treatments for recurrent genital herpes, such as oral anti-HSV nucleosides, which do not appear to have a posttreatment benefit. However, phase III clinical trials were suspended due to the lack of efficacy of resiquimod gel in recurrent genital herpes lesions. It may make a comeback, however, as a vaccine adjuvant for viral infections that require a strong Th1 immune response.

4.2.1.5.2 CpG Oligodeoxynucleotides

Local vaginal delivery of CpG-containing oligodeoxynucleotide (ODN), a synthetic mimic of bacterial DNA and TLR9 agonist, held substantial promise as a strong inducer of innate immunity against genital herpes infections in animal models of the disease.

TLRs are responsible for recognition of conserved molecular structures named PAMPs such as LPS, bacterial DNA, and viral double-stranded RNA in microbes. Interaction between CpG motifs in microbial DNA and TLR9 in APCs stimulates the responding cells to produce proinflammatory cytokines such as IFN-γ and IL-12 through the Toll/IL-1-receptor signaling pathway and to activate B cells for proliferation and antibody production. Among PAMPs, synthetic analogs of bacterial DNA, termed CpG ODN, have shown a great promise in mobilization of protective immunity against different pathogens. In a

mouse model, a single intravaginal dose of CpG ODN induced production of Th1-type cytokines IFN-γ, IL-12, and IL-18; CC chemokines RANTES, MIP-1α, and MIP-1β; and CXC chemokines IP-10 and MIP-2 in the genital tract mucosa as well as dramatically increased the total cell numbers of B cells, NK cells, NKT cells, and T cells in the genital lymph nodes. Studies have proven a protective effect of prophylactic delivery of CpG ODN against primary genital herpes in mice and have shown that the observed protection can lead to the development of a HSV-2-specific memory response affording sterilizing immunity against reinfection. In addition, a therapeutic effect of topical application of CpG ODN on genital herpes was demonstrated in both mouse and guinea pig models of the disease.

Interestingly, several experiments have been performed to determine whether intravaginal immunization with recombinant glycoprotein B (rgB) of HSV-2 plus CpG ODN can induce specific immunity and protect against genital HSV-2 challenge. Mice immunized with rgB + CpG had higher levels of anti-gB IgA and IgG in the vaginal washes and serum compared to mice immunized with rgB alone. Mice immunized with rgB + CpG showed higher survival and lower pathology scores following genital HSV-2 challenge than mice immunized with rgB + non-CpG ODN or rgB alone.

Intranasal immunization with CpG ODN plus rgB of HSV-1 resulted in significantly elevated levels of specific anti-gB IgA antibodies in vaginal washes that remained high throughout the estrous cycle. Additionally, dramatically elevated numbers of specific IgA-secreting cells were present and persisted in the genital tract in response to intravaginal HSV-2 challenge. Strong CTL responses were observed locally in the genital tissues of both CpG and non-CpG ODN-immunized mice following intravaginal HSV-2 challenge. Interestingly, mice immunized intranasal with rgB and CpG ODN, but not non-CpG ODN, were significantly protected following intravaginal HSV-2 challenge. In conclusion, these results indicate that intranasal immunization with CpG ODN plus protein mediates immunity in the female genital tract capable of

protecting against a sexually transmitted pathogen. Comparing the effectiveness of CpG ODN
and resiquimod for topical immunotherapy of
intravaginal HSV-2 infection in mice demonstrated some efficacy for CpG ODN but less so
for resiquimod. Intravaginal administration of
GpG ODN resulted in a strong local but weak
systemic immune response, as determined by the
levels of chemokines as IP-10, whereas intravaginal administration of resiquimod resulted in high
levels of plasma IP-10 and weaker local immune
responses. These findings provide a basis for further intervention studies of the efficacy of CpG
ODN in humans.

4.2.1.6 Vaccination Strategies

Despite antiviral therapy, HSV-2 is a suitable target for a vaccine because the virus causes life-
long infection and significant medical morbidity.
Vaccination to prevent HSV infection, or to
reduce reactivation frequency and severity,
would reduce morbidity, the risk of dissemination to newborns, and the risk of HIV acquisition.
Vaccines may be sought for two independent purposes; prophylaxis in uninfected individuals and
therapy in those already infected. The history of
HSV vaccine development goes back almost 80
years. HSV vaccines may be divided into two
groups of live or inactivated vaccines. Live vaccines contain organisms capable of at least limited replication in vivo, whereas inactivated
vaccines contain viruses that are incapable of
replicating. The vaccines may be further subdi-
vided into the categories: attenuated HSV vaccines, replication-limited HSV vaccines, vaccines
consisting of live nonpathogenic replicating vectors engineered to express HSV gene products,
inactivated HSV vaccines, subunit vaccines, and
nucleic acid (plasmid) vaccines.

Many types of vaccines have been evaluated in
clinical trials of immunogenic and prophylactic or
therapeutic efficacy. Some of the early vaccines
showed either low immunogenic or safety flaws;
some did appear immunogenic but the trial design
then precluded interpretation of efficacy. Efforts
to develop vaccines to protect women against
HSV-2 and other sexually transmitted pathogens

would be facilitated by a better understanding of
the immune mechanisms that protect the female
reproductive tract against such infections.

4.2.1.6.1 Vaginal Versus Nasal/Parenteral Immunization

In the progestin-treated adult mouse model, intravaginal inoculation of WT-HSV-2 caused infection of the vaginal epithelium followed by lethal
neurological illness. Intravaginal inoculation of
an attenuated strain of TK-depleted HSV-2
induced an epithelial infection but did not lead to
neurological illness. Importantly, vaginal infection with the attenuated strain induced protective
immunity to subsequent lethal challenge with the
WT-virus. These observations indicated that
intravaginal immunization with the attenuated
virus induced mucosal immunity in the vagina
that prevented reinfection.

Others have studied immunization at IgA-
inductive sites including the intestine, nasophar-
ynx, and pelvis at least partly with a view toward
the induction of S-IgA responses in the female
genital tract. Parr compared nasal and vaginal
immunization using attenuated HSV-2 for protection against vaginal infection with WT-HSV-2.
Compared to vaginal immunization, nasal
immunization neither increased IgA plasma cell
numbers in the vagina nor elicited a higher IgA
titer in vaginal secretions. Vaginal immunization
increased the number of vaginal IgG plasma cells
and the secretion/serum titer ratio of IgG, indicating a local production of virus-specific IgG. Both
T and B lymphocyte numbers were rapidly
increased by about 20-fold in the vagina after
virus challenge in immune mice but not in nonimmune mice and lymphocyte recruitment was
mediated by IFN-γ. Data clearly indicated that
the IFN-γ secreted by memory T cells in the
vagina of immune mice after virus challenge was
responsible for the rapid recruitment of large
numbers of additional T and B lymphocytes to
the vagina. In addition, the expression of endothelial addressins in the vagina and their regulation by IFN-γ in immune mice after vaginal
inoculation with HSV-2 was investigated, as
lymphocyte recruitment into tissues requires the

presence of adhesion molecules on vascular endothelial cells. ICAM-1 and VCAM-1 may be involved in the rapid IFN-γ-mediated recruitment of lymphocytes to the vaginal mucosa of immune mice.

The titer of viral IgG in vaginal secretions of mice that were immunized in the vagina with attenuated HSV-2 may be higher than can be accounted for by passive transudation from serum. The number of IgG plasma cells in the vaginae of immunized mice was markedly higher than in nonimmune mice, suggesting that IgG may be produced locally in vaginae of immune mice. This is also an important issue considering the route of immunization in vaccination strategies that would best protect against reinfection. The results summarized above indicate that vaginal immunization of mice with attenuated HSV-2 elicits a strong protective immune response in the vagina consisting of cell-mediated immunity, IFN-γ, and viral IgG antibody in vaginal secretions.

The question is whether parenteral immunization with attenuated HSV-2 would protect against vaginal challenge infection as effectively as vaginal immunization. One of the paradigms of mucosal immunity is that immunization at a mucosal surface provides stronger immunity against challenge at that surface than does parenteral immunization. However, the basis of enhanced immune protection at sites of mucosal immunization is generally thought to be the local production of specific S-IgA antibody, and vaginal immunization with HSV-2 induces mainly IgG viral antibody.

Immunity resulting from local immunization in the vagina to that induced by parenteral immunization with attenuated HSV-2 has been compared. Interestingly, vaginal immunization induced sterilizing immunity against challenge with a high dose of WT-virus, whereas parenteral immunizations protected against neurological disease but did not entirely prevent infection of the vagina. Vaginal immunization caused 86-fold and 31-fold increases in the numbers of IgG plasma cells in the vagina at 6 weeks after immunization, whereas parenteral immunizations did

not increase plasma cell numbers in the vagina. Vaginal secretion/serum titer ratios and specific antibody activities in vaginal secretions and serum indicated that IgG viral antibody was produced in the vagina and released into vaginal secretions at 6 weeks and 10 months after vaginal immunization but not after parenteral immunizations. In contrast to plasma cells, the numbers of T and B lymphocytes in the vagina were increased similarly by vaginal challenge with HSV-2 in both vaginally and parenterally immunized mice. Thus, local vaginal immunization with attenuated HSV-2 increased the number of IgG plasma cells in the vagina and increased vaginal secretion/serum titer ratios 3.0- to 4.7-fold higher than in parenterally immunized groups but appeared to cause little if any selective homing of T and B lymphocytes to the vagina.

4.2.1.6.2 HSV Protein Targets for Vaccine Construction

As mentioned above, studies have shown that recurrent disease is prevented by virus-specific Th1 cytokines, i.e., IFN-γ, and activated innate immunity. Th2 cytokines, i.e., IL-10, and regulatory (suppressor) T cells downregulate this immune profile, thereby allowing unimpeded replication of reactivated virus and recurrent disease. Accordingly, an effective therapeutic vaccine must induce Th1 immunity and be defective in Th2 cytokine production, at least of IL-10. In different approaches, the most immunogenic HSV proteins were tried to be identified as possible targets for vaccines (Fig. 4.6).

One approach was directed at identifying the Th2-polarizing proteins so that they can be deleted from a potential vaccine. The functionally independent protein kinase (PK) domain of the HSV-2 large subunit of ribonucleotide reductase which is known as ICP10 has Th2-polarizing activity. In infected cells, ICP10PK upregulates the Th2 cytokines IL-6, IL-10, and IL-13 and downregulates RANTES, which is a chemoattractant for Th1 but not Th2 cells. Significantly, ICP10PK is required for virus replication and latency reactivation, suggesting that its deletion will interfere with virus replication and latency

Fig. 4.6 HSV protein targets for CD4 and CD8 T cells as potential vaccine candidates. *ICP* infected cell protein, *g* glycoprotein, *UL* unique long, *VP* viral protein (Cunningham AL, Mikloska Z. The Holy Grail: immune control of human herpes simplex virus infection and disease. Herpes. 2001;8 Suppl 1:6A–10)

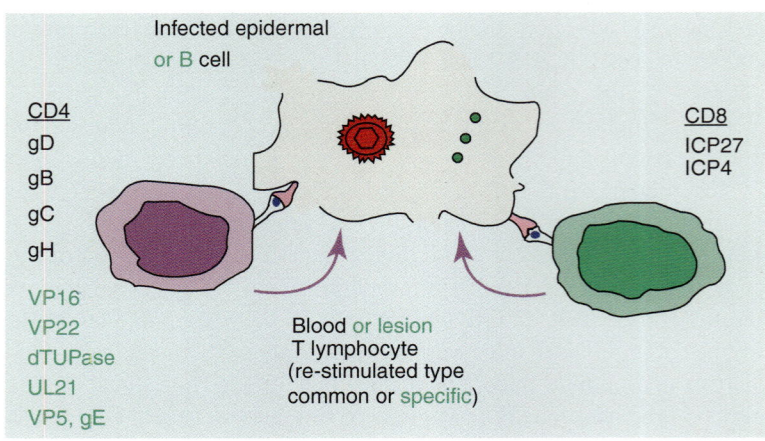

establishment while reducing or eliminating Th2 polarization and toleragenic potential. Therefore, the vaccine candidate ICP10ΔPK with deleted ICP10PK was developed. It was shown to be growth and latency compromising, and in the mouse, ICP10ΔPK vaccination inhibited HSV-2 replication and provided virtually absolute protection from fatal and cutaneous HSV-2 disease.

Other approaches using blood lymphocytes taken from infected patients and restimulated with whole virus in vitro identified the viral glycoproteins gD and gB as key targets for the activation of CD4+ T cells and viral ICP27, a protein present only at early stages in infected cells, as the key target for activation of CD8+ T cells. Another method is to clone T lymphocytes out of current herpes simplex lesions and react them against B lymphocytes infected with HSV-1 and HSV-2 and combinations thereof. With this method, several tegument proteins were identified as major T-cell targets.

Based on these targets, the original goal was to develop a prophylactic vaccine that induces local mucosal and systemic immunity which prevents infection and, thereby, virus transmission. The objective of a prophylactic vaccine is to induce sterilizing broad and durable immunity effective at all portals of HSV entry. A vaccine providing effective immunity against HSV must produce a response more powerful than the response produced by natural infection. This goal was predicated on the belief that neutralizing antibody and activated T cells at mucosal surfaces are the likeliest means to prevent infection, and its construction targets the viral glycoproteins D and B, which are involved in cell entry. However, it is becoming increasingly evident that the original vaccination goals may be unrealistic. Accordingly, the more recent goals of prophylactic vaccination are to prevent or reduce the clinical symptoms of primary infection and to shift the titer of virus necessary to give a primary infection and establish latency. In this context, efforts focus on the selection of ideal adjuvants and the definition of optimal immunization routes and protocols.

4.2.1.6.3 Subunit HSV-2 Vaccines

Subunit HSV-2 vaccines using glycoproteins B and D prepared from infected cells or immune-stimulating complexes (ISCOM) consisting of glycoproteins provided protection from lethal HSV infection and decreased severity and frequency of disease in animal models. In humans, a Chiron vaccine consisting of glycoproteins B2 and D2 with the adjuvant MF-59 was only transiently effective in two double-blind, placebo-controlled phase III studies that assessed prevention of HSV-2 infection. The first study enrolled 531 persons and the second 1,862 individuals who were at high risk for HSV-2 infection. During the first 5 months of the studies, the acquisition rate of HSV-2 among vaccine recipients was 50 % lower than in the placebo group, but after one year, the overall efficacy was only 9 %. In both studies, the vaccine failed to reduce the likelihood or severity of symptomatic disease. Interestingly, the HSV-2 antibody titers did not differ between vaccinated-uninfected and vaccinated-infected individuals. These results suggest that neutralizing antibody alone is not sufficient to protect against genital HSV-2 infection and that the vaccine failed to induce critical cell-mediated immune responses against HSV-2 infection. Possible explanations for the loss of efficacy could be that the protective immune response was only of short duration or that initial protection was lost with frequent exposure to the virus.

In another trial by GlaxoSmithKline (GSK), a vaccine consisting of glycoprotein D and a mixture of alum and 3-deacylated monophosphoryl lipid A (3-dMPL) as adjuvant was tested. In a phase I trial, the vaccine was well tolerated and induced both cellular and humoral immune responses. In two double-blind, placebo-controlled trials with 847 and 2,491 partners of HSV-2-infected individuals, respectively, the vaccine's efficacy was 38 % in seronegative male and female in study 1 and 42 % in seronegative females of study 2. This vaccine was effective in preventing symptomatic genital HSV-2 disease in women in about 73 % if they were initially HSV-1 and HSV-2 seronegative. The vaccine was shown to induce both gD-specific neutralizing antibodies and a Th1 cell-mediated immune response. This is the most promising approach of creating a vaccine preventing genital herpes and is currently further investigated in another trial on 7,550 HSV-2 seronegative women.

The partial effectiveness of this vaccine compared to the Chiron vaccine suggests that the adjuvant may be critical in facilitating the induction of protective immune responses (Fig. 4.7). The MF59 adjuvant induces a Th2 pattern of response, whereas the MPL adjuvant induces a Th1 pattern of cytokine response. However, in vitro studies have shown that MPL alone is not sufficient to induce CD8-lymphocyte cytotoxicity. MPL plus the Quil A derivative, QS21, significantly enhanced cytotoxicity, via induction of IL-12 from APCs and IFN-γ from T lymphocytes.

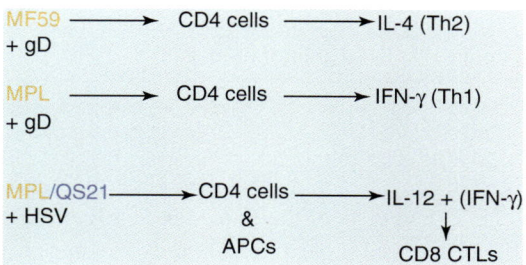

Fig. 4.7 Postulated mechanisms of action of adjuvants for HSV vaccines (Cunningham AL, Mikloska Z. The Holy Grail: immune control of human herpes simplex virus infection and disease. Herpes. 2001;8 Suppl 1:6A–10)

The difference between herpes disease and herpes infection is crucial in interpreting the studies. The primary endpoint of the GSK study was the occurrence of genital herpes disease and no distinction was made between HSV-1 and HSV-2 as causes. As HSV-1 is responsible for a high rate of primary genital herpes, recipients may be protected against disease caused by either virus. An effective HSV vaccine might mimic the immunological process underlying the phenomenon that previous HSV infection protects against HSV disease by reducing its severity. It appears that in HSV-1 seropositive, HSV-2 seronegative persons, the GSK vaccine provided no additional protection over their presumed HSV-1 induced immunity. There might also be hints in statistical analysis of the GSK studies that the study was insufficiently powered to detect a difference in infection rates between placebo and vaccine. In addition, the significantly different results in efficacy for men and women raise questions.

4.2.1.6.4 Live Attenuated HSV Vaccines

Attenuated live virus vaccines cause a primary infection but do not reactivate after establishing latency in ganglia. Two strategies were used to develop live HSV-2 vaccines. The first strategy used viral vectors that express HSV glycoproteins. R7020, constructed from a HSV-1 strain by replacing a deleted portion with a fragment of HSV-2 genome encoding glycoproteins D, E, G, and I, was poorly immunogenic and caused adverse events in clinical trials despite reduced latency results in animal models.

4.2.1.6.5 Viral DNA Vaccines

Concerning viral DNA vaccines, results are inconsistent. Plasmid DNA encoding glycoproteins D and/or B or the immediate-early protein ICP27 induced protective immunity in some animal models, whereas immunity was incomplete in other models.

Therapeutic vaccines aim to prevent HSV recurrence or minimize disease severity and duration and reduce transmission. A vaccine must augment the host's specific immune responses, but as immune mechanisms, controlling outbreaks seem to be different from those required to prevent initial infection; therapeutic vaccines will have to boost different immune responses to that of a prophylactic vaccine.

Therapeutic vaccines probably need to stimulate strong virus-specific cell-mediated immune responses. The challenge in developing a therapeutic vaccine is to identify the HSV antigens that induce a greater protective response than infection with the whole virus. Therapeutic vaccines could be an alternative to antiviral therapy as well.

The above-mentioned ICP10ΔPK has shown therapeutic activity in phase I and phase II clinical trials with a reduced recurrence rate, total days of disease, and disease severity compared to placebo group. At 6 months after treatment, HSV-2 recurrences were completely prevented in 37.5 % of the vaccinated patients but were prevented in none of the placebo-treated patients. Vaccinated patients who experienced disease had a significantly lower frequency of episodes, reduced severity of episodes, and a lower mean total illness days relative to the placebo group.

The second strategy used to develop live vaccines is to generate mutants rendered nonvirulent by the deletion of one or more genes while retaining the viral glycoproteins previously identified as immunogenic targets.

An HSV-2 mutant deficient in glycoprotein H, known as DISC (disabled infectious single cycle), reduced HSV-2 replication and provided protection from HSV-2-induced disease. DISC also caused a 36 % reduction in recurrent lesions in the guinea pig when given systemically but not when administered by the mucosal route. In phase I clinical trials, DISC was well tolerated and induced neutralizing antibody and lymphoproliferative T-cell responses. Eighty-three percent of the vaccine recipients also developed HSV-specific CTL. However, clinical endpoints were not met in phase II trials to assess DISC's efficacy as a therapeutic vaccine, and further development was halted.

An overview of double-blind placebo-controlled clinical trials on different therapeutic HSV vaccines is provided in Table 4.3.

4.2.2 Human Immunodeficiency Virus

HIV-type 1 is the etiological agent of AIDS, a disease characterized by progressive immune deterioration and disappearance of CD4+ T cells from peripheral blood and lymphoid organs. It is estimated that over 40 million people currently live with HIV-1, most of them in sub-Saharan Africa and Asia, and that about 28 million have already died of the pandemic. As the mean incubation period from seroconversion to AIDS is about 8–10 years and many HIV-infected persons are unaware of their infection status, the chance for further dissemination of HIV through sexual contact is very high. Therefore, HIV/AIDS has the potential to become an even more serious health problem than it already is today.

On the African continent, women living with HIV/AIDS make up 60 % of the number of HIV-infected people. Heterosexual transmission of HIV-1 is the major route of infection on a worldwide basis and accounts for 70–80 % of new infections. Although female-to-male transmission of HIV can occur, the vast majority of cases (80 %) involve transmission of virus or virus-infected cells from male to female. Nonetheless, only one in 200 to one in 1,000 encounters results in productive infection that emphasize the effectiveness of structural and cellular barriers to virus entry. Genital tract infection is also linked to mother-to-child transmission of HIV.

Table 4.3 Results of therapeutic human HSV vaccination trials

Therapeutic vaccines	n (vaccine/placebo)	Results
Nonspecific live vaccines		
Bacillus Calmette-Guérin (BCG) (339)	83/72	Mean rate of recurrence 0.528/month vs 0.392/month (placebo)
		No influence on duration of lesions
Whole inactivated virion vaccines		
Whole virus, formalin-inactivated (689)	16/23	Fewer recurrences in 70 % vs 76 % of placebo group
Whole virus, heat-killed (Lupidon G/H) (1,490)	28/34	Cure/reduced disease severity/prolongation of interval length in 80 % vs 30 % of placebo group
Whole virus, heat-killed (Lupidon G/H) (881)	142/50	Reduced number and duration of recurrences increased interval length and reduced length of active disease
Inactivated subunit vaccines		
Subunit, lectin-purified (758)	18/24	Fewer recurrences in 43 % vs 35 % of placebo group
Skinner vaccine, formalin-inactivated (11,315)	148/144	Reduced number of recurrences in women
		Reduced number of lesions per recurrence in men
Recombinant glycoprotein vaccines		
gD2-alum vaccine (1,360)	98	24 % fewer clinical and 36 % fewer culture recurrences per month vs placebo group
gD-gB-MF59 vaccine (1,361)	101/101	No effect on recurrence rate
		Reduced symptom duration/new lesion formation/lesion duration
Disabled infectious single cycle (DISC) virus vaccines		
TA-HSV2 vaccine (1,339)	483	No significant differences between vaccine and placebo groups

M. Wirth 2006, Personal communication

As the genital mucosa is the site of initial contact with HIV-1 for most exposed individuals, study of the virus from the genital tract is critical for the development of vaccines and therapeutics. Therefore, a better understanding of the immunological mechanisms in the genital tract mucosa occurring during HIV infection is essential. It is currently not clear which factors contribute to the establishment of HIV-1 infection within the female reproductive tract. The establishment of HIV-1 infection seems to be dependent on the virus concentration, the presence of other genital tract infections, and the effectiveness of the immune system in the reproductive tract.

In recent years, significant progress has been made in understanding anti-HIV immunity in the vagina by using the simian immunodeficiency virus (SIV)/rhesus monkey model of heterosexual HIV transmission. Both HIV and SIV are retroviruses of the lentivirus family. They have a high degree of nucleotide sequence homology and similar organization of viral genes. It has been shown that vaginal inoculation of SIV in rhesus macaque results in systemic infection. The reproductive physiology of rhesus monkeys is remarkably similar to that of humans with both having menstrual cycles with an average length of 28 days. In addition, the similarity of the immune cell populations of the human and rhesus macaque lower female reproductive tract suggests that the biology of the closely related SIV and HIV viruses is likely to be very similar in their respective species. Thus, the rhesus macaque has become a widely accepted animal model for studying anti-HIV immunity in the female genital tract.

Dysregulation of the immune system is seen in association with HIV infection, with a fall in the CD4+ lymphocyte count and a reversal of the CD4/CD8 ratio now being well-recognized systemic manifestations of infection. However, alterations in mucosal immunity in the presence of HIV infection have been clearly documented in both the gut and the lungs, whereas in contrast, the female lower genital tract has not been as extensively studied.

4.2.2.1 HIV Transmission and Shedding in the Genital Tract

HIV-1 is present as free virus and virus-infected cells in semen from HIV-1-infected men and is deposited within the vagina in close proximity to the cervix during sexual intercourse. Which cells become infected and how the virus replicates is still not exactly clear. Other aspects that are not well understood are the mechanisms of viral transmission within the female reproductive tract, the mode of viral spread to the periphery, and whether susceptibility to infection varies under different hormonal and inflammatory conditions. Although HIV can be recovered from the vagina of women who have had a total hysterectomy, genital virus arises from the cervix and possibly the upper genital tract. The proximity to the vaginal lumen of cervical stroma lymphocytes, which compose the genital-associated lymphoid tissue, probably contributes both to HIV shedding and to susceptibility to mucosal transmission.

The cervix and especially the transformation zone has been identified as the major inductive and effector site for cell-mediated immunity in the genital tract which favors the cervix as a primary infection site of HIV-1. Expression of HIV receptors and coreceptors is likely to correlate with susceptibility to viral infection. In defining whether the ectocervix or the uterus serves as the first site of HIV infection, studies on the expression of HIV receptors CD4 and GalCer and coreceptors CCR5 and CXCR4 in the female genital tract have given important clues; these studies are discussed below.

4.2.2.1.1 HIV Receptors

The envelope glycoprotein gp120 of HIV-1 binds to cell surface receptors on target cells. The primary receptors are CD4, which is mainly expressed on a subset of T cells and on macrophages, and galactosyl ceramide (GalCer).

Furthermore, it is evident that the chemokine receptors CCR5 and CXCR4, which are expressed by most leukocyte subsets and ECs, function as HIV coreceptors and are important for HIV infection of cells. There are T-cell-tropic strains of HIV that are specific for CXCR4 and can infect continuous CD4+ T-cell lines and primary CD4+ T cells. Macrophage-tropic strains are specific for CCR5 and can infect primary macrophages and primary CD4+ T cells. The CCR5 ligands MIP-1α, MIP-1β, and RANTES block infection by macrophage-tropic strains of HIV-1, and, similarly, the CXCR4 ligand stromal cell-derived factor-1 blocks infection by T-tropic strains of HIV-1. However, the designation of HIV-1 phenotype is revised to indicate coreceptor usage. Accordingly, HIV-1 variants are designated as either X4 (CXCR4-specific) or R5 (CCR5-specific).

It has been shown that HIV-1 infects viable tissue sections and isolated cells from both the lower and upper female genital tract, suggesting that both ECs and submucosal leukocytes may be targets for initial HIV-1 infection. Moreover, it was also demonstrated that uterine EC lines can be productively infected with X4 strains of HIV-1 and that these cells express CD4, GalCer, and CXCR4, but not CCR5. CCR5 and CXCR4 expressing primary human uterine ECs are able to internalize both X4 and R5 strains of HIV but can only become productively infected by X4 strains. HIV-1 strains that utilize the CXCR4 chemokine receptor for infectivity are able to undergo reverse transcription, integration, viral DNA transcription, and viral release, whereas viral strains that utilize CCR5 do not undergo these early replicative events and are only released unmodified from these cells. Endometrial ECs have been shown to express all four receptor types, and altered expression of these receptors as a function of menstrual cycle stage could serve to either enhance or inhibit HIV-1 infection.

Three potential mechanisms of virus transmission in the female genital tract have been suggested. One mechanism seems to occur only with X4-tropic strains of HIV-1 and supports the development of a productive viral infection by the EC. Infection with the R5 strain of HIV-1 in which replication is not supported appears to lead to a gradual release of unmodified infectious virus. The

Fig. 4.8 Structure of squamous epithelium in the ectocervix (Yeaman GR, Asin S, Weldon S, Demian DJ, Collins JE, Gonzalez JL, Wira CR, Fanger MW, Howell AL. Chemokine receptor expression in human ectocervix: implications for infection by the human immunodeficiency virus-type 1. Immunology. 2004;113:524–33)

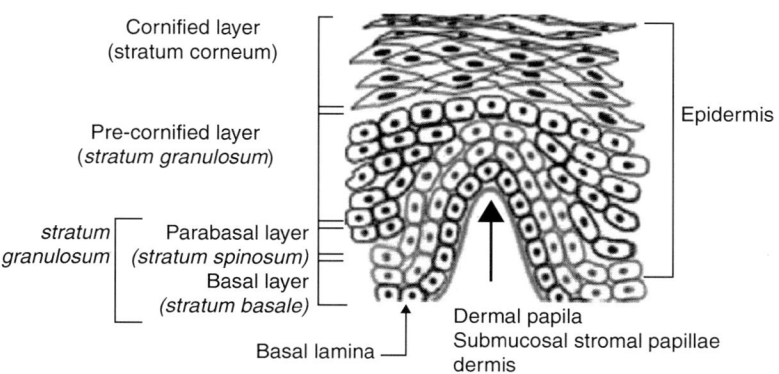

Cornified layer
(stratum corneum)

Pre-cornified layer
(*stratum granulosum*)

stratum granulosum
Parabasal layer
(*stratum spinosum*)
Basal layer
(*stratum basale*)

Epidermis

Dermal papila
Basal lamina
Submucosal stromal papillae
dermis

results indicated that uterine ECs could preferentially bind the R5 strain during the proliferative phase, whereas during the second half of the cycle, they may be more susceptible to X4. In addition, HIV-1 infection is transmitted after cell-to-cell contact between the infected ECs or stromal fibroblasts and the susceptible target cell. An alternative mechanism of HIV infection of the lower female genital tract involves the transcytosis of endosome-internalized HIV through the epithelium barrier, without EC infection. This approach may allow HIV to transverse directly to the submucosa, where it can infect susceptible immune cells.

To characterize the frequency of potential targets of HIV infection within the female genital tract, a study of the expression of HIV receptors and coreceptors on ECs and leukocytes from the ectocervix was performed.

Results demonstrated expression of CCR5 and CD4 on basal and parabasal epithelium and a clear compartmentalization of chemokine receptor expression between the squamous mucosa and submucosal stroma (Fig. 4.8, Table 4.4). CCR5- and CXCR4-expressing leukocytes were found exclusively in the submucosal stroma adjacent to the basal lamina. GalCer was expressed by cells of the parabasal and cornified layers and as such is likely to be the only HIV receptor readily accessible to virus. Moreover, studies show that CD4+ and chemokine receptor-expressing cells are proximal to the lumen in the dermal papillae. Given the phenotypes present in the papillae, it is proposed that these structures serve as a potential first site of encounter with infectible leukocytes and, given the large number of HLA-II positive macrophages within the stromal papillae

Table 4.4 HIV receptor/coreceptor expression in the human ectocervix in different phases of the menstrual cycle

	Basal	Parabasal	Midzone	Superficial
CCR5	++/+	+/+	–	–
GalCer	–	+++/+++	+/+	+++/+++
CD4	++/+	++/+	–	–
CXCR4	–	–	–	–

Adapted from Yeaman GR, Asin S, Weldon S, Demian DJ, Collins JE, Gonzalez JL, Wira CR, Fanger MW, Howell AL. Chemokine receptor expression in human ectocervix: implications for infection by the human immunodeficiency virus-type 1. Immunology. 2004;113:524–533

and HLA-II positive DCs as APCs present, may represent an antigen sampling structure for the ectocervix and vaginal mucosa.

The lack of CCR5-, CXCR4-, and CD4-expressing cells accessible to HIV in the lumen of the ectocervix contrasts with previous findings of HIV-1 receptor and coreceptor expression in the uterus, where all three of these receptors are expressed on the luminal aspect of the glandular and columnar epithelium. Results suggest that HIV infection of cells in the ectocervix could most likely occur through GalCer and CCR5, which were both expressed on ectocervical ECs throughout the menstrual cycle.

Based on findings of HIV-1 infection and HIV-1 receptor and coreceptor expression on uterine ECs, it appears that in comparison to the ectocervix, the uterus is a more likely first site for infection and transmission of virus after vaginal intercourse. In the uterus, HIV-1 transmission could involve secretion of newly synthesized infectious virus from the uterine ECs or viral transmission by cell-to-cell contact between the infected EC and a susceptible leukocyte. In contrast, the lack of CD4, CCR5, and CXCR4 expression on ectocervical ECs and the inability of these cells to develop a productive infection by HIV-1 suggest that HIV-1 transmission in the ectocervix is more likely to occur through the gradual release of infectious unmodified virus that is then able to infect susceptible submucosal leukocytes. An alternative mechanism of HIV infection in the lower female genital tract involves the transcytosis of endosome-internalized HIV through the epithelium barrier, without EC infection. It is also known that mutations in chemokine receptors markedly reduce the likelihood of acquiring HIV infection following exposure to virus. The well-described deletion in CCR5 has been shown to protect against HIV transmission among discordant couples.

4.2.2.1.2 Mediators of HIV Transmission

Enhanced detection of HIV in CVL is often correlated with decreased CD4+ count and increased viral load. Additional correlates of enhanced HIV in the female genital tract include oral contraceptive use, pregnancy, cervical ectopy, and STDs (Table 4.5).

The exact mechanism of STD-mediated enhanced shedding of HIV is still unknown. Enhanced recruitment of activated immune cells, disruption of the epithelium barrier (which can be induced by either agents in contraceptives or microbicides or infectious agents), reduction of T-helper and CTL function, which are all associated with STDs, may contribute to this STD-mediated enhancement of HIV detection in the female genital tract. Inflammation associated with STDs may also lead to increased proinflammatory cytokine production such as IL-1, IL-6, and TNF-α, which can potently upregulate HIV replication.

Growing evidence suggest that not only the presence of STDs but also bacterial vaginosis (BV) supports HIV transmission in the genital tract. Cultured bacteria such as mycoplasma or streptococci from CVL of HIV-positive women with BV have been shown to induce HIV-1 expression in vitro. These studies point to a direct role of BV-associated microorganisms in the

Table 4.5 Causes of increased predisposition of individuals with other STDs to HIV and vice versa

Associations between HIV and STDs
Increased shedding/replication of HIV as a result of the local inflammation produced by the STD
Recruitment of activated (HIV-susceptible) immune cells (e.g., CD4+ T cells)
Increase of proinflammatory cytokine production
Increased susceptibility to HIV as a result of the macroscopic/microscopic breaks in mucosal barriers caused by the STD
Higher prevalence of STDs among HIV infected individuals as a result of common risk factors for both infections
Increased susceptibility to STDs due to immunosuppression associated with HIV infection

M. Wirth 2006, Personal communication

induction of HIV replication, which may increase genital tract viral load and possibly affect horizontal and vertical transmission of HIV. BV also causes an increased vaginal pH, which may prolong the survivability of HIV in this lower genital tract microenvironment. Additional mediators of HIV transmission may also exist. There has been described an HIV-inducing factor isolated from the CVL of women, independent of HIV serostatus, that potently upregulated the expression of HIV. This factor induced HIV-LTR transcription in a NF-κB-dependent pathway and is closely correlated with abnormal vaginal pH and BV. This HIV-inducing factor in the genital tract of women may have a role in enhanced replication or horizontal or vertical transmission of HIV.

4.2.2.1.3 Compartmentalization

One of the main questions in understanding HIV replication in the genital tract is whether HIV is locally produced within the female genital tract or whether the virus is circulated through peripheral/tissue-infected cells to the genital tract. Therefore, the question of compartmentalization, the occurrence of distinct, yet phylogenetically related HIV-1 genotypes within different anatomical sites, is a very important one. Mucosa-associated lymphoid tissues may provide a source of HIV infection in the female genital mucosa, but limited studies have addressed this compartmentalization question.

Viral sequence analysis of HIV isolated from the periphery and the genital tract of infected women indicated that these viruses are similar between the blood and the CVL.

However, other studies supported compartmentalization between genital tract and periphery. HIV-1 variants in genital secretions of chronically infected transmitters differed from those in the blood and variants in cells differed from those in cell-free plasma, indicating sequence heterogeneity as well as compartmentalization of the virus in different body sites. Some of those differences can be attributed to differences in the techniques used to detect HIV-1 in the lower genital tract compartment and the significantly higher short-term variations in HIV-1 load in the genital tract compartment than in that of blood. Another study documented significant differences in the mean number of glycosylations on viruses derived from the genital tract and plasma, underscoring the importance of considering HIV-1 and immune response in the genital tract when designing vaccines. In addition, by quantifying the proportion of R5 and X4 viruses in each site, it was found that coreceptor usage often varied significantly between genital tract and plasma. Moreover, the study demonstrated a significant association between higher CD4+ cell counts and compartmentalization of both viral genomes and density of gp120 glycosylation sites, suggesting that the immune response influences the development of viral genotypes in each compartment.

4.2.2.2 Innate Immune Responses in HIV Infections

4.2.2.2.1 Antimicrobial Peptides

HNP1-3 inhibited both laboratory and clinical isolates of HIV in vitro and notably, although it is not as well characterized, HNP-4 shows even greater anti-HIV activity than HNP1–3 and was more effective in protecting human PBMC from infection by both R5 and X4 HIV-1 strains. HBD-2 and HBD-3 inhibited HIV-1 replication and downregulated CXCR4 expression. Interestingly, a recent study showed a significant correlation between a single-nucleotide polymorphism in the untranslated region of the DEFB1

gene, which probably regulates the gene expression of HBD-1, and the risk of perinatal HIV infection supporting a potentially important role for defensins in innate immunity of HIV infection. However, further studies are needed to further elucidate their role in HIV immunity in the female genital tract.

Another factor that is likely to control HIV infection within the female reproductive tract is SLPI. SLPI protects human macrophages and CD4+ T cells from HIV-1 infection, demonstrated that SLPI blocks HIV infection through interactions with a cellular target, annexin II, a cofactor for macrophage HIV-1 infection. There is mounting evidence suggesting that SLPI may be an important host defense. Higher SLPI concentrations in vaginal fluid samples correlate with a reduced rate of perinatal HIV transmission. Hormonal regulation of SLPI together with its anti-HIV activity may also be an important factor in the susceptibility of women to HIV infection.

4.2.2.2.2 Dendritic Cells and Macrophages

Several reports have identified DC, NK cells, resting and activated CD4+ T cells, and macrophages as the earliest cell populations to become positive for SIV- and HIV-RNA following a nontraumatic exposure to the virus. Although in chronically HIV-1-infected women, T cells, macrophages, and LCs in cervical tissue are infected with HIV-1, analysis of lymph nodes in HIV-infected men indicates that active virus replication occurs in activated and resting CD4+ T cells. However, there are no in vivo data to indicate the cell types that first become infected in the reproductive tract of women.

DCs are considered important target cells in HIV infection and transmission. In the SIV rhesus monkey model, there are controversial data on which cells are first infected during sexual transmission. CD4+ T cells might be the first cells to become infected after intravaginal inoculation of SIV, whereas the presence of SIV RNA in DCs can be observed shortly after intravaginal exposure of SIV. The latter authors found that infected DCs appear first in the mucosa and within 18 h they are in the draining lymph nodes, where they efficiently transmit the virus to CD4+ T cells. Cervical biopsies from HIV-positive women have shown significantly reduced levels of LCs but increased numbers of macrophages. The epithelium of the cervix from HIV + subjects showed a significant increase in both numbers of macrophages (CD68+) and proportions of activated macrophages (CD68+ HLA-DR+) compared to healthy persons, which could act as APCs for lymphocytes. The stroma contained increased proportions of inductive (D1+) and suppressive (D1+ D7+) macrophages but decreased effector phagocyte (D7+) proportions and LCs. In HIV-infected individuals, viral infection of DCs isolated from peripheral and lymphoid tissues has been immature DCs (iDCs) as well as LCs express both CD4 and the HIV chemokine coreceptors CCR5 and CXCR4 at their surface. Their surface receptor DC-SIGN is also thought to be one of the receptors to bind and internalize virus prior to its transmission to CD4+ T cells. However, they are infected with lower efficiency than are CD4+ T cells and macrophages. In contrast, mature DCs (mDCs) do not efficiently replicate the virus and may therefore represent an important reservoir of latent virus infection. Once bound, HIV is internalized and retains its infectivity for several days, a time also required for migration of DCs to regional lymph nodes, their differentiation to mDCs and the transfer of virions (transinfection) to CD4+ T cells. However, several functional impairments and a reduction of DCs have been reported. Ex vivo cultured DCs from HIV-infected persons are impaired in their ability to stimulate T-lymphocyte proliferation. NK cell function and numbers are also impaired in terms of cytolytic activity, mainly by the capacity to secrete CCR5-binding chemokines. This results in impaired elimination of infected cells and limited virus replication. However, further studies need to be done to evaluate these findings and if results are relevant to the genital tract mucosal immune system.

It has been proposed that HIV binds to DC-SIGN on DCs in the genital tract and is internalized into nonlysosomal compartments where it retains infectivity, before being transported to lymph nodes and presented to T cells. However,

DC-SIGN is not expressed on LCs, the most superficially located DCs. It seems likely that other types of HIV receptor are expressed by DCs.

One problem in studying HIV-1 transmission in humans is the lack of a suitable in vitro model. A cervical tissue-derived organ culture model was used to provide the natural tissue architecture and identified memory CD4+ T cells as the first cells that became infected during HIV-1 transmission across the cervical mucosa. This would imply a higher replication of HIV in T cells which would allow the virus to expand and be transferred to DCs. DCs are considered important target cells in HIV infection and transmission, as the cell surface receptor DC-SIGN is thought to be one of the receptors to bind and internalize virus prior to its transmission to lymph nodes where the infection would be passed to CD4+ T cells. Although HIV can be recovered from the vagina of women who have had a total hysterectomy, most genital virus arises from the cervix and possibly the upper genital tract. Studies on leukocyte populations in the human cervix showed leukocytes in the squamous mucosa and submucosal stroma to be predominantly T lymphocytes and DC that did not vary in numbers or distribution during the menstrual cycle.

4.2.2.3 Specific Immune Responses in HIV Infection

4.2.2.3.1 Cytotoxic T Lymphocytes

CTLs have been shown to be the major means by which an immune response eliminates systemic viral infections. In studies with mice, it has been shown that virus-specific CTLs, generated in the genital lymph nodes, can participate in effective genital immune responses against a sexually transmitted viral pathogen, for example, HSV. Systemic HIV-1-specific CD8+ T lymphocytes have been associated with protection against HIV-1 infection and improved host control immune control of HIV-1. In the acute phase of infection, the CTL response initially follows the rise of HIV in the blood, and when that response reaches a peak, the virus level falls (Fig. 4.9). There is an inverse relationship between CTL response and virus load. Quantification of the early

Fig. 4.9 Early CTL responses (*mauve line*) and virus load (*red line*); further observations were influenced by the initiation of antiretroviral drug therapy (*blue bands*) (McMichael AJ, Rowland-Jones SL. Cellular immune responses to HIV. Nature. 2001;410:980–7)

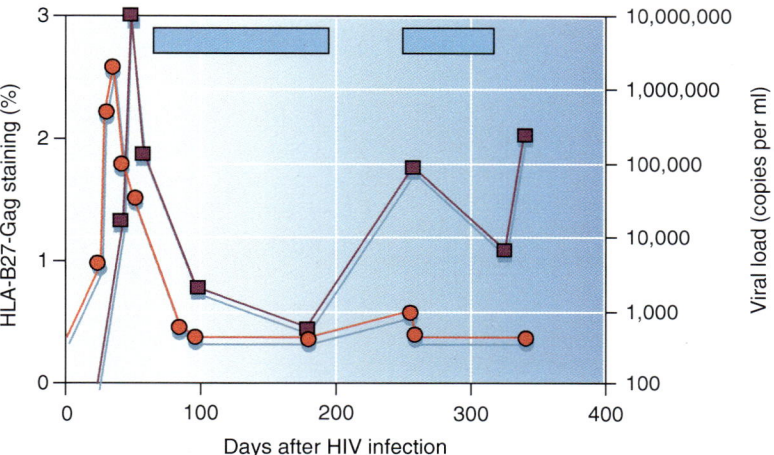

T-cell response can be made with HLA tetramers (Fig. 4.9). HIV-specific CTLs produce cytokines such as IFN-γ and TNF-α and the chemokines MIP-1α, MIP-1β, and RANTES which can suppress viral replication. However, less than 15 % of HIV-specific CTLs contained perforin which may result in poor target-cell death. Analyzing their surface glycoproteins compared to CMV-specific T cells, HIV-specific CD8+ T cells may be immature rather than end-stage effectors. The cellular immune response to HIV, mediated by T lymphocytes, thus seems strong but fails to control the infection completely. HIV undermines this control by infecting key immune cells, thereby impairing the response of both the infected CD4+ T cells and the uninfected CD8+ T cells. The failure of the latter to function efficiently facilitates the escape of virus from immune control and the collapse of the whole immune system.

In the uterus, CD8+ T cells were found to be noncytolytic during the secretory phase, and CTL activity was higher in postmenopausal women than in premenopausal women. One could postulate that this would lead to a higher viral susceptibility at the uterine level during the secretory phase. Furthermore, the decrease in percentage of CD4+ T cells typically seen in HIV-infected persons is also detectable in the lamina propria of the genital tract in monkeys and humans.

The relative importance of local HIV-specific antibodies and CD8+ CTL immune responses is presently not clear. Animal models suggest that virus-specific CD8+ T cells, together with adequate help from CD4+ T cells, can efficiently suppress replication of SIV and HIV-1 and slow down disease progression. It may be that mucosal CD8 lymphocytes play a particularly important role in protecting against mucosal virus challenge. Therefore, it is important to assess the function as well as the frequency of HIV-1-specific CD8+ cell responses in the genital tract. One study showed that SIV-specific CTL activity is present in the CD8+ T-cell population in the vaginal epithelium of SIV-infected animals. The SIV-specific CTL in the vaginal epithelium may be recognizing SIV-infected DCs present in the vaginal epithelium of acute and chronically infected rhesus macaques. The generation of antiviral CTL activity in vaginal IEL appears to be part of the normal immune response to infection with SIV and HIV. It is also possible that SIV-specific CD8+ CTLs are homing to the vaginal epithelium as part of a normal pattern of lymphocyte recirculation, unrelated to the presence of virus-infected cells. The immune cell population in the ectocervical and vaginal epithelia is immunophenotypically similar, and it is likely that similar CTL activity is present in the CD8+ T cells in the ectocervical squamous epithelium.

A similar population of anti-HIV CD8+ CTL has been found in brushings of the endocervical canal from HIV-infected women and in the genital tract of highly exposed persistently seronegative sex workers. Genital HIV-1-specific CD8+ cell responses of HIV-positive women were present at similar or higher levels than in the blood. HIV-positive women had significantly increased numbers of CD8+ lymphocytes resulting in reversal of the CD4/CD8 ratio compared with the control group which is in keeping with systemic events. However, the elevated numbers of CD8+ cells seen in the ectocervix of HIV-positive women demonstrates the active recruitment of nonresident CD8+ lymphocytes rather than an expansion of the resident intraepithelial population.

As elsewhere, these cells do not appear to be capable of mounting an adequate immune response to the virus. There was a significant increase in the proportion of activated CD8+ HLA-DR+ and CD4+ HLA-DR+ lymphocytes, but not in CD8+ TIA-1+ cells. The monoclonal antibody TIA-1 identifies cytotoxic granules in cells. Although the majority of CD8+ T cells express TIA-1 in low-risk women, the lack of a significant increase in the proportions of CD8+ TIA-1+ cells in HIV-infected women provides circumstantial evidence that there is no increase in the cytotoxic capacity of these CD8+ cells. The increased proportion of activated CD4+ HLA-DR+ cells seen in the female genital tract despite declining CD4 T-cell numbers suggests that this mucosal immune system of HIV-positive women exists in a more activated state than that in seronegative individuals.

4.2.2.3.2 Anti-HIV Antibodies in Genital Tract Secretions

Anti-HIV antibodies in vaginal washing samples include antibodies from serum transudates, local vaginal production, and cervical mucus. Anti-HIV antibodies have been found in CVS of seropositive individuals. Cervicovaginal Igs were significantly increased with IgG as the predominant isotype of anti-HIV antibodies in CVS of HIV-1-infected women and SIV-infected rhesus macaque. Low levels of anti-HIV-1 IgA associated with large increases in anti-HIV-1 IgG in CVS are common in HIV-infected women. A significantly higher HIV-1-specific IgG activity than that of IgA in CVS, saliva, and breast milk of HIV-infected individuals was demonstrated. Correlation studies suggested that IgG, IgM, and

HIV-1-specific IgG in CVS is mostly serum derived. CVS IgA seems to be both locally produced and serum derived, while IgA, IgM, and HIV-1-specific antibodies in saliva and breast milk are mostly locally produced. IgA antibodies are also either absent or present at very low levels in urine, intestinal fluid, and tears.

In the rhesus macaque, the relative levels of anti-SIV IgG and IgA in the serum seem to reflect the relative levels of anti-SIV IgG and IgA in vaginal secretions. This is most easily interpreted as an indication that the bulk of anti-SIV antibody in vaginal secretions is due to serum transudation. However, the results in hysterectomized animals are consistent with anti-SIV Ig production in the vaginal mucosa. Thus, it seems that both local production and transudation of serum antibodies are sources of anti-SIV antibodies in the vaginal secretions.

The relative contributions of serum-derived and locally produced antibodies need further study. It has been demonstrated that plasma-derived IgG antibodies are functional in the prevention of vaginally induced SIV infections in monkeys. Thus, there is hope that intensive systemic active immunization with relevant HIV-1 antigens may provide long-term protection against genitally encountered HIV-1 infection.

4.2.2.4 Cytokine Profiles

Proinflammatory cytokines may stimulate the replication and spread of HIV. TNF-α, IL-1β, and IL-6 concentrations in paired serum and CVL from 45 HIV-negative and 50 HIV-positive women were investigated to evaluate to what extent the female genital tract represents a source of proinflammatory cytokines in normal conditions and during the course of HIV infection. Expression of cytokine mRNA in cervicovaginal fluid and the proportion of inflammatory cells was increased in advanced stages of HIV infection. Levels of TNF-α and IL-6 correlated positively with the homologous serum cytokine levels in HIV-infected women. A transudation of cytokines from serum to the cervicovaginal fluid may have occurred in HIV-infected patients, but local production of cytokines was assessed by detection of cytokine mRNAs.

Elevated levels of IL-1β and MIP-1α in genital secretions of HIV-infected persons compared to uninfected women have been also described, suggesting an inflammatory state of the genital tract.

IL-2, IL-10, and IL-12 concentrations were evaluated in cervical secretions of female adolescents in order to determine how cytokine levels are influenced by infection with HIV and coinfection with other sexually transmitted pathogens. Compared with HIV-negative patients, HIV-positive patients had higher concentrations of IL-10. Coinfection of HIV and HPV predicted the highest IL-10 concentrations; coinfection of HIV, human papillomavirus, and other sexually transmitted pathogens predicted the highest IL-12 concentrations. In contrast, HIV infection, HPV infection, or infection with other STIs was not associated with differences in IL-2 concentrations. The data indicate that concomitant infection of the genital tract with HIV and other viral, bacterial, or protozoan pathogens influences the local concentrations of immunoregulatory cytokines. The review of Fauci summarized that IL-2, TNF-α, IL-1, and IL-6 can upregulate HIV replication, whereas IFN-α, TGF-β, IL-10, and β-chemokines (MIP-1α, MIP-1β, RANTES) can downregulate HIV. The balance between HIV-inducing and HIV-inhibiting cytokines may impact the viral load in the mucosa and, subsequently, the sexual transmission of the virus.

The above-mentioned results parallel reports demonstrating increased concentrations of Th2-type cytokines, IL-6 and IL-10, in the systemic circulation and at mucosal surfaces of HIV-positive adults. They also correspond to reports of increased IL-10 mRNA expression in cervical biopsy specimens from HIV-positive patients compared with those from HIV-negative patients. Moreover, they parallel findings of increased levels of these cytokines in serum and digestive tract mucosa in HIV-infected persons.

As these cytokines are present in CVS in healthy women as well, they could enhance HIV replication as soon as the virus enters the vagina. This hypothesis is in keeping with the higher risk of male-to-female transmission in cases of female genital tract infection or inflammation, a situation likely associated with increased local production of proinflammatory cytokines. As indicate above, data indicate that concomitant infection of the genital tract with HIV and other viral, bacterial, or protozoan pathogens influences the local concentrations of some immunoregulatory cytokines, for example, IL-10. In adults, systemic IL-10 concentrations increase with HIV disease progression. Most of the analyzed patients had CD4+ T-cell counts >400/μL, and increased IL-10 concentrations were detected in female adolescents who had been infected relatively recently, suggesting that the local immunoregulatory mechanisms of the cervix are altered early in the course of infection, long before systemic CD4+ T-cell counts decline.

4.2.2.5 Impact of Hormones and Menstrual Cycle on HIV

Female hormones may impact HIV replication not only in the genital tract but also in the periphery. Steroid hormones can bind to hormone-responsive elements within the long terminal repeat (LTR) of HIV which leads to an upregulation of HIV transcription. Studies using the SIV–macaque model of vaginal infection indicated that progesterone implants enhanced HIV transmission, presumably by thinning of the vaginal wall, whereas estrogen inhibited HIV infection, inversely, by thickening of the vaginal wall.

The impact of the menstrual cycle on genital tract shedding of HIV is controversial. Genital tract HIV-1 RNA levels from CVL fluid and endocervical cytobrush specimen were highest during menses and lowest immediately thereafter. The menstrual cycle had no effect on blood levels of HIV-1 RNA. A significant positive correlation between serum levels of progesterone and serum levels of HIV-1 RNA was detected. The lowest levels of cervical virus levels were present at the midcycle surge in LH, which was followed by an increase in virus levels that reached a maximum before the start of menses. Other studies, however, were unable to detect a menstrual cycle pattern to HIV genital tract shedding. Variation in assay methods, other influencing factors, and differences in the number of women sampled may account for this discrepancy.

The length of the menstrual cycle also seems to be independent of HIV serostatus.

Women demonstrated a significant increase in the prevalence of HIV-1-infected cells and a slight increase in HIV-1 RNA detection in CVS after initiating hormonal contraception whereas no changes were observed in concentrations of HIV-1 RNA. This may have implications for the HIV infectivity of women using hormonal contraception.

Expression of HIV-1 receptors and coreceptors in the female genital tract varies as a function of menstrual cycle stage, suggesting that sex hormone levels may influence a women's susceptibility to HIV-1 infection. The expression of HIV receptors and coreceptors was evaluated on uterine epithelia at different stages of the menstrual cycle. CD4, CCR5, and CXCR4 were found on glandular and luminal ECs. Both CD4 and CCR5 expressions on uterine ECs were high throughout the proliferative phase of the menstrual cycle; CXCR4 expression increased gradually during the proliferative phase. During the secretory phase of the cycle, CD4 and CCR5 expression was reduced, whereas CXCR4 expression remained elevated. Expression of GalCer on endometrial glands is higher during the secretory phase than during the proliferative phase.

This variation in receptor expression suggests that receptors are regulated by estradiol and progesterone and that a woman's susceptibility to HIV infection may vary due to this hormonal regulation of HIV receptor expression. Progesterone also causes a decrease in IL-2-mediated induction of the two main coreceptors for HIV entry, CCR5 and CXCR-4, on activated T cells, leading to reduction in HIV infection.

Several results suggest that, in contrast to the uterus, expressions of CD4, CCR5, CXCR4, and GalCer in leukocyte populations from the ectocervix do not greatly vary with the stage of the menstrual cycle. Moreover, ECs from tissues at early and mid-proliferative stages of the menstrual cycle express CD4, although by late proliferative and secretory phases, CD4 expression was absent or weak. In contrast, GalCer and CCR5 expression on ectocervical ECs was uniform in all stages of the menstrual cycle

(Table 4.4). A study of 55 HIV-positive women with a CD4 count <350 cell/μl examined over the course of eight consecutive weeks found that vaginal IL-1β, IL-2, IL-4, IL-6, IL-10, MIP1β, TGF, and TNFRII were all increased during menses whereas peripheral cytokines were not altered. Increased cytokine levels during menses of HIV-positive women may be correlated with the increased numbers of granulocytes and macrophages in the genital mucosa at menses which in the case of HIV may be hyperactivated, leading to enhanced cytokine production. In HIV-seropositive women with advanced HIV disease and a CD4 count <200 cells/μl, TNFα, IL-1β, and IL-6 are enhanced in comparison to patients with early HIV disease and a CD4 count >500 cells/μl or HIV-seronegative women. Phenotypic and functional analysis of systemic lymphocytes was not altered by the menstrual cycle as evaluated in HIV-positive or HIV-negative women.

4.2.2.6 Summary

In summary, HIV-1 infection leads to a dysregulation of the immune system of the genital tract mucosa (Table 4.6). As in the periphery, HIV-1 infection causes a disruption of the CD4/CD8 ratio in cervical mucosa. The increased CD8+ T cells are predominately primed/memory T cells; however, these CD8+ T cells are functionally impaired, as indicated by a decrease in or lack of perforin and TIA-1 (cytolytic granule-associated protein) expression. In the systemic compartment, HIV infection leads to an alteration in the cytokine pattern, most prominent in advanced

Table 4.6 Features of immune system dysregulation in the female genital tract caused by HIV infection

T lymphocytes	Increase in CD8+ T cells
	Decrease in perforin/TIA-1 production in CD8+ T cells
	Shift in CD4+/CD8+ ratio
DCs	Reduced levels
Igs	Decrease in plasma cells
	Decrease in S-IgA production, predominance of IgG
Cytokines	Increased production of proinflammatory cytokines (e.g., IL-6, IL-10)

M. Wirth 2006, Personal communication

stages of HIV disease. Likewise, in the CVL of HIV-positive women, proinflammatory cytokines are enhanced and at least one study, using mRNA in situ hybridization techniques, pointed to a shift toward Th2 cytokines (IL-4, IL-5, IL-10), which were significantly higher among HIV-positive women than HIV-seronegative women. LCs are lost or decreased in the cervical epithelium of HIV-positive women, which may be caused by direct HIV infection of LCs or redistribution of these primed LCs to lymphoid tissues. Plasma cells are also reduced in the submucosa of HIV-positive women, which may account for the impaired local production of IgA. HIV infection in women is often associated with chronic viral infection, candidiasis, syphilis, pelvic inflammatory disease, and bacterial infections. These conditions are seen in the genital tract before any manifestation in the periphery, which suggests that breakdown in the genital mucosal immune system may occur before immune system dysregulation.

That some individuals become HIV positive after a single virus exposure whereas others remain resistant to repeated challenge indicates that there are factors involved beyond the simple viral contact with particular mucosal cells. Sex hormones and cytokine levels in the environment of the virus and target cells may influence infectivity. It has been hypothesized that in frequently HIV-exposed but uninfected individuals, HIV-specific mucosal antibody responses may exist and play a role in resistance to HIV. It has been reported that HIV-1-resistant sex workers have HIV-specific IgA in their genital secretions, whereas other studies described an absence of HIV-specific antibodies in genital secretions of HIV-resistant sex workers. So far, a condition that mimics the reports of HIV infections that produce genital anti-HIV antibodies without exposures of a systemic immune response could not be reproduced in monkeys. Seronegative sex workers also have higher frequencies of CD8+ T cells in the cervical mucosa than in blood, whereas HIV-infected individuals have higher CTL responses in blood than in mucosal tissues, which would again suggest a more important role for cell-mediated responses in the immunity against HIV. A vaccine that can elicit strong antiviral immunity may provide protection from heterosexual HIV-1 transmission. Further trials of anti-HIV vaccines should include an analysis of potential genital mucosal immune responses induced by the vaccine candidates.

4.2.3   Human Papillomavirus

HPV is a heterogenous group of DNA viruses from the Papovaviridae family. With at least 100 different genotypes, it can infect and replicate in skin epithelium (cutaneous HPV) and in mucous membranes (mucosal HPV) and induce epithelial proliferation resulting in warts. More than 40 anogenital genotypes have been associated with STD, which makes HPV the most common viral STD in the world.

Two out of three people having sexual contact with an HPV-infected partner will develop an infection within the next months that will be asymptomatic in almost three out of four cases. Most HPV infections regress spontaneously with HPV DNA persisting for about 6–12 months in the genital tract and then spontaneously disappearing in the majority of patients.

The correlation between genital HPV infections and cervical cancer was first documented in the early 1980s by the study group of *zur Hausen*. HPV infection is now generally accepted as being involved in the development of anogenital precursor neoplasia, i.e., cervical, cervical glandular, vulval, vaginal, and anal intraepithelial neoplasia. Approximately 30 % of high-grade CIN will progress to invasive cervical carcinoma over a period of 10–20 years which makes persistent HPV infection the major risk factor for developing cervical carcinoma (Fig. 4.10). HPV types 16, 18, 31, 33, 35, 45, and 58, and about 8–10 other minor types, are oncogenic and are found in almost all cervical cancer biopsy samples and in 90 % of high-grade intraepithelial precursor lesions (Fig. 4.11). HPV types 16 and 18 are the most commonly detected HPV types in biopsy samples.

HPV types which infect the genital tract can be classified into three groups (Table 4.7). The low-risk group includes HPV 6 and 11 which are

Fig. 4.10 Etiology of cervical carcinogenesis as the result of HPV infection (Wirth 2006)

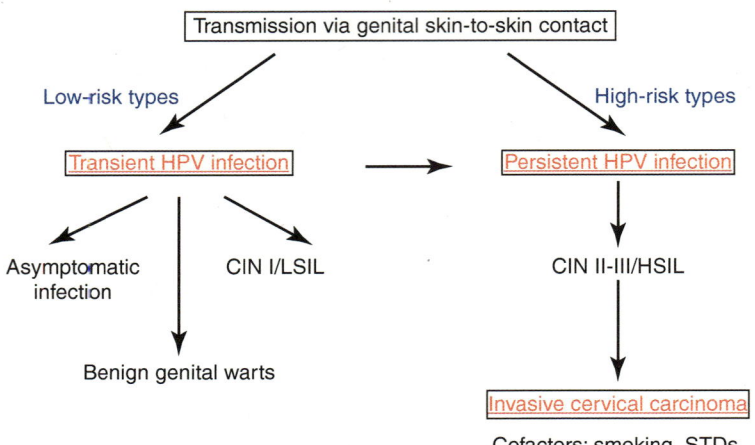

Fig. 4.11 Prevalence of different HPV types in cervical cancer biopsies (Stanley MA. Human papillomavirus (HPV) vaccines: prospects for eradicating cervical cancer. J Fam Plann Reprod Health Care. 2004;30:213–215)

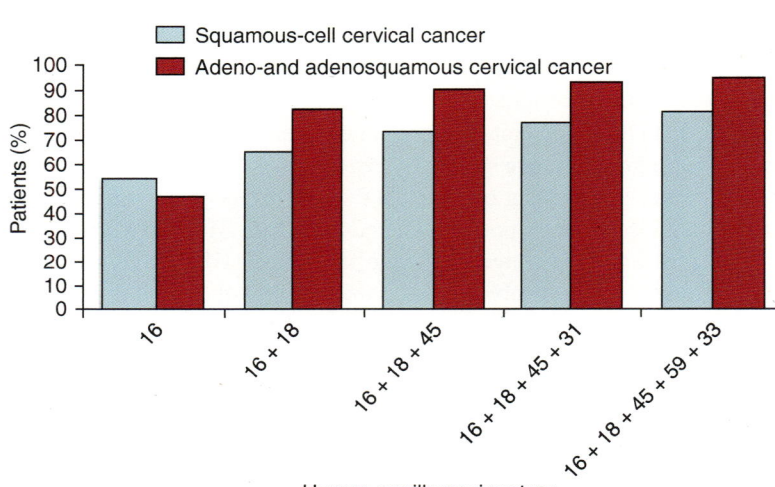

Table 4.7 Classification of HPV types according to oncogenic potential and clinic

Risk type	HPV type	Association with
Low risk	HPV 6/11/41/42/43/44	Condylomata accuminata Low-grade CIN (CIN I)/LSIL
Intermediate risk	HPV 31/33/34/35/39/51/52	High-grade CIN (CIN II-III)/HSIL
High risk	HPV 16/18/45/51/52/56/58/59/61/62/64/ 66/67/68/69/70	High-grade CIN (CIN II-III)/HSIL Invasive carcinoma of cervix, vulva, anus, or penis

M. Wirth 2006, Personal communication

commonly associated with condylomata accuminata and low-grade squamous intraepithelial lesions (LSIL or CIN I). The high-risk group includes HPV 16, 18, 45, and 56 which are commonly found in patients with high-grade squamous intraepithelial lesions (HSIL or CIN II/III)

or invasive carcinoma of the cervix, vulva, anus, or penis. The intermediate risk group is associated with high-grade CIN but less commonly with invasive cancer; this group includes HPV 31, 33, 35, 51, and 52. Low-risk types remain extrachromosomal or episomal, whereas the genomes of high-risk HPV types 16 and 18 are found integrated into the cellular host DNA in most human cervical carcinomas. The differences in oncogenicity between high- and low-risk HPV result from their different ability to integrate into the host DNA and to cause genetic instability.

Cervical carcinoma constitutes a major public health problem worldwide with 500,000 new cases per year. It is the most common female malignancy in developing countries and the second most common in Western countries following breast cancer. The latest cancer statistics for the year 2006 reported 9,710 estimated new cases and 3,700 estimated deaths of cervical cancer in the United States. Despite optimal management with options like radical surgery, radiotherapy, and chemotherapy, the overall 5-year survival for patients with cervical carcinoma is still only 58 %. This suggests a need to develop novel approaches not only to treatment, for example, immunotherapy, but also to the strong need for prophylactic or therapeutic vaccines.

4.2.3.1 Composition and Mechanism of HPV Infection

4.2.3.1.1 The HPV Genome

The HPV genome can be divided into a coding and a noncoding region. The noncoding region, the long control region (LCR), contains the origin of viral DNA replication and the enhancer/promoter elements regulating the viral transcription. The coding region consists of open reading frames (ORFs) and encodes the early (E) and late (L) viral proteins. The late genes encode structural proteins, the viral capsid proteins (L1 and L2) which self-assemble into the viral capsid interacting with a receptor of the target cell facilitating entry of the viral DNA. The early proteins E1 and E2 are involved in regulation of viral transcription and DNA replication. The E6 and E7 genes of high-risk HPV types encode for oncoproteins that can immortalize human keratinocytes. This potential appears to be limited to high-risk types, because E6 and E7 from HPV6 or HPV11 are nontransforming. E6 will bind, inactivate, and degrade the host's oncosuppressor protein p53, which results in loss of p53-induced

apoptosis and G1 arrest of the cell cycle. The binding of E7 to retinoblastoma gene product (Rb) will lead to the transcriptional deregulation of cell-cycle control and results in uncontrolled cell proliferation. When viral DNA integrates into the host genome (malignant transformation), it will cause successively the disruption of the E2 ORF, loss of E2 protein expression, the overexpression of E6 and E7, uncontrolled cell proliferation, and in the end oncogenic transformation of the cell. The HPV genome is usually present in an episomal (circular and nonintegrated) configuration in CIN, whereas in invasive cervical cancer, the genome is commonly integrated into the host DNA. HPV DNA integration appears to be the critical event in the development of cervical neoplasia, since HPV E6 and E7 are conserved intact and show persistent and increased expression in carcinomas.

4.2.3.1.2 Molecular Pathogenesis

HPV penetrates the suprabasal cells in the cervical epithelium and tightly maintains a program of viral transcriptional repression of its late genes L1 and L2, which are potentially the most powerful immunogens that HPV synthesizes. This repression allows escape from immune surveillance and recognition. This is different from certain animal models where papillomavirus infections are rapidly eradicated due to the expression of L1 and L2 in all layers of the infected epithelium, which attracts more immune effector cells to the infected area. As HPV progresses through the layers of the epithelium, the replicative program of its genes changes in an orderly fashion. The HPV early proteins E6 and E7 are produced through most of the phases of the HPV life cycle, making them better candidates for therapeutic vaccines. On the other hand, the HPV L1 and L2 late proteins are not produced until the virus is located in the most superficial layers of the epithelium, correlating with the assembly of infectious virions and their release from the epithelium with the desquamated-infected superficial cells.

Human HPV infections are exclusively intraepithelial, and, theoretically, HPV infection should be detected by the APC of squamous epithelia, the LC. The activated LC should then migrate to the draining lymph node, processing HPV antigens en route, and present antigen to naïve T cells in the node. The T cells should then differentiate into armed effector cells, migrate back to the infected site, and destroy the infected keratinocytes.

4.2.3.2 Mechanisms of HPV to Evade the Immune Response

HPVs, unlike other recurrent or persistent human viruses such as influenza or Epstein–Barr virus, do not provoke strong humoral or cellular immune responses. The diagnosis of HPV still relies on the cytological detection of cellular abnormalities and the histopathological confirmation of epithelial lesions. In addition, the chronic nature of HPV infection, especially with oncogenic types, suggests that the virus has apparently evolved to avoid the mammalian immune response.

A number of immune evasion mechanisms have been proposed, and these are employed especially by the cancer-associated HPV types (Table 4.8).

4.2.3.2.1 Low Profile

HPV infection per se does not elicit any major damage likely to evoke the principle innate immunity danger signals. The virus infects only ECs and encodes nonsecreted proteins expressed at low levels, with virus production within cells, which are sloughed off at the end of their lifespan. There is no viremia and the infected cells are not lysed, limiting the production of antigens for systemic presentation. The infectious cycle of HPV is itself an immune evasion mechanism inhibiting host detection of virus. The virus replication cycle is conducted within the maturing keratinocytes (KC) and mature virions escape from the infected epithelial surface within desquamating KCs, so there is little local or systemic presentation of HPV antigens to the immune system by professional APCs during infection. HPV replication and release do not cause cell death, since the differentiating KC is already programmed to die, which does not present a danger signal to the immune system. Thus, for most of the HPV infectious cycle, there is little or no release of the proinflammatory cytokines important for DC activation and migration into the local milieu, and the essential signals required for immune responses in squamous epithelia are absent. Another level of immune evasion derives from the tropism of genital HPVs for KCs. Unlike the so-called professional APCs such as DCs, KCs have low levels of HLA class I and class II molecules and costimulator molecules such as B7.1. Exposing CD4+ T-cells to KCs in vitro has

Table 4.8 Mechanisms of HPV to evade the host's immune responses, resulting in increasing viral persistence

	Mechanisms of HPV to evade host's immune response	Results in
Low profile	KC as priviledged site for HPV infection	Little local/systemic HPV antigen presentation by APCs
	Low HLA I/II expression	Little release of proinflammatory cytokines
	No lysis of infected cells	Resistance to CTL-mediated lysis
	No viremia	
Early proteins	Interference with IFN pathways	Limitation of HPV antigen presentation by LC
	Downregulation of activity of MCP-1/IL-18/TGF-β2	Inhibition of cytokine release
	Interference with MHC II antigen maturation on KC	
T cells	Downregulation of TCR signaling components	Resistance of KC to CTL-mediated killing
	Predominance of Th2 lymphocytes and Treg cells	Reduction of cell-mediated immunity
	Downregulation of TNF-α	
	Upregulation of IL-10	
LCs	Reduction in number	Interference with antigen presentation
	Inhibition of EC-DC interaction	

Adapted from Frazer IH, Thomas R, Zhou J, Leggatt GR, Dunn L, McMillan N, Tindle RW, Filgueira L, Manders P, Barnard P, Sharkey M. Potential strategies utilised by papillomavirus to evade host immunity. Immunol Rev. 1999;168:131–42 led to nonresponsiveness, a mechanism which could be operating in vivo to render HPV-specific T cells functionally inert.

4.2.3.2.2 Immunosuppression by Early Proteins

However, even in the absence of viral-induced cytolysis and cell death, HPV-infected KCs should activate secretion of type 1 IFNs, IFN-α and IFN-β. As is the case with most DNA viruses, HPVs have evolved mechanisms for inhibiting IFN synthesis and signaling by downregulating IFN-α-inducible gene expression. HPV 16 E6 and E7 oncoproteins directly interact with components of the IFN signaling pathways. It is also apparent that these viral genes regulate other factors likely to influence the survival of virus-infected cells including TGF-β2 as important components of any local inflammatory response. Another strategy for immune evasion stems from the ability of HPV 16 E6 to downregulate the IFN-promoting factor, IL-18. Other immunosuppressive actions of HPV early proteins include the inhibition of EC interactions with DCs by E6. E6 and E7 further inhibit the activity of the important MCP-1. Thus, activity of E6 and E7 provides the molecular basis for promoting viral persistence and avoiding innate immunity and the consequential activation of adaptive immunity. E5, another early protein of HPV, prevents the efficient pH-dependent processing of peptidic antigens. Other relevant influences include the modulation of antigen processing pathways through E5-mediated MHC expression

4.2.3.2.3 Downregulation of HLA

A further level of immune evasion is also related to the KCs in that HLA class I molecules on HPV-transformed cells are often expressed at a low level or are absent altogether. It is not known if this is of functional consequence for CTLs, but the downregulation of certain HLA-B alleles does correlate with a poorer prognosis for some patient populations with cervical dysplasia. The MHC molecular expression is usually upregulated by cytokines associated with an inflammatory response, so this will be suboptimal in an HPV-infected target cell. However, the genetics of HLA may also influence susceptibility to HPV infection or ability to clear the virus and thus avoid persistence, which is the key risk factor for progression.

4.2.3.2.4 Activation of T-Cell Subsets

Another potential mechanism of immune evasion is the suppression of immune responses by HPV-transformed KCs, through the production of either inhibitory cytokines or proteins that can inactivate stimulatory cytokines. HPV-transformed KCs might resist CTL killing either by producing proteins that interfere with CTL-lytic mechanisms or by inducing apoptotic cell death in the CTLs themselves. As a consequence, HPV infection is not accompanied by inflammation resulting in persistent infections as the host remains ignorant of the pathogen for long periods.

It is possible that HPV has evolved to exploit the endogenous tissue responses utilized by innate immunity to disfavor induction of a more threatening Th1 response which would favor the development of CTLs. Indeed, it has been shown that in CIN lesions there is a relative downregulation of TNF-α by the epithelium and upregulation of the Th2 cytokine IL-10 compared to normal cervix. The migrating LC may thus be inappropriately activated, skewing any subsequent immune activation of T cells, which might include the induction of anergic or Treg cells. Recent studies have documented a predominant Th2 polarity (instead of a Th1 response) of tumor-infiltrating lymphocytes in human cervical cancer and the draining lymph node in cervical cancer appeared to have an increased proportion of Treg cells. Immune evasion by HPV-transformed cells can also be considered at the level of the effector T cells. Immune responses in patients with advanced cancer are often diminished as a result of disease or treatment. One mechanism that has been proposed for their decreased immune responsiveness is the downregulation of signaling components of the TCR such as CD3 zeta chain. These alterations were associated with reduced cellular functions such as the production of TNF-α. Studies also propose a role for FasL expression in cervical carcinoma, which allows the tumor cells to evade host immune surveillance.

4.2.3.2.5 Suppression of Langerhans Cells

Disturbances in the afferent phase of the immune response are suspected. The analysis of inflammatory infiltrates in cervical dysplasia has revealed reduced numbers of LCs in CIN II and III lesions. This may result in changes in cell surface E-cadherin expression in the basal and suprabasal layers. For example, E6 can downregulate epithelial E-cadherin expression, which could modulate their contacts with LCs, not allowing optimal antigen capture or activation necessary for the initiation of antiviral T-cell responses. In addition, the change in tissue architecture is more permissive for the expansion and spread of immortalized and/or transformed cells.

The interaction of HPV with LCs which are the first APCs that the virus comes into contact with during infection has been further explored. In contrast to DCs, LCs are not activated by HPV virus-like proteins (VLPs), which is illustrated by the lack of upregulating activation markers, secreting IL-12, stimulating T cells in a mixed lymphocyte reaction, and inducing HPV-specific immunity and migrating from epidermal tissue. Since DCs or LCs are generally accepted as being the most efficient APCs of the immune system, their lack could probably result in an inefficient primary immune response which also delays the activation of the adaptive immune response in HPV infection.

Moreover, capsid entry is usually an activating signal for DCs, but there is evidence that LCs, unlike stromal DCs, are not activated by uptake of HPV capsids, a phenomenon that would inhibit both LC migration and maturation, and the priming of the immune response against the capsid proteins.

4.2.3.3 Cell-Mediated Immunity in HPV Infection

As HPV transmission and subsequent infection is a local event in the lower female genital tract, local immunity seems to be of crucial importance in the outcome of an HPV infection. The local immune status might determine whether the virus infection will be cleared or will be persistent, finally resulting in the development of cervical neoplasia. Although a very high percentage of young sexually active women are positive for genital HPV, most HPV infections are subclinical in immunocompetent patients or manifest intermittently as self-limiting warty lesions. Most HPV infections are transient with a median duration of about 8 months which means that HPV is successfully attacked by the immune system after transmission. A small but medically important fraction of the lesions, however, will progress to HSIL, CINs, and, if left untreated, invasive and metastatic carcinomas. Thus, infection with oncogenic HPV types is a necessary but not a sufficient cause of cervical cancer; other risk factors probably include smoking, genetic factors, cervical inflammation, and immune system dysfunction.

Cervical carcinogenesis includes HPV infection, viral persistence, progression to precancer lesions, and invasion. HPV persistence and progression involve a complex interaction between viral and host factors, such as viral variants, viral load, susceptibility genes, immune response against HPV, and molecular events associated with progression. The host immune response is essential for restraining both HPV infections and HPV-related cervical cancer.

The peak prevalence of genital HPV infections is soon after the onset of sexual activity in women. Thereafter, the prevalence declines, indicating that long-term protection can be acquired. Supportive to this is the fact that up to 65 % off all CIN1 lesions in women between 15 and 34 years of age will regress. Cell-mediated immunity is likely to be important since in immunocompromised individuals like HIV-infected women and organ transplant recipients, the presence of HPV infections and anogenital neoplasia is higher than in the general population. In addition, HIV-1-infected patients have lesions that progress more rapidly. Furthermore, the regression of HPV-induced warts is associated with lymphocytic infiltration in both patients with genital warts and animal papillomavirus models, whereas non-regressing warts are characterized by a lack of immune cells.

Clues to the nature of the cellular immune response to HPV infection have come from immunohistological studies of spontaneously regressing genital warts. Non-regressing genital warts are characterized by a lack of immune cells at the site of infection; the few intraepithelial lymphocytes are CD8+ cells, and mononuclear cells are present mainly in the stroma. Histological examination of regressing genital warts reveals a large infiltrate of both CD4+ and CD8+ T cells and macrophages in the warts' stroma and epithelium. The infiltrating lymphocytes express activation markers, the cytokine milieu is dominated by proinflammatory cytokines such as IL-12, TNF-α, and IFN-γ, and there is upregulation of the adhesion molecules required for lymphocyte trafficking on the endothelium of the wart capillaries. This is characteristic of a Th1-based immune response.

Moreover, the detection of HPV-specific circulating T cells in healthy individuals substantiates the role of a cell-mediated response as well as the detection of anti-HPV IgG1 and IgG2, IFN-γ, and IL-4 in individuals with cleared infection. The role of specific or nonspecific cell-mediated immunity in the clearance of HPV is not exactly known, largely because immune parameters after primary HPV infection have not been studied to a large extent. In women with preinvasive cervical neoplasia, the spontaneous regression of lesions occurs in 30–65 % of cases. The question if HPV-specific immunity influences this process and if the development of cancer results from a failure of the immune system is still unclear.

The investigation of the role of natural immunity to HPV infection is problematic as HPV infections can be transient and often asymptomatic. Studies have been carried out largely on patients with established HPV-associated disease and have focused on the oncogenic HPV types, in particular responses against the viral transforming proteins, E6 and E7, the only viral antigens constitutively expressed in transformed cells. Also studies have focused on systemic rather than mucosal immunity, so a substantial component of the host response against HPVs could be missed.

The link between HPV16 and cervical carcinoma opens up the possibility of immune T-cell intervention, either against the preinvasive lesions from which tumors arise or against the virus antigen-positive tumor cells themselves. This requires a better understanding of the spectrum of T-cell responses induced by HPV16 antigens during the course of natural infection, and of their role in disease clearance and progression. Cell-mediated responses comprise both CD4+ and CD8+ T cells which take part directly as CTL or indirectly as T-helper cells for CTL or antibody production in HPV immunity. In almost all studies of cell-mediated immunity against HPV, peripheral blood rather than local T cells have been used due to the low yield of T cells from surgically removed cervical cancer tissue and the low availability of relevant cervix tissue.

4.2.3.3.1 CD4+ T-Cell Responses

There are several studies providing information about CD4+ T-cell responses to HPV16 where proliferative responses to either peptides or soluble HPV proteins have been demonstrated in patient groups. In early studies, PBMCs from patients with a history of skin warts were able to proliferate in vitro against crude wart antigen preparations but also PBMCs from individuals with no history of warts responded specifically to the same wart antigen preparations.

Serological T-cell responses against peptides derived from HPV 16 E7 and HPV 16 L1 were not, however, significantly associated with HPV disease as T-cell responses were also seen in healthy asymptomatic controls. It is not clear if the results in healthy control group represent in vitro artifacts or memory responses based on a prior exposure to HPV.

However, results suggested that a Th1 pattern of response was predominant among healthy adults but reduced in women with cervical dysplasia. Indeed, immunohistological studies have indicated that regression of HPV-infected lesions is associated with a Th1 response.

T-cell proliferative responses to HPV16 E7 peptides in women with mild dyskaryosis demonstrated the strongest T-cell responses in women with persisting HPV infection and progressive disease (99 % reactive) compared to those who cleared the infection (44 % reactive).

Other studies on HPV 16 E7 peptides have shown that the T-cell responses correlated with both the stage of disease and the presence of HPV 16 DNA. Women with CIN I or II demonstrated that the cell-mediated responses to E7 peptide significantly correlated with disease regression and resolution of viral infection within 12 months.

Persistence of HPV infection has been reported to be correlated with a lack of CTL responses to HPV 16 E6. Failure of the immune system to eliminate HPV was reflected by the absence of type 1 T-cell immunity against HPV 16 E2 and E6 in patients with cervical lesions. This is also consistent with trials on vaccination against HPV E6 and E7 in experimental animals which induced cell-mediated immunity. Regression of skin papillomas in rabbits and tumors formed by HPV16 E7-transformed cells in mice has been observed.

In summary, these studies suggest a relationship between T-cell responses against HPV and cervical disease, with a decreased response in cancer patients and an increased response in women with high-grade CIN and viral persistence.

4.2.3.3.2 CD8+ T-Cell Responses

The role of naturally occurring CTLs in mediating the regression of HPV-related disease has not been proven. There has been an increasing interest in CD8+ CTLs as vehicles for immunotherapy in human cancers, using either vaccines capable of inducing CTLs or adoptive therapy protocols which has been based on clear demonstrations of antitumor immunity. The expression of E6 and E7 proteins by HPV-transformed cells provides attractive tumor-specific targets for immunotherapy.

The search for human memory CTL responses was initially difficult because of the lack of well-defined viral reagents for in vitro testing. HPV16 E2-, E6-, and E7-specific CTLs can be detected in patients with previous or ongoing HPV infections using whole HPV proteins to restimulate CTL responses, either in a soluble form or expressed by recombinant viral vectors. Results suggest that naturally occurring HPV E6- and E7-specific CTLs do exist in patients with HPV-associated disease, for example, HPV16 E7-specific CTLs that exist in the peripheral blood of women with high-grade CIN and cervical carcinoma, but are extremely rare.

The difficulties of obtaining memory T-cell responses from patients have resulted in the use of DCs to generate primary responses. HPV-specific CTL responses could be generated from healthy asymptomatic donors and cervical cancer patients using DCs pulsed with recombinant HPV 16 or HPV 18 proteins. The successful processing and presentation of exogenous HPV antigens in vitro raises the possibility that antigens released from HPV-infected cells during the disease process or by surgical procedures could be stimulating HPV immunity in vivo.

CTL responses in asymptomatic subjects appear to be rare, suggesting that CTL responses are associated with HPV-induced disease. Preliminary studies have not, however, addressed whether CTLs have a role in the prevention, control, or treatment of disease. Furthermore, although CTLs have been operationally defined as HPV specific, based on their reactivity against recombinant HPV proteins, few as yet have been shown to recognize tumor cells.

4.2.3.3.3 Further Evidence on CD4+ and CD8+ T-Cell Responses

To date only a limited number of prospective studies have been carried out. Obviously, failure to develop effective cell-mediated immunity to clear or control infection results in persistent infection and, in the case of the high-risk HPVs, an increased probability of progression to HSIL or invasive carcinoma. Therefore, there is the need for further studies on T-cell responses in longitudinal studies and at sites of disease.

More recent studies indicated that a majority of both patients with cervical lesions and healthy persons display HPV16 L1 peptide-specific type 1 T-cell responses with a similar magnitude. These responses covered a broad range of peptides within L1, which suggests that during persistent or repeated exposure to HPV16 L1, the immune system maximizes its efforts to counter the viral challenge. Unlike type 1 T-cell responses against HPV 16 E2 and E6, type 1 T-cell immunity against L1 does not correlate with health or disease. This is in contrast to the previously mentioned finding that such patients lack such type 1 T-cell immunity against HPV16 early antigens E2 and E6.

The frequency of CD4+ responders was far lower among those with progressive disease, indicating that the CD4+ T-cell response might be important in HPV clearance. CD8+ reactivity to E6 peptides was dominant across all disease grades, implying that E6-specific CD8+ T cells are not vitally involved in disease clearance.

Concerning the production of cytokines by CD4+ T-helper cells, a decreased level of IL-2 production but elevated levels of IL-4 and IL-10 were observed in patients who had extensive HPV disease compared with those suffering from localized HPV disease or healthy controls. Production of cytokines that mainly enhance potentially protective cell-mediated immunity is defective in women with extended HPV disease. Moreover, a pronounced shift from type 1 to type 2 cytokine production is associated with more extensive HPV infection. This suggests a shift toward the T-cell production of cytokines associated with the suppression of cell-mediated immunity. Another study showed significant IL-2 production against HPV peptides in patients with CIN and persistent HPV infection, as well as to a significantly lesser extent in patients with cervical cancer; this suggests a correlation between IL-2 responses and disease.

4.2.3.4 Antibody Responses in Genital HPV Infection

Circumstantial evidence suggests a role for the humoral immune system, e.g., antibodies to capsid proteins, as well as the cellular immune system, e.g., CTLs versus oncogenes, in the clearance of HPV infections. Neutralizing antibodies may be an effective way of preventing early viral infection and spread, but cell-mediated antiviral immune responses may mainly be important in the resolution of infection and associated disease. HPV infections induce both systemic and local humoral immune responses manifested by the presence of IgG and IgA antibodies to HPV-associated antigens. Although low levels and frequencies of anti-HPV antibodies are present in serum and CVS of apparently healthy women, women with cervical cancer present these antibodies at higher levels and frequencies.

The generation of serum-neutralizing antibody is observed in most, but not all, infected individuals and is directed against conformational epitopes on the L1 protein displayed on the outer surface of the intact virus particle. Serum-neutralizing antibody levels following natural HPV infections, even at peak titers, are low. This probably reflects the exclusively intraepithelial infectious cycle as well as the production of virus particles in the superficial ECs distant from APCs and patrolling macrophages. These factors limit antigen uptake, delivery to the lymph node, and presentation to naïve B and T cells.

Increased local levels of HPV 16 E7-specific IgG antibodies in cervicovaginal washes of women with cervical cancer indicate local inflammation, perhaps due to invasive tumor growth that results in transudation of IgG from plasma to the vaginal secretion. The majority of women with cervical HPV-16 infections generate a systemic IgG Ab response to the major HPV-16 capsid protein as detected by ELISA, using VLPs as antigens. Systemic IgA and IgG responses against HPV-16 VLP were more frequently observed in women with HPV DNA than in the controls and the presence of HPV-16 VLP-specific IgG in plasma is correlated with persistent viral infection. In contrast, systemic IgG response to HPV-16 E7, as determined by peptide-based ELISA, is correlated with viral clearance in a subset of CIN. However, the presence of serum Abs to HPV-16/18 VLP L1 as well as antigens E6 and E7 is not correlated with occurrence or prognosis of cervical cancer. Similarly, local HPV-16 VLP-specific IgA and IgG responses do not correlate with viral clearance in patients with CIN and healthy women. Rather, the mucosal HPV-16 VLP-specific IgA and IgG responses reflect current HPV infection and development of cervical lesions. Results suggest a selective downregulation of local HPV-specific IgA responses in women with cervical cancer. Gene expression profiling also indicated downregulation of genes associated with Ig synthesis including gene encoding the heavy chain of IgA2 in cervical tumor tissue as compared to that in the normal tissue of the same patient. Previously, it was also reported that the number of IgA plasma cells infiltrating invasive cervical carcinoma was altered when compared to normal cervix specimens. This was supported by data obtained from cytokine analysis. Th2-type cytokines, including IL-4, IL-5, and IL-10, that play important roles in B-cell differentiation and subsequent Ab production were not detected in the vaginal washes.

So far, several studies have reported on the local antibody response to HPV. IgA antibodies against HPV capsids from HPV 6, 11, 16, 18, 31, 33, and 35 could be demonstrated in cervical mucus from patients with cervical neoplasia and controls. In other studies, local antibodies have been detected against E2, E7, L1, and L2 of HPV 16 in cervical secretions and in CVL of patients with cervical neoplasia, patients with condylomata and women with normal cervical cytology. IgA against HPV 16 E2 was found in 49 % of cervical secretions from patients with CIN, whereas IgA against E2, E7, L1, and L2 from HPV 16 was observed in 15–32 % of secretions in healthy women. Local IgG against HPV 16 E2 was reported in 46 % of patients with CIN and in 15 % of healthy controls. A recently published study showed IgA, IgG, and S-IgA antibodies to HPV 16 capsids in cervical samples in, respectively, 11, 24, and 9 % of the subjects. IgG, IgM, IgA, and S-IgA in CVS of healthy and HPV-infected women were quantified. IgG, IgA, and S-IgA were significantly higher in CVS of HPV-infected patients with a lower S-IgA/IgA ratio compared to the control group, which suggests that HPV could be responsible for an increase in local production of nonsecretory IgA.

There are also some observations relevant to development and persistence of humoral responses to HPV. HPV-specific local antibodies are apparently induced several months after the initial HPV infection and the persistence of these antibodies is dependent on the concomitant presence of HPV. Conization of CIN lesions was shown to be followed by a gradual decline in serum and cervical mucus antibodies. Mucosal IgG and IgA also display different kinetics of appearance and persistence in the cervical mucus. IgA responses are more frequent and reflect current HPV infection, whereas IgG appears to parallel the development of cervical lesions. Moreover, local IgA responses are elicited earlier than IgG responses with rare detection of IgG in preclinical HPV infection.

Systemic as well as mucosal IgA and IgG responses to HPV-16 oncoprotein E7 in women who underwent radical hysterectomy for cervical cancer (HCC) compared to those in women who underwent loop excision for cervical dysplasia or had hysterectomy for other reasons have been also analyzed. It was demonstrated that the levels of HPV16 E7-specific IgA and IgG were relatively, but not significantly, higher in sera of patients undergoing HCC as compared to those in patients of other noncancerous groups. These results indicate that serum antibodies to oncoprotein E7 were not a specific marker for diagnosis or prognosis of cervical cancer which is in agreement with other studies on large populations. Another interesting finding in this study was that the local mucosal immune response, as determined by levels of HPV-16 oncoprotein E7-specific IgA in the genital tract of women with cervical cancer, was downregulated. The gene expression profiling also indicated downregulation of genes associated with Ig synthesis including the gene encoding the heavy chain of IgA2 in cervical tumor tissue as compared to that in the normal tissue of the same patient.

4.2.3.5 Vaccination Strategies

The role of HPV in cervical carcinogenesis and their cellular immune response have created expectations for prevention. A primary preventive strategy which also includes vaccination aims to reduce the incidence of disease and generally targets the entire population without symptoms or disease.

It is widely expected that a vaccine that would prevent HPV infection, which is mediated by antibodies at the site of infection, and restrict the spread of HPV from infected KCs, which depends on the induction of CTLs, would greatly reduce the incidence of cervical cancer and associated mortality.

Compared to developing countries, considerably lower incidences of cervical cancer are observed in Western Europe, the United States, and Japan probably due to the widely available screening in these regions. Screening methods comprise the conventional Papanicolaou test, liquid cytology, and HPV DNA testing.

Unfortunately, no trials have shown reduction of cancer incidence in populations where HPV testing was added to cytologic screening and, currently, despite all the screening and treatment facilities, the incidence of invasive cervical cancer remains stable or even increases.

Two types of HPV vaccine have been or are currently under development:

- First, there are therapeutic vaccines which induce cellular immunity targeted against ECs infected with HPV and induce regression of precancerous lesions or remission of advanced cervical cancer.

- Second, there are prophylactic vaccines inducing virus-neutralizing antibodies protecting against new but not against established infections. The prophylactic vaccines are focused on the generation of neutralizing antibodies against L1 and in a lesser extent on L2. In therapeutic chimeric vaccines, the targets are E6 and E7, which have no shared epitopes with human cellular proteins; therefore, the risk of inducing an autoimmune response is theoretically eliminated.

4.2.3.5.1 Prophylactic Vaccines

Decades of investigation and immunological research have led to the development of two prophylactic vaccines in 2007. Although these investigations are milestones regarding the HPV infection and probably also cervical carcinogenesis, there are still several unresolved issues. Additionally the development of these vaccines represents itself several novel and important aspects in this search of vaccination strategies against infectious agents. Therefore, the major novelties are being discussed in this section to elucidate and enlighten further research.

Most viral vaccines are based on an attenuated form of the virus. But the development of an attenuated HPV vaccine is not possible, as there is no effective culture system. Secondly, such a vaccine would be ethically unacceptable, because it would expose healthy subjects to potentially harmful viral oncogenes. The observation that the major papillomavirus capsid protein L1 has the intrinsic ability to self-assemble into VLPs when expressed in specific expression vector systems in the absence of other gene products has provided a major technical advance in the field.

VLPs contain empty virus capsids containing the major HPV capsid antigen and, possibly, the minor capsid antigens but lack viral DNA. Therefore, they mimic the natural structure of the virion and are immunogenic but not harmful as they do not contain the viral genome. VLPs were found to bind very well to human and mouse immune cells that expressed markers of APCs such as MHC class II, CD80, and CD86, including DCs, macrophages, and B cells. DCs were found to internalize and present VLP-derived antigens to CD4+ and CD8+ T cells in vitro, suggesting that DCs initiate immune responses to the VLP in vivo. Both monocyte-derived DCs and plasmacytoid DCs bind and acquire papillomavirus VLP, but only monocyte-derived DCs undergo phenotypic activation after exposure to the VLP and induce primary T-cell responses. Together with the observation that cutaneous LCs are not activated by papillomavirus VLP, these findings underscore the heterogeneity of DC populations and strongly suggest that monocyte-derived DCs are the principal cells in the T-cell response to VLP observed in individuals vaccinated with VLP. However, HPV16 VLP induced plasmacytoid DCs to secrete IFN-α and IL-6, both cytokines that play a role in the generation of antibody responses, as well as TNF-α and IL-8.

In several animal papillomavirus models, the parental injection of VLPs elicited high titres of type-specific neutralizing antibodies and subsequent protection against virus challenge which made L1 VLPs clear candidate immunogens for prophylactic vaccination in humans. Other studies have shown oral, intranasal, or intravaginal vaccination to be more effective in inducing mucosal immunity and also in producing serum IgG antibodies of higher affinity than parental vaccination routes.

The vaccines are generally well tolerated and highly immunogenic. Current clinical data indicate that prophylactic vaccines are very effective against new persistent infections and the development of cervical intraepithelial lesions. The protection is type specific although some cross-reaction has been reported. Overall, the vaccines show a good safety profile and an almost universal induction of high titers of virus-specific antibody by VLP-based vaccines. Further follow-up is needed to see whether the high levels of virus-specific antibody induced by VLP-based vaccines remain after decades or whether booster vaccination is needed.

4.2.3.5.2 Arising Problems in HPV Vaccine Development

Some further problems should be briefly discussed here. Levels of specific antibodies in the human female genital tract are likely to be an important determinant of vaccine efficacy. All examined participants developed detectable titers of anti-HPV16 VLP IgGs in their cervical secretions after immunization; however, cervical titers of specific IgG and total IgGs and IgAs among participants in the contraceptive group were relatively constant throughout the contraceptive cycle. In contrast, the cervical titers of specific IgG and total IgGs and IgAs among participants in the ovulatory group varied during the menstrual cycle, being highest during the proliferative phase and decreasing approximately ninefold around ovulation.

Another consideration is the preferred delivery route for vaccine administration in order to induce effective mucosal immune responses. The vaccination should induce a local mucosal immunity in the form of S-IgA in the lower genital tract in addition to systemic immunity to adequately prevent HPV infection. Mucosal antibodies are induced by systemic delivery of VLPs. Obviously, a single dose with mucosal delivery would be the preferred route for vaccine delivery; if nasal or oral delivery can induce antibodies still has to be further investigated.

Interestingly, different vaccination schemes were evaluated: escalating doses of HPV16L1 VLPs via nasal nebulization, bronchial aerosolization, or a combination of intramuscular and aerosol vaccination. The alternative routes of vaccination were well tolerated and many of the volunteers who received aerosol vaccinations exhibited serum antibody titers that were comparable to those induced by intramuscular vaccination. A mucosal immune response was induced by aerosol vaccination as demonstrated by the induction of anti-HPV16 VLP IgA-secreting cells in PBMC and S-IgA in secretions.

The choice and the number of HPV types included in the vaccine is an important issue as there are geographic differences in the prevalence of HPV types involved in CIN and cancer. In order to be effective for at least 80 % of the population, the vaccines should theoretically consist of VLPs of the four or five most common types of HPV of that country or region but combining multiple types in one vaccine may be problematic. A pentavalent vaccine with VLPs of HPV types 16, 18, 45, 31, and 33 would potentially prevent 83 % of all cervical carcinomas, whereas a heptavalent vaccine that also included types 52 and 58 could potentially prevent 87 % of the overall cervical cancer burden internationally. Whether such a polyvalent vaccine would result in immunological equivalence such that each component virus-like particle induces an antibody response that correlates with protection is unclear.

Finally, all trials to date of HPV vaccines have enrolled women, but genital HPV infections are mainly sexually transmitted and men will also need to be vaccinated if the whole population is to develop immunity. In infected patients, targeting already infected basal cells that do not express capsid antigens remains a major challenge. Therefore, chimeric VLP vaccines are being developed which contain not only structural viral L1 or L2 proteins but also functional E-proteins. In preclinical data, these chimeric VLP vaccines elicited both neutralizing antibodies to the VLP and T-cell responses to L1 and E7 and could therefore be prophylactic and therapeutic.

4.2.3.5.3 Therapeutic Vaccines

Therapeutic vaccines for HPV are at a much earlier stage of development than their prophylactic counterparts. In contrast to preventive vaccines, HPV therapeutic vaccines would need to include some antigenic determinants derived from the early HPV proteins as E6 or E7 rather than the late proteins that VLPs use to self-assemble. For therapeutic vaccines L1/L2 would be a poor target because of its restricted expression in patients already having cervical neoplasia, whereas both E6 and E7 proteins are continuously expressed in cervical lesions and tumors. This has proved to be a much more challenging task in terms of biodelivery and response.

E7 is probably the best studied; it induces protective cellular immunity against cervical dysplasia and prevents tumor growth in animal models. Anti-E7 antibodies have been correlated with more advanced stage of disease and worse prognosis, but do not seem to denote an effective host immune response against cervical cancer. Indeed, it seems that immune responses in patients with cervical cancer are marginal and functionally ineffective, making this a less attractive group for immunomanipulative strategies. Given that E6 and E7 expression increases as the HPV infection progresses in establishing a dysplastic process, they seem ideal targets for immune attack. Therapeutic vaccines consisting of E6 and/or E7 have been tested in patients and have proven to be safe and effective against benign warts; however, they have had limited therapeutic effect so far in cases of cervical cancer.

In general, there are several broad categories of therapeutic vaccine strategies: chimeric VLPs, peptides, proteins, nucleic acid-based, and cell-based. The major challenge in infected patients remains the targeting of already infected basal cells that do not express capsid antigens. Therefore, chimeric VLP vaccines with structural viral L1 or L2 proteins and functional E proteins are being developed. In preclinical data, these chimeric VLP vaccines elicited both neutralizing antibodies to the VLP and T-cell responses to L1 and E7. Chimeric VLPs comprised of a fusion of HPV16 E7 to the L1 or L2 capsid proteins have been shown to initiate a potent E7-specific CTL response in vaccinated mice. The vaccine was found to be sufficient to protect mice against challenge with an E7-containing tumor cell line. This vaccine's high immunogenicity is a result of the interaction of chimeric VLPs with potent APCs residing at or near the vaccination site which are able to induce an efficient antigen-specific immune response after interaction with naïve CD8+ T cells. These vaccines could therefore be prophylactic and therapeutic and would eliminate any breakthrough infection that escaped antibody neutralization.

On the results of a randomized, double-blind, placebo-controlled, clinical trial with HPV16/E7 chimeric VLPs, HPV DNA was cleared in vaccinated individuals and placebo group although there were more responders in the vaccine group. Serum IgG to HPV16 L1 developed in all who were vaccinated but not in placebo recipients whereas only some vaccinated subjects showed CTLs. Antibody responses and CTL generation, however, did not correlate with clinical outcome. Chimeric capsomeres may be more stable and less expensive than chimeric VLPs and HPV16 L1/E7 capsomeres were immunogenic, generating both anti-L1 antibody and E7-specific CTLs in mice. In another study, DCs and LCs are activated by three different therapeutic vaccination strategies including heterologous papillomavirus VLPs and HPV VLP immune complexes. DCs and LCs incubated with these VLP upregulated surface activation markers and increased secretion of IL-12 p70 and IL-15. The activated cells are then able to initiate an immune response against chimeric VLP-derived antigens. Other therapeutic vaccination strategies based on using heterologous chimeric VLP or chimeric HPV VLP immune complexes may be more effective in generating an immune response against HPV-induced diseases such as cervical cancer.

Only a few animal studies and preliminary clinical trials have been performed with either peptide-based or protein HPV vaccines, so it is too early to reach conclusions on whether they are a viable alternative. In animal models, CTLs can be generated using E6 and E7 peptide-based vaccines that are protective against subsequent challenge with lethal doses of E6- and E7-containing tumors. Stimulation of peripheral blood lymphocytes from patients with HPV16-positive cervical cancer with synthetic HPV-16 E7 peptide generates specific CTLs capable of tumor recognition and lysis of cervical cancer cells. A clinical trial using a peptide-based vaccine was performed on 18 patients with high-grade dysplasia. Ten of 16 subjects mounted primary CTL responses to the E7 peptides, and a complete clinical response was observed in three subjects.

Protein-based vaccinations have been used in early-phase clinical trials. A randomized, placebo-controlled phase I study with E6/E7 fusion protein plus adjuvant was tested in women with CIN. Antibody and CD8+ T-cell responses were significantly greater in immunized subjects than in placebo recipients.

Various attempts are currently in progress to develop DNA vaccines, which tend to be more effective in the generation of both humoral and cellular protective immunity responses. DNA vaccines usually involve intramuscular injection of plasmid DNA or DNA delivery into the epidermis via a gene gun. Polynucleotide and recombinant viral vaccines encoding nonstructural viral proteins show therapeutic efficacy in animal models and are candidate immunotherapies for established low-grade benign genital infections. Immunization of rabbits with the nonstructural viral proteins E1 and E2 induced a CD4+ T-cell response; fewer papillomas developed and they regressed more rapidly than those in non-vaccinated animals. The canine oral papillomavirus (COPV) model has provided evidence that immunization with codon-modified early proteins will be effective in preventing the development of lesions postexposure to virus. Animals challenged orally with COPV and immunized subsequently with a COPV E2 polynucleotide vaccine remained free of oral warts. Immunization of rabbits with established papillomas with an E1, E2, E6, and E7 gene cocktail reduced the development of carcinoma by 75 % and suppressed papilloma growth substantially. In high-grade intraepithelial lesions, there are only two possible antigenic targets, E6 and E7. Tolerance to viral antigens, modulation of the cytokine milieu, and downregulation of MHC class I alleles on the neoplastic KCs are associated with progressive CIN and possibly invasive cancer, which pose strong barriers for immunotherapies. It is possible and also supported by a few studies that there is a spectrum of responses to therapeutic vaccination ranging from complete through partial up to no regression of the clinical disease. For example, studies with a recombinant vaccinia virus encoding modified E6/E7 genes of HPV 16 and 18 in patients with high-grade vulval intraepithelial neoplasia showed complete clearance in less than 10 % of the patients, partial regression in at least 50 %, and no clinical change in 10–30 %. Lesion regression did not correlate with T-cell responses in all cases. This method for delivering antigenicity using a DNA vaccine involves the use of viral vectors as delivery carriers into the body.

Vaccines designed to elicit CTLs specific for the HPV oncoproteins E6 and E7 show immunogenicity and inhibition of tumor growth in transplantable tumor models in rodents. However, human HPV-induced CTLs tumors have been largely refractory to the approaches successful in rodents. All the vaccines tested have been safe and well tolerated and have induced T-cell responses which did not necessarily correlate with clinical responses.

A previous trial with a L1 DNA vaccine evidenced only weak immune responses to HPV. Recently, a modified version DNA vaccine targeting HPV6 L1 and L1-E7 was constructed and tested to determine if this DNA vaccine would elicit an immune response in mice.

In summary, other potential delivery systems for HPV immunogens besides recombinant viral vectors include recombinant bacterial vectors such as Listeria monocytogenes, viral DNA, proteins, and peptides alone or tagged to immune adjuvants such as CpG oligonucleotide and DCs; some of these experimental strategies have already even been tested clinically with promising results. An overview of the different strategies with candidate biologics for HPV vaccines is shown in Table 4.9. Despite the current enthusiasm about the future prospects of preventive HPV vaccines, limitations concerning restricted coverage to only a few HPV types, expenses, and potential barriers to wide availability and acceptability in both developed and developing countries and the potential epidemiological shift of HPV disease to currently less frequent types and variants have to be taken into consideration.

4.3   Bacterial Infections of the Genital Tract

4.3.1   Gonorrhea

Gonorrhea, a bacterial STD, is caused by *Neisseria gonorrhoeae*, a gram-negative diplococcus. It is an exclusive human pathogen that primarily infects the urogenital epithelia but can

Table 4.9 Different strategies with candidate biologics for HPV vaccines

Virus-like particles (L1 based)	Prophylactic
Chimeric virus-like particles (both late and early proteins expressed)	Prophylactic/therapeutic
Viral DNA	Therapeutic
Fusion proteins	Therapeutic
Recombinant viral vectors	Therapeutic
Recombinant bacterial vectors	Therapeutic
Peptides (alone or with adjuvants such as CpG oligodeoxynucleotide)	Therapeutic
Dendritic cells	Therapeutic

Adapted from Padilla-Paz LA. Human papillomavirus vaccine: history, immunology, current status, and future prospects. Clin Obstet Gynecol. 2005;48:226–40; Steller MA. Cervical cancer vaccines: progress and prospects. J Soc Gynecol Investig. 2002;9:254–264

also lead to infection of other EC surfaces. Gonococcal infection, with over 60 million cases, is a major global health problem with the highest incidences in less developed countries. However, more than 300,000 cases are reported to the Centers for Disease Control and Prevention in the United States each year, and an estimated 600,000 people are infected. Teenagers and young adults are at high risk for infection, which is unsettling in view of the increased risk associated with gonorrhea for infection with HIV-1.

Gonococcal infections usually remain localized to the site of primary infection in men. In contrast to the inflammatory response generated predominately with gonococcal infection of the male urethra, 50–80 % of women with lower genital tract *N. gonorrhoeae* infection are asymptomatic. However, despite the tendency of gonococcal cervicitis to remain asymptomatic, it subsequently tends to spread to the upper genital tract, inducing chronic complications. Ascending infection occurs in up to 45 % of infected women and can result in pelvic inflammatory disease (PID) which can cause infertility and ectopic pregnancies due to fallopian tube blockage. Repeated infections are rather common, which suggests antigenic variations in the organisms or an ineffective immune response to infection. Furthermore, the gonococcus-induced increase in the local expression of viral RNA together with the loss of mucosal integrity due to an acute inflammatory response is associated with increased susceptibility to HIV-1 infection. Despite the presence of effective antibiotic treatment, these health concerns demand the need for further investigation on the mechanisms of the infection in order to develop a vaccine against gonorrhea.

4.3.1.1 Mechanisms of *N. gonorrhoeae* to Evade the Immune Response
4.3.1.1.1 Virulence Factors
Only recently, it has been shown that *N. gonorrhoeae* can invade mucosal ECs and are intracellular during human infection. A repertoire of virulence factors have been identified and allow this bacterium to successfully adapt to variable microenvironments within its sole human host and are thought to play a role in EC invasion. These virulence factors are responsible for gonococcal evasion of the immune system. These factors consist of outer membrane constituents such as porin, pili, opacity-associated outer membrane proteins (Opa), reduction modifiable protein (Rmp), and lipooligosaccharides (LOS).

Pili seem to modulate host cell signaling mechanisms to aid gonococcal epithelial invasion and participate in forming an initial attachment with host cells. They may also provide a mechanism by which nonmotile gonococci are able to colonize and to ascend mucosal surfaces through their ability to exhibit twitching motility. The transmembrane protein CD46 involved in regulation of complement activation has been demonstrated to serve as a receptor for gonococcal pilus in human cells.

Opa proteins are thought to contribute to the cellular tropisms exhibited by gonococci and are divided into two classes based on their ability to differentially recognize host cell surface molecules. Opa50 recognize host cell heparin sulfate proteoglycans and Opa52 recognize carcinoembryonic antigen-related family of cell adhesion molecules (CEACAM or CD66).

LOS play a role in attachment of the pathogen to epithelial tissues and are a target for bactericidal antibodies found in normal human serum. Variations of LOS molecule structure in the outer membrane of *N. gonorrhoeae* are observed within and between strains which results in constant antigenic variation. This spontaneous conversion of oligosaccharide determinants can change the manner in which the gonococcus associates with host tissues and, hence, can potentially alter the course of gonococcal disease.

Porin, a water-filled channel through which small molecules traverse the gonococcal outer membrane, is thought to play multiple roles in potentiating disease caused by *N. gonorrhoeae*. Porin molecules trigger variable functional responses within host cells depending upon the particular porin and the host cell type under study. A unique feature of gonococcal porin is its ability to translocate into eukaryotic cell membranes and form a voltage-gated channel. By demonstrating the ability of porin to induce apoptosis in ECs, it is proposed that porin plays a role in the cytotoxicity observed in fallopian tube organ culture and in the shedding of ECs which occurs in vivo during mucosal infection. In contrast, gonococcal infection of primary human male urethral ECs results in antiapoptotic events. It is hypothesized that the enhanced survival of the urethral EC may allow the bacterium to proliferate within an intracellular, protective environment and, consequently, promote gonococcal colonization. Porin may also facilitate the cytoskeletal rearrangements required for actin-mediated entry of the gonococcus into its target host cell.

These virulence factors together with the high heterogeneity and adaptability with repeated phase and antigenic change may be a way to downregulate the functional immune response of the host. Pathogens use at least two basic strategies to survive the host's immune response. Some avoid provoking specific host defenses and others induce immune responses but possess the ability to evade the consequences. The high rate of reinfection despite the presence of anti-gonococcal antibodies leads to the assumption

that *N. gonorrhoeae* evades the host's immune response. Indeed, *N. gonorrhoeae* possess several mechanisms which could potentially thwart the effects of immune responses directed toward this organism in vivo, including hypervariation of surface antigens, resistance to complement-mediated bacteriolysis, and the production of IgA1 protease.

4.3.1.1.2 Resistance to Complement-Mediated Bacteriolysis

Gonococci possess several potential mechanisms to avoid complement-mediated bacteriolysis, including sialylation of LOS, induction of blocking antibody to Rmp, and binding of complement downregulating proteins such as C4bp to particular porin domains. However, it seems unlikely that complement-mediated, IgG-dependent bacteriolysis operates at mucosal surfaces, where a fully functional complement system is not usually present and IgA may interfere with complement activation. Both IgA and IgG in genital secretions have been shown to inhibit adherence of gonococci to ECs.

4.3.1.1.3 IgA1 Protease

Vaginal washes from patients infected with *N. gonorrhoeae* have been found to contain IgA1 protease activity demonstrable in vitro and were able to cleave exogenous IgA1 in a manner suggestive of IgA1 protease activity. However, despite the presence of substrate, and contrary to expectations, some studies have failed not to detect any evidence of IgA1 cleavage fragments by gonococcal IgA1 protease in cervical mucus or vaginal wash samples. Nevertheless, all of the clinical isolates of *N. gonorrhoeae* infecting these patients produced IgA1 protease in vitro.

These apparently contradictory results may be explained by two linked hypotheses. First, *N. gonorrhoeae* may not be present in the lumen or on the mucosal surface in sufficiently high numbers but rather may colonize a subepithelial niche. This hypothesis is supported by the lack of significant local immune or cytokine responses in women infected with *N. gonorrhoeae*. Therefore, the lack of detectable IgA1 protease activity in cervical mucus, in addition to the lack of local host responses, may simply be due to small numbers of bacteria at that site. Secondly, *N. gonorrhoeae* may require IgA1 protease for survival within, as well as outside, the host tissues. In addition, there is evidence that the lysosomal–phagosomal protein LAMP-1 on ECs is cleaved by neisserial IgA1 protease. Growth of gonococci within ECs was enhanced by cleavage of LAMP-1, which may contribute to intracellular gonococcal survival and facilitate escape from antibodies and complement.

4.3.1.1.4 Differences in Gonococcal Infection in Males and Females

Interestingly, there are important differences between gonococcal genital infection in men and women and *N. gonorrhoeae* has evolved variable pathogenic mechanisms to ensure its survival in the distinctly different microenvironments found within the male and female (uro)genital tracts. In male urethral epithelium, the interaction of gonococcal LOS with the asialoglycoprotein receptor present on the urethral EC mediates invasion and results in production of the cytokines IL-1, IL-6, IL-8, and TNF-α. Cytokine release contributes to the usually symptomatic nature of gonococcal disease in men and is accompanied by a large influx of PMNs, which in turn contribute to the observed cytokine release and inflammation. The interaction of gonococci with PMNs is mediated by the interaction of Opa gonococcal proteins and CEACAM host cell proteins. The specific interactions occurring between these two families of proteins may dictate specific host cellular responses and the survival or death of phagocytosed gonococci. The PMN response to gonococci is further modulated by gonococcal porin, which inhibits PMN degranulation and the production and release of toxic oxidants from the host cell to the extracellular milieu. Transmission of gonococci to a sexual partner is then partly aided by the ability of gonococci to bind to human sperm which also were found to express asialoglycoprotein receptor.

In contrast to the inflammatory response generated predominately with gonococcal infection of the male urethra, 50–80 % of women with lower genital tract *N. gonorrhoeae* infection are asymptomatic, and 70–90 % of women with disseminated infection lack signs of genital tract involvement. The clinical findings that there is neither an antibody response nor elevated local cytokine levels in women with gonococcal infection are consistent with the ability of the gonococcus to evade and subvert host immune function. Cervical epithelia provide a source of alternative pathway complement activity, yet, at a level comparable to only approximately 10 % of that observed for human serum. Within minutes of infection of primary cervical ECs, complement protein C3b is deposited on the lipid A portion of gonococcal LOS and is rapidly inactivated to iC3b. This is supported by the predominance of iC3b in comparison to C3b on the surface of clinically isolated gonococci. Analysis of clinical biopsies obtained from women with culture-documented gonococcal cervicitis and infection studies performed with primary human cervical ECs indicate that complement receptor 3 (CR3) on female genital epithelia serves as the primary receptor for *N. gonorrhoeae* adherence to and invasion of the ectocervix and endocervix. Binding of gonococcal pilus to the I domain of CR3 probably allows the gonococcus to overcome the electrostatic repulsion between its own cell surface and that of the cervical cell and may juxtapose the gonococcus at the cervical cell surface, where complement concentrations would be expected to allow efficient opsonization for the subsequent intimate adherence of iC3b, i.e., converted C3b, and gonococcal porin to the I domain. Binding of the gonococcus to CR3 requires the cooperative action of iC3b bound to the gonococcal surface in conjunction with gonococcal porin and pilus. This ligand binding to the I domain of CR3, however, does not invoke a proinflammatory response in professional phagocytic cells, and cellular fate of gonococci is not clear. Interestingly, menses is associated with an increased risk to women for PID and for disseminated infection. C3 production by the cervical epithelium exhibits cyclic variability, and the highest levels of C3 are detected during menses. Additionally, a correlation can be made between the presence or the absence of Opa and the site of gonococcal infection. Opa- gonococci are predominate within the fallopian tubes and in the cervix at the time of menses while Opa + gonococci are found predominately within the male urethra and within the cervix at the time of ovulation. Ascent to the upper female genital tract might be facilitated through the ability of gonococci to exhibit twitching motility, in conjunction with hormonal changes which influence the mucosal epithelium and the expression of complement and molecules serving as gonococcal receptors within the female genital tract. Microscopic analysis of tissue biopsies indicates that the expression of CR3 progressively decreases in an ascending manner from the ectocervix to the fallopian tubes. But expression of the lutropin receptor (LHr) which might serve as gonococcal receptor in upper genital tract epithelia increases in an ascending manner to fallopian tubes with highest levels at menses. The presence of LHr on the human uterus, placenta, decidua, and fetal membranes may partly contribute to the fact that the increased risk of spontaneous abortion associated with *N. gonorrhoeae* infection is due to a gonococcus-LHr interaction occurring on deciduas and placental membranes.

4.3.1.2 Immune Responses to Gonococcal Infection

4.3.1.2.1 Immunoglobulins

Early studies using enzyme immunoassay determined the presence of IgM, IgA, and IgG antibodies to gonococcal pili antigens in serum. In all Ig classes, a significantly higher mean antibody activity and a higher percentage of positive sera were found in men and women with *N. gonorrhoeae* than in controls. The magnitude of antibody response was higher among infected women than men, especially in the IgM class. Another study found serum and local IgG and IgA to be produced against several antigens during gonococcal infection, although the quantity of antibody was greater in serum.

As mentioned earlier, preliminary evidence indicated, however, that while antigonococcal antibodies were detected in infected patients, the levels of both serum and antigonococcal antibodies in genital secretions were surprisingly low. A follow-up study measured the concentrations of total IgA1, IgA2, IgG, and IgM in cervical mucus, vaginal wash, and serum samples from volunteers without demonstrable infection, from volunteers in whom only *N. gonorrhoeae* was detected, and from volunteers infected with other pathogens (*C. trachomatis* or *T. vaginalis*) with or without *N. gonorrhoeae*. There were no differences between the concentrations of total IgA1, IgA2, IgG, and IgM in genital tract secretions in patients with different STDs compared with noninfected women. Moreover, levels of IgA1, IgA2, IgG, and IgM antibodies specific for *N. gonorrhoeae* MS11, a widely studied gonococcal strain, in female mucosal secretions and serum were found at low levels in both uninfected and infected women. IgA1 antibody levels in serum, but not in secretions, were higher in female patients infected with *N. gonorrhoeae* than in noninfected patients while the levels of IgG and IgM antibodies in serum and secretions were not different between gonococcus-infected and noninfected patients.

A history of previous infections with *N. gonorrhoeae* did not alter the antibody levels in patients with a current infection except for arising levels of serum IgA1 antibody. These results further support the possibility that repeated infections with *N. gonorrhoeae* are common because there is little development of immune memory and therefore only minimal levels of protective immunity. One potential explanation for the paucity of antibody responses to *N. gonorrhoeae* in uncomplicated genital tract infections may be related to the absence of organized mucosaassociated lymphoid tissue, such as the Peyer's patches of the small intestine, which are recognized as major sites for the uptake and processing of antigens leading to generalized disseminated mucosal immune responses as described earlier. Although in some studies local vaginal antibody responses were recorded, intravaginal immunization in humans appeared to be inefficient in inducing either circulating or generalized mucosal antibody responses compared to oral or nasal immunization. In contrast to the genital tract, the rectum contains lymphoid follicles resembling Peyer's patches that likely serve as an inductive site of the common mucosal immune system. In addition, it has been suggested that these sites may preferentially supply specific antibody-secreting cell precursors to the adjacent genital tract which shares the same lymphoid drainage. Therefore, it seemed likely that persons infected at both the rectum and genital sites might be expected to display enhanced antibody responses to the infecting organism, both in the genital tract and perhaps also in remote secretions. Due to the prevalence of rectal infections with *N. gonorrhoeae*, it was examined whether more pronounced antigonococcal antibody responses were generated by gonococcal infection at a site known to contain organized inductive lymphoid tissue.

There was a small effect of rectal infection on the levels of isolate specific IgG in cervical mucus, but overall only little difference in antibody levels in patients with cervical compared with cervical and rectal infections was found, suggesting that rectal infection was no more efficient than the genital tract infection for inducing humoral responses to *N. gonorrhoeae*. Moreover, *N. gonorrhoeae* via its Opa protein has the ability to suppress antibody production by killing CEACAM1-expressing B cells.

4.3.1.2.2 Cytokines

This relative paucity of antibody response provokes the question as to whether there is a cytokine response to gonococcal infection as is seen in female urinary tract infection and experimentally infected men. Therefore, the levels of IL-1, IL-6, IL-8, IL-10, and TGF-β in sera and genital tract secretions from women with gonococcal cervicitis and other genital infections were examined. Surprisingly, the local levels of all these cytokines in genital secretions were not elevated in women with gonococcal cervicitis compared with levels of uninfected persons. In contrast, serum IL-6 levels, but not IL-8 and IL-1 levels, were significantly elevated in gonococcus-infected women. Serum, but not local, IL-1 and IL-6 levels were elevated in patients concomitantly infected with *Trichomonas vaginalis* or *Chlamydia trachomatis* in addition to *N. gonorrhoeae* compared with levels in patients infected with any single organism.

However, increased IL-1, IL-6, and IL-8 expression with immortalized vaginal, endocervical, and ectocervical epithelia was demonstrated.

Experiments with whole gonococcal lysates revealed that the IL-8 and IL-6 response of cervical and vaginal ECs was not restricted to the interactions with viable gonococci. Similarly, viable *N. gonorrhoeae* is not essential for a proinflammatory response by innate immune cells, since mature human macrophages generate an array of cytokines and chemokines in response to purified gonococcal surface antigens. These findings suggest that gonococcal components can stimulate proinflammatory responses, which are independent of gonococcal metabolic activity, i.e., viability or entry into the host cells.

4.3.1.2.3 T Lymphocytes

Gonorrhea typically correlates with a transient reduction in T-cell counts in blood, and these populations recover when gonococcal infection is resolved. Opa proteins have been shown to bind CEACAM1 expressed by primary CD4+ T cells and suppress their activation and proliferation.

On the basis of the absence of cytokines and the low levels of antigonococcal antibody detected during uncomplicated cervical infections by *N. gonorrhoeae*, it is proposed that in addition to their ability to evade the consequences of immune responses, gonococci fail to either induce or possibly actively suppress the host's immune and inflammatory responses.

4.3.1.3 Development of Vaccines

The production of an effective vaccine against *N. gonorrhoeae* should be an important goal, also due to increasing antibiotic resistance, but there is still minimal success despite a long list of potential candidate proteins. As *N. gonorrhoeae* is an obligate human pathogen, the development of a vaccine has been hampered by the unavailability of a convenient and simple animal model. Attempts to infect or colonize the genital tracts of different animal species have been unsuccessful. Certain vaccines have been evaluated in human males, but earlier prototype gonococcal vaccines have shown limited or no protection against reinfection with *N. gonorrhoeae* despite the generation of serum antibody responses against the vaccine antigens. A trial with gonococcal pilus vaccine, which has been shown to be safe as well as antigenic and resulted in the production of specific antibodies, failed to protect men. A second vaccine consisted of porin protein as a systemic immune response to porin protein was shown after endocervical and urethral infection. This vaccine failed to provide protection but it was later recognized that the vaccine was contaminated with Rmp. Rmp leads to production of blocking antibodies capable of preventing the function of bactericidal antibodies against porin. This suggests that vaccination endeavors should therefore be directed toward exploiting novel concepts and strategies of mucosal or systemic immunizations. Examples include nasal immunization, which has been shown to generate antibody responses in genital secretions and which has been studied to determine if it could elicit an immune response capable of preventing vaginal colonization of gonococci in a mouse model. Bacterial clearance was significantly faster for mice immunized intranasally with gonococcal outer membrane preparations than control mice. The development of systemic and local vaginal antibodies directed mainly against a number of these outer membrane proteins was induced. Intranasal immunization in mice with gonococcal transferring binding receptor proteins showed promise owing to the induction of local and systemic antigen-specific IgA and IgG antibodies, which is also consistent with the earlier trials in the mouse model. An improved mouse model of gonococcal female genital tract infection was developed, which will facilitate testing of topical microbicides and experimental vaccines for mucosal gonococcal infection.

4.3.2 *Chlamydia trachomatis*

Chlamydia trachomatis is one of three major species within the genus *Chlamydia* and an etiological agent for several common genital tract syndromes such as urethritis, cervicitis, and PID in women as well as urethritis and epididymitis in men. Genital tract infection with *C. trachomatis* is often chronic and is associated with few symptoms and a scant inflammatory exudate.

Despite continuous improvement of screening and treatment programs, approximately 4 million new genital chlamydial infections occur

per year. It is the most common bacterial STD in the United States. There are about 90 million new cases per year worldwide and it is a major health problem. The prevalence rates for chlamydial infection among sexually active individuals range from 3 to 25 %. The highest rates of chlamydial infection occur among adolescent women who are also at the greatest risk to develop complications arising from untreated infection.

C. trachomatis is an obligate intracellular bacterium, and, therefore, efficient antimicrobial therapeutics have to achieve adequate intracellular concentrations. Most patients are free from infections after a 2- or 3-week treatment with tetracyclines or macrolides. However, approximately 70 % of initial chlamydial infections remain asymptomatic, which results in the lack of seeking medical help and in further spreading of the disease. *Chlamydia* specifically infects ECs in the reproductive tract where the organism ascends from the cervix to the fallopian tubes. The lack of antibiotic treatment and the ability of *Chlamydia* to evade immune defense mechanisms results in persistent fallopian tube infection. An ongoing infection eventually leads to scar formation and occlusion of the fallopian tubes which consequently results in pregnancy loss, infertility, or ectopic pregnancy.

In order to fully appreciate the development of a local immune response against *Chlamydia*, it is important to understand its life cycle with respect to host–parasite interactions. Chlamydiae have a unique developmental cycle among obligate intracellular bacteria that involves two distinct morphological forms called the elementary body (EB) and the reticulate body (RB). Protective immunity might include responses directed at EB, such as neutralizing antibody, or at infected cells, such as CTLs or ADCC. The infectious but metabolically inactive EB particle enters host cells by first binding to a number of proposed ligands on *Chlamydia*, which induces the internalization of the pathogen. EBs are finally differentiated to RBs within the cell and start replication. After the developmental cycle is completed after 40–72 h, RBs differentiate back into infectious EBs which are released from the host cell and infect neighboring cells. The most common cellular host in the reproductive tract is the superficial columnar EC.

With the exception of *Chlamydia* serovar L which causes lymphogranuloma venereum, infections are mainly local. *Chlamydia* exits the apical end of the EC preventing the spread of infection to cells underlying the basement membrane. Currently there have been detected 18 serovars of *C. trachomatis* based on immunoepitope analysis using monoclonal antibodies directed against the major outer membrane protein (MOMP) of chlamydiae. Most efforts at elucidating the pathophysiology of chlamydial infections have focused on two protein antigens. The first is MOMP which is almost certainly involved in the earliest interactions of this organism with leukocytes during the course of natural infection. MOMP, an immunodominant molecule, constitutes almost 60 % of the outer membrane protein of *C. trachomatis* and appears to evoke a protective humoral response to infection. A second protein produced by *C. trachomatis* is the 60 kDa heat shock protein (hsp-60), which induces proinflammatory immune system activation.

Despite progress in the past decade, the current understanding of mucosal immunity to this pathogen in the human host remains limited. Most of our current knowledge comes from studies in women or female animal models.

4.3.2.1 Early Cell-Mediated Immune Response to Chlamydia

The immune-mediated eradication of chlamydiae from the genital mucosa appears to occur in two distinct phases and most likely by different mechanisms.

4.3.2.1.1 Neutrophils

One early mechanism that appears to reduce the number of organisms soon after infection is an influx of neutrophils. Shortly after the vaginal inoculation of guinea pigs with *Chlamydia*, neutrophils were found in the uterine horns and oviducts. In vitro experiments have shown that neutrophils have the capability to destroy chlamydiae. Also in mice that were depleted of neutrophils by antibody treatment, the number of organisms isolated from the genital tract were approximately tenfold greater the day after infec-

tion. In addition, a greater number of mice that were depleted of neutrophils were culture positive during the first week of infection compared to controls. However, neutrophils were not critical for eradication of chlamydiae since all mice were able to resolve the infection within the same time frame. Thus, neutrophils appear to play a role in reducing the initial amplification of *C. trachomatis* and possibly limit the spread locally within the genital tract.

4.3.2.1.2 NK Cells

NK cells also seem to play an important role in the initial control of chlamydial infection as they not only are responsible for the production of IFN-γ early in the course of chlamydial genital tract infection but are also, via IFN-γ, a significant factor in the development of the Th1 CD4+ response and in the control of the infection. Mononuclear cells isolated from the genital tract of infected mice demonstrated YAC cell cytotoxicity in vitro, which is a measure of NK cell function. This response peaked as early as 3 days after vaginal inoculation. Although the antibody-induced depletion of NK cells in mice did not reduce the number of pathogens isolated from the genital tract within the first week after infection, continued depletion throughout the course of infection resulted in delayed clearance of chlamydiae.

In experiments performed by the enzyme-linked immunospot assay, high numbers of cells producing IFN-γ were found in the genital tract, concomitant with resolution of the infection; however, in addition, an increase in IFN-γ-producing cells which were CD4-negative was seen early in the infection. Both IL-12 and IL-18, which synergize to stimulate NK cells to produce IFN-γ, are produced following the infection of DCs and ECs by live *C. trachomatis*.

4.3.2.1.3 Dendritic Cells

The recruitment of cells with a DC phenotype was demonstrated in the genital tract during *Chlamydia* infection of mice. These cells expressed the costimulatory molecules CD86 and CD40 and stimulated allogeneic T cells, suggesting that these mononuclear cells are a population of APCs and that they may play a role in clearing antigen and protecting against inflammatory disease.

4.3.2.2 Specific Immune Response to Chlamydial Infection

Knowledge of the processes that influence the induction of an acquired immune response against *Chlamydia* within the genital mucosa is still limited. Although *C. trachomatis* primarily utilizes ECs to complete the developmental cycle, the organism can also enter other cell types such as DCs and monocytes. In monocytes, chlamydial EBs were found to colocalize in lysosomal compartments containing MHC class I molecules and, upon activation with IFN-γ, in vesicles containing both MHC classes I and II. Thus, during a chlamydial infection, the production of both CD8+− and CD4+−specific T cells can occur. In DCs, the internalized bacteria appeared in lysosomes expressing MHC class II molecules. These cells most likely play a role in initiating a Th1 immune response needed to eradicate the organism. *C. trachomatis* infection of APCs reduced the ability of these cells to stimulate T-cell proliferation through defects in antigen processing but not presentation. This has been shown to be mediated via a chlamydial protein that induces degradation of transcription factors that control IFN-γ-induced expression of both MHC classes I and II antigens. While the ability of *Chlamydia* to manipulate the host cell response to infection is obviously a survival advantage, it may also contribute to observations that immunity to *Chlamydia* is weak, resulting in persistent or recurrent infection.

4.3.2.3 CD4+ T Cells

The first studies implicating a role for T cells in clearing infection in the local genital mucosa were performed in nude mice. An infection in nude mice was chronic and persisted over 200 days, whereas normal mice could resolve the infection within 18–21 days after vaginal inoculation. These findings have been confirmed by showing that the transfer of CD4+ or CD8+ lymphocyte lines specific for chlamydial antigens could clear infection in nude mice where the CD4-enriched cell line was much more efficient.

Interestingly, mice lacking MHC class II molecules were unable to clear *Chlamydia* from the genital tract, demonstrating the necessity of CD4+ cells in the resolution of chlamydial infection. In addition, mice with disrupted CD4 expression (fewer CD4 lymphocytes) also showed significantly delayed clearance. Consequently, a critical number of antichlamydial CD4+ cells appeared necessary to eradicate infection. This is also consistent with the postulated interactions between *Chlamydia* and genital tract DCs. Although recognition of chlamydial antigens on genital ECs by CD4+ and also CD8+ T cells has not been demonstrated, recognition of antigens that have been processed by DCs is very likely. Following phagocytosis of *Chlamydia* by DCs in the genital tract of immune animals and processing of chlamydial antigen in the MHC II pathway, CD4+ Th1 memory cells are probably located in the mucosa, where they rapidly begin to secrete IFN-γ. Several authors had originally suggested that mainly genital ECs present chlamydial antigen to T cells.

The local mononuclear cytokine response by examining IFN-γ and IL-4 production has been also analyzed. The biphasic appearance of IFN-γ-producing cells at 1 and 3 weeks after infection was attributed on the one hand to NK cells at week 1 and on the other hand to the time when T-cell proliferative responses against chlamydial antigens and the influx of CD4+ lymphocytes were observed. In contrast, only small numbers of IL-4-secreting cells could be found throughout the course of infection. The dominant production of IFN-γ-producing cells was also observed in draining iliac lymph nodes as well as the mesenteric lymph nodes and spleen during the course of infection.

It has been shown that a *Chlamydia*-specific CD4 Th2 clone is unable to clear organisms from the genital mucosa of nude mice for up to 2 months after infection. In addition, it has been found that if the immune response was manipulated to favor a Th2 response, the local clearance of organisms was delayed. For example, the absence of IL-6 during a *C. trachomatis* respiratory infection did prolong the clearance of organisms from the lung and resulted in higher titers of antichlamydial IgG1 antibody in the serum. The authors also noted increased levels of IL-10 in these mice and were able to restore a dominant Th1 response by administering anti-IL-10 during infection.

From these studies it appears that a predominately Th1 CD4+ lymphocyte response is required to clear chlamydiae from the local genital mucosa.

4.3.2.3.1 CD8+ T Cells

Over the past few years, reports have been published examining the role of chlamydial-specific CD8+ lymphocytes in the resolution of genital infection. Cytotoxic killing of chlamydial-infected cells was demonstrated in targets transfected with ICAM-1 and classical MHC class I restricted cytolysis from the spleens of infected mice.

Summarizing the various studies, it may be concluded that Th1-type CD4+ cells are the main effectors in the resolution of genital infection and clearance of challenge infections, whereas CD8+ lymphocytes are neither sufficient nor necessary to confer optimal levels of protective immunity. However, immune CD8+ T cells can confer a limited level of immunity to naïve mice and display measurable cytotoxicity for *Chlamydia-infected* cells in vitro.

4.3.2.3.2 Interferon-γ

There is strong evidence indicating that IFN-γ is a major effector mechanism of the cell-mediated immune response, and the majority of the antichlamydial activity for both CD4+ and CD8+ lymphocytes is associated with the production of high levels of IFN-γ. This was initially demonstrated in vivo by administering anti-IFN-γ to mice prior to vaginal inoculation which interfered with the clearance of *Chlamydia* from the genital mucosa. In addition, a protective CD4+ Th1 clone was shown to produce high levels of IFN-γ and TNF-α, whereas the ability of a cytotoxic CD8 cell to eliminate *Chlamydia* infection was largely due to the production of IFN-γ. Direct evidence for rapid IFN-γ secretion in Th1-immune mice after vaginal challenge with *Chlamydia* has been reported. Besides some minor mechanisms of cytotoxicity such as perforin-mediated lysis, it is proposed that IFN-γ is a primary mechanism for eradication of *Chlamydia* by CTL and CD4+ T cells.

IFN-γ, however, also has bacteriostatic effects on *Chlamydia* via NO, as has been demonstrated in murine models in vitro where chlamydial growth inhibition was mediated by the induction of NO. Although NO inhibits chlamydial replication in vitro and is induced following infection, it does not contribute to the resolution of genital infection in vivo. Another possible role for IFN-γ in vivo may include the activation of local macrophages which may be necessary to stimulate antichlamydial activity from local Th1 lymphocytes within the genital mucosa. While IFN-γ clearly plays an important role in immune-mediated killing of *Chlamydia* in vivo, studies in IFN-γ−/− mice have revealed an additional, IFN-γ-independent mechanism for eradication of *Chlamydia* from the genital tract. The large majority of chlamydial burden in the genital tract is cleared in IFN-γ −/− mice and these mice did not develop dissemination of the organism following a second vaginal inoculation. In the respiratory model, results showed that immunity in IFN-γ −/− mice was associated with increased levels of TNF-α and GM-CSF in the lungs.

4.3.2.3.3 Adhesion Molecules

Besides high concentrations of cytokines such as IFN-γ delivered in close proximity to infected cells, activation and cell-to-cell contact are required for the inhibition of growth by a specific CD4+ T-cell clone. Bearing in mind the extensive surface area of the genital tract mucosa and the small numbers of CD4+ lymphocytes present during infection, it may be concluded that immune effector cells must be directed to infected ECs in order to be effective in eradicating the infection. Indeed, it may be said that the key to understanding cell-mediated immunity to chlamydial genital infection lies in defining the mechanisms by which lymphocytes traffic to the genital tract. The recruitment of leukocytes into tissue sites depends on interactions between adhesion molecules on ECs and integrin receptors on leukocytes. However, the role of homing molecules in lymphocyte recruitment to and retention in genital tract mucosa, which lacks the organized lymphoid structures present in the gut, has not been defined.

Predominantly CD4+ T cells with a peak at 3 weeks after infection were recruited to the genital mucosa following chlamydial vaginal inoculation in mice. In the genital tract of mice, recruitment of CD4+ cells is mediated through the interactions between homing receptors on CD4+ T cells, such as α4β7, and adhesion molecules ICAM-1, VCAM-1, and MadCAM-1. The latter were both temporarily induced in genital tract of mice due to chlamydial infection. During *Chlamydia* infection, cellular recruitment differs in the upper genital tract, i.e., oviduct and uterine horn, compared to the lower genital tract, i.e., cervix and vagina. It was found that CD4+ cells were recruited mainly to the upper genital tract during a primary genital infection with mouse pneumonitis (MoPn), a biovar of *C. trachomatis*, whereas neutrophils and monocytes were recruited to all regions of the genital tract. This was unexpected given that *Chlamydia* initially infect ECs in the cervix and then ascend to the oviducts. The study group also discovered a differential regulation of adhesion molecules on endothelial cells in the lower tract compared to the middle or upper tract. ICAM-1 was found to be expressed in the lower tract of uninfected mice; VCAM-1 and MAdCAM-1 were induced early after infection in the lower genital tract. In contrast, no adhesion molecules were expressed in the upper genital tract of uninfected mice, but all three were induced later in the course of infection which correlates with the appearance of CD4+ cells in these tissues. It is to be noted that the mucosal address in MAdCAM-1 is not expressed by human female genital tract tissue.

Other data suggest that the IFN-γ-inducible protein-10 (IP-10) and monokine induced by interferon gamma (MIG) are responsible for recruiting Th1 cells to the genital tract during infection. The binding of these chemokines to specific receptors activates integrin homing receptors on leukocytes, which in turn facilitates adhesion and directed migration within the tissue parenchyma. Focusing on chemokines that would attract Th1 cells, it was found that protein levels of IP-10 and MIG were elevated in the upper but not the lower genital tract early after infection. These data showing differential chemokine expression in the upper and lower genital tracts support increasing evidence that the inflammatory response in the lower genital tract may be prematurely terminated even in the presence of an active *C. trachomatis* infection.

Some investigators have tried to identify the antigen specificity of the B cells that traffic to the sites of human mucosal chlamydial infection. IgG- and IgA-secreting B cells with specificity for chlamydial MOMP, hsp-60, and a chlamydial plasmid encoded protein accumulate at sites of chlamydial genital tract infection.

4.3.2.4 Cytokine and Chemokine Response to Chlamydial Infection

Several studies in vivo and in vitro have shown the release of proinflammatory mediators including IL-1β, TNF-α, IL-6, and IL-12 upon chlamydial infection. However, studies demonstrated that *C. trachomatis* can enter host ECs without inducing the immediate production of inflammatory cytokines. Peak levels of IL-8 were delayed until 2–4 days after the initiation of infection suggesting that neither physical entry of *C. trachomatis* nor cell surface contact with molecules such as chlamydial LPS was capable of inducing IL-8 secretion. Transcription of IL-8 mRNA was also delayed and was first observed 2 h after infection, most likely through the translocation of NF-kB. These data suggest that the initiation of the chlamydial developmental cycle is responsible for inducing IL-8 secretion. Other proinflammatory cytokines such as IL-1, IL-6, and GM-CSF were also released following chlamydial infection of EC lines as well as primary endocervical ECs. However, unlike other invasive bacteria, the entry of *Chlamydia* was not responsible for the cytokine release.

The relatively small size of infectious EBs compared to other invasive bacteria was one factor allowing *Chlamydia* to enter without stimulation of cellular cytokine production. Chlamydial LPS has a weaker stimulatory ability compared to other LPS-containing bacteria, for example, gonococcal LOS. Others illustrated the ability of live *Chlamydia*, but not of heat-killed organisms, to induce IL-1β, TNF-α, and IL-6 from a monocyte cell line.

The dynamics of chemokine and chemokine receptor expression in genital mucosae during genital chlamydial infection in a murine model has been also analyzed to determine how these molecular entities influence the development of immunity and the clearance of infection in an increase in the levels of expression of RANTES, MCP-1, IP-10, MIP-1, and ICAM-1, which are involved in the recruitment of Th1 cells after genital infection with the *C. trachomatis* agent of mouse pneumonitis. Peak levels of expression of RANTES, MCP-1, and MIP-1 occurred by day 7 after primary infection, while those of IP-10 and ICAM-1 peaked by day 21. After 6 weeks and resolution of infection, the expression of these molecules as well as of chemokine receptors CCR5 and CXCR3 (known to be preferentially expressed on Th1 cells and DCs) decreased but was upregulated again after secondary infection.

While in vitro studies have revealed that chlamydiae can enter ECs without signaling the immediate production of proinflammatory cytokines, a similar result is also seen in the genital mucosa in vivo.

Peak levels of TNF-α were not seen until 5 days into the infection of *C. trachomatis* after the pathogen was inoculated into the mouse vagina. Overall, the local cytokine response appears to be weak and does not follow serum levels. IL-1, IL-6, IL-8, IL-10, and TGF-β were evaluated in genital secretions of women with bacterial STD. The genital secretions of women with *C. trachomatis* or *N. gonorrhoeae* were not consistently elevated compared to uninfected controls. However, increased levels of IFN-γ were found in endocervical secretions compared to uninfected women, and TNF-α expression was found in cultures of fallopian tubes that were infected in vitro with *C. trachomatis*.

All Th1 and Th2 cytokines analyzed in their study, i.e., IFN-γ, TNF-α, IL-10, and IL-12, were upregulated. As both CD4+ and CD8+ cells contribute to the production of and IL-10, these results confirm again that CD4+ and CD8+ lymphocytes may be important for local regulation of Th1/Th2 responses in the genital tract during *C. trachomatis* infection. Thus, the predominant cytokines produced following chlamydial genital infection in animal models are also found in humans.

APCs play a central role in shaping the cytokine profile of an immune response to *Chlamydia* through production of IL-12, IL-18, and IL-10. Both IL-12 and IL-18 are important for producing Th1 responses and are induced following infection with *Chlamydia*. IL-12 appears to play a dominant role over IL-18 since the chlamydial burden was only slightly increased following infection in IL-18 knockout mice. Anti-IL-12 prolongs the course of infection while IL-12 administration shortens infection. Finally, IL-10 appears to reduce the frequency of IFN-γ-producing T cells and resulted in an increase in chlamydial burden.

Depletion of TNF-α in genital secretions early after infection did not alter chlamydial burden or tissue pathology following vaginal inoculation of guinea pigs. However, there was an increased influx of inflammatory cells in TNF-α-depleted animals. Surprisingly, earlier studies had found that TNF-α displays antichlamydial properties in vitro.

Table 4.10 shows a summary of the different immune parameters and their functions in primary and secondary chlamydial infection.

4.3.2.5 Persistence of Chlamydial Infection

A number of studies have documented that within a year after treatment of a previous *Chlamydia* infection, individuals have persistent or recurrent infections at a rate of 13–26 %. In fact the mean time to reinfection is 6–7 months in a sexually active adolescent population. Nearly one-third of individuals became reinfected with the same serovar and that this was associated with continued contact with the same partner. As an explanation, selective immune pressure has been postulated to induce point mutations in the MOMP which have been shown to abrogate the binding of antibodies to epitopes that can neutralize infectivity in vitro.

Given the frequent reinfection with *Chlamydia* in humans, the question arises as to whether protective immunity against chlamydial infection can develop. There are several studies that support this concept. For instance, the incidence of chlamydial infection was significantly reduced in both women

Table 4.10 Summary of relevant immune parameters in immunity against *C. trachomatis* infection

Immune effectors	Role in immunity against genital *Chlamydia* infection	Importance
Factors of adaptive immunity		
CD4+ T cells	Th1 cytokines (IFN-γ, TNF, IL-2)	Obligatory
	Eradication of infection	
	Protective immunity	
CD8+ T cells	Th1 cytokines (IFN-γ, TNF, IL-2)	Contributory
	Synergistic role together with CD4+	
B cells/Igs	Faster clearance of infection	Contributory; obligatory in reinfection
Factors of innate immunity		
DCs/macrophages	Phagocytosis and antigen presentation, stimulation of T cells, cytokine costimulation, ADCC	Obligatory
NK cells	Production of IFN-γ	Contributory
Neutrophils	Reduction of amplification and focal spread	Contributory
Cytokines/chemokines	Immunostimulation	Obligatory

Adapted from Igietseme JU, Eko FO, Black CM. Contemporary approaches to designing and evaluating accines against Chlamydia. Expert Rev Vaccines. 2003;2:129–146

and men with a history of STDs. In addition, older women with an equivalent number of sexual contacts became infected less often than younger women. Also, immunosuppressed women with HIV infection had both an increased prevalence and risk of reinfection. However, the immunity that develops appears to last for only a short time. The rate of reinfection significantly increased in those individuals whose last reported *Chlamydia* infection was more than 6 months previous, as compared to those with more recent infection. In another study, a proportion of women who had not received antimicrobial therapy were shown to resolve infection. A short-term and serovar-specific immunity against chlamydial infection in female sex workers has been also reported.

Animal models of chlamydial genital infection exhibited short-term immunity against subsequent infection. Using a second vaginal inoculation of chlamydiae at various times after resolution of the primary infection, guinea pigs demonstrated immunity against reinfection with a shortened course of infection and reduced numbers of viable chlamydiae when the animals were challenged 30 days later. However, if the guinea pigs were reinfected on day 77, the level of immunity was reduced. In addition, a protective response was associated with the more rapid recruitment of CD4+ cells to the genital tract upon reinfection.

Studies have also observed a more rapid increase in the number of venules expressing adhesion molecules when mice were challenged shortly after the resolution of infection. Peak levels of adhesion molecules were seen 7 days after a challenge infection in the lower genital tract, similar to the kinetics following a primary infection. In the oviducts and uterine tissues, however, the number of venules expressing VCAM-1 peaked 3 days after infection compared to the peak on day 21 in VCAM-1-positive venules observed following a primary infection. A reason may be that low numbers of antichlamydial memory T lymphocytes recirculate through the genital mucosa following resolution of infection. Upon activation with chlamydial antigens, these lymphocytes could release cytokines and chemotactic factors to facilitate the rapid recruitment of CD4 lymphocytes.

It is likely that cellular immunity is primarily responsible for clearing the initial infection; however, it appears that antibody plays a role in protection from reinfection. It was shown that IFN-γ receptor knockout mice resolved infection only after a prolonged time period while high levels of antichlamydial IgA and IgG antibodies were present in genital secretions. Antibodies against *Chlamydia* are found in genital secretions and serum after infection and the resolution of a primary infection coincides with the appearance of antichlamydial antibody in genital secretions. A few proposed antibody-mediated mechanisms of control include neutralization of the entry of *C. trachomatis* into ECs; opsonization, which enhances the uptake of *Chlamydia* by macrophages; and antibody-dependent cell-mediated cytotoxicity via antichlamydial IgA. A less intense infection was noted in guinea pigs that were challenged as long as 825 days after a primary infection which was correlated to serum IgG levels but not IgA levels in genital secretions since IgA antibodies were undetected 75 days after infection.

Murine studies have provided evidence that the delayed appearance of antichlamydial IgA antibodies in CVS correlated with a delay in the resolution of infection. Women with antichlamydial IgA antibodies in CVS shed significantly fewer infectious chlamydiae than women without IgA in CVS; this effect was not observed with high serum antibodies. Moreover, the presence of IgA in CVS seems to accelerate the clearance of infection with antibiotic therapy. Equally convincing results from murine models put forward the hypothesis that antibodies are not required for protective immunity against *Chlamydia*. B-cell-deficient mice have been shown to resolve chlamydial genital tract infection as effectively as intact mice. The presence of antichlamydial IgA in mouse CVS alone seems to be insufficient to resolve infection which clearly points to a synergistic role of antibody- and cell-mediated immunity in protection.

A study by Morrison and Morrison in antibody-deficient mice confirmed that antibodies contribute to a high degree to immunity to chlamydial genital tract reinfection, and that antibody-mediated protection is highly dependent on CD4+ T-cell-mediated adaptive changes that occur in the local genital tract tissues during primary infection. However, a study by Johansson and Lycke in B-cell-deficient mice indicated that long-term protection in the genital tract against *C. trachomatis* infection is conveyed by IFN-γ-producing CD4+ memory T cells, which appear to be maintained in the absence of antibodies and local antigen deposition.

One serious problem with repeated chlamydial genital infections is, as already mentioned

above, tissue damage followed by tubal scarring, chronic salpingitis, and distal tubal obstruction. Studies proposed the hypothesis that at least some component of the immune response in form of a delayed-type hypersensitivity reaction could be responsible for causing tissue damage. By characterizing the inflammatory infiltrate, Patton found only mononuclear infiltrates during repeated infection compared to both mononuclear and polymorphonuclear infiltrates after a primary infection. Moreover, a lack of *Chlamydia*-specific T lymphocytes may enhance tubal pathology. Studies observed oviduct ectasia, hydrosalpinx, and marked acute inflammatory infiltrates in mice that lacked an antichlamydial CD4+ lymphocyte response.

Recurrent or chronic chlamydial infections, which are associated with damage to the reproductive tract, may result from an insufficient number of antichlamydial Th1 CD4+ cells or possibly factors that interfere with the effector mechanisms of Th1 cells, for example, IL-10. *Chlamydia* was eradicated more rapidly following infection in IL-10 knockout mice and that antichlamydial Th1 responses were enhanced in IL-10 knockout mice. IL-10 is a potent counter-regulatory cytokine that suppresses Th1 immune responses by many mechanisms such as inhibiting IL-12 production from APCs or suppressing transcription of the chemokine IP-10, which attracts Th1 CD4 cells. Another factor that may dampen Th1 responses during *Chlamydia* infection is the anti-inflammatory cytokine TGF-β which is elevated in the genital tract late in the course of MoPn infection in mice.

Neutrophils or their products might also play a significant role in tubal pathology and infertility since they have the potential to cause damage through the release of proteinases and hydrolases. Furthermore, neutrophils primed by exposure to cytokines such as GM-CSF, IL-8, and TNF-α can release large quantities of ROI and granule enzymes upon activation with soluble immune complexes. In addition, a shift from a Th1-dominated response to a mixed Th1/Th2 response may further dampen antichlamydial responses. Unfortunately, cytokines characteristic of Th2 responses are associated with increased collagen deposition, a measure of fibrosis, which may contribute to reproductive tract dysfunction. In contrast, IFN-γ inhibited this process.

In vitro, the production of most chlamydial components is extremely downregulated when *C. trachomatis* is in its persistent, non-replicative form. However, synthesis of chlamydial heat shock protein (c-hsp60) is upregulated under these conditions. Immunity to this protein, which only results from a persistent infection, seems to contribute to the development of tubal occlusion and adverse pregnancy outcome. A study showed that detection of antibody to c-hsp60 did not correlate with a positive *C. trachomatis* genital culture but with tubal occlusion, PID, and adverse pregnancy outcome. There is a human hsp60 (h-hsp60) homologue to c-hsp60 which is expressed by ECs of the decidua and embryo during early pregnancy. Therefore, a chlamydial fallopian tube infection can induce the development of autoantibodies to h-hsp60 and in women already sensitized to c-hsp60; the exposure to h-hsp60 will reactivate the c-hsp60 lymphocytes. This may lead to immune rejection of the embryo.

The immunological components that contribute to the production of tubal pathology may also be associated with many factors, including the genetic background of the individual. Another question is whether individuals become reinfected with the same serovar or perhaps develop persistent infections. Although the large majority of women infected with *Chlamydia* are effectively treated and reinfection commonly occurs, it is difficult to document persistence in vivo. However, some less prevalent serovars, such as serovars I, J, K, and H, show increased rates among those with repeat infections. More studies are needed to understand whether these serovars have an increased ability to escape recall responses against *Chlamydia* or whether these organisms can persist in a latent state.

4.3.2.6 Chlamydial Vaccine Development

A major challenge in designing antichlamydial vaccines is to develop an immunization regimen capable of inducing and retaining a mucosal Th1 CD4+ response in order to foster long-term

protective benefits. This type of immunity would help to resolve infections rather than prevent them and could therefore influence the consequences of asymptomatic infections ascending from the cervix.

Studies to develop a safe and protective vaccine against chlamydial infection are still ongoing. In the 1960s, a vaccine for trachoma was developed and tested in humans but the protection was short-lived and induced immunopathologic scarring in a few individuals. Several vaccination methods have since been described that target antigens into the endocytic MHC II pathway of DCs and elicit a Th1-type CD4+ immunity. These include immune-stimulating complexes (ISCOMS), alphavirus vectors, opsonized liposomes, and conjugation of antigen to lysosome-associated membrane protein-1 (Sig/LAMP-1). The antigens that would be the most effective targets for a Th1 cellular immune response have not been identified, but chlamydial MOMP is a suitable candidate. T-cell epitopes appear to be found in association with many HLA alleles and for the most part are directed against nonpolymorphic constant regions of the MOMP. Thus, cellular immunity could be generated to nonvariable segments of the organism for protection against an array of serovars. Support for this approach has been generated in mice, where infection with MoPn provides subsequent protection against human serovars of *C. trachomatis*.

Different routes of immunization have been examined for stimulating protective immune responses against chlamydial infection within the reproductive tract. Thereby it is possible to eliminate disturbances on immune responses coming from reproductive hormones, for example. Chlamydiae were recovered from the upper genital tract of significantly more mice when infected during the luteal phase with increased levels of progesterone and estradiol than follicular phase. However, progesterone increases and estradiol decreases susceptibility to intrauterine chlamydial infection, at least in a rat model.

In the mouse model, various mucosal versus parenteral routes of immunization were compared. In mice which were given live *Chlamydia* by mucosal routes, i.e., oral, intranasal, and vaginal,

Table 4.11   Vaccine design strategies in development against chlamydia infection

Immunmodulatory approach	Vaccine effect	Research status
Selection of antigens with T and B cell epitopes	Induction of required T- and B-cell response	In progress
Multisubunit vaccines	Furnishing adequate B- and T-cell epitopes for elevated immune responses	In progress
Use of delivery vehicles (adjuvants, vectors)	Boost of immune responses; vehicles for subunits	In progress
Modulation of cytokine chemokine expression	Up regulation of Th1 cytokines; downregulation of Th2 cytokines	Experimental stage
Modulation of costimulatory factors	Induction of high T-cell response	Experimental stage
Vaccine targeting specific inductive sites	Mucosal immunity	Active

Adapted from Igietseme JU, Eko FO, Black CM. Contemporary approaches to designing and evaluating accines against Chlamydia. Expert Rev Vaccines. 2003;2:129–146

the course of infection was significantly shortened and of less magnitude compared to mice injected subcutaneously with live *Chlamydia*. Examination of the cytokine profile produced after immunization showed a dominant Th2 response in the draining iliac lymph nodes following parenteral immunization, whereas a dominant Th1 response was noted in mice immunized via mucosal routes. Mice first given live *Chlamydia* intranasally or vaginally had greater levels of IFN-γ in the genital tract after a challenge infection compared to mice immunized via a subcutaneous route. Oral immunization has been shown to elicit antibodies in other mucosal tissues, such as the reproductive tract and mammary glands, as well as the intestine. However, the intranasal route was found to produce the greatest amount of IgA and IgG in genital secretions for the longest period of time. For instance, both IgA and IgG, specific for the immunizing antigen, could be found in genital secretions following immunization via the nasal, oral, rectal, and vaginal routes. However, both the nasal and vaginal routes consistently produced the greatest increase in IgA and IgG compared to other routes in humans. Immunization via the nasal route elicited the highest level of antichlamydial IgG antibody titers in the genital tract even in comparison with a vaginal immunization. Moreover, immunization by the nasal route has been shown to protect mice from infertility following a challenge infection.

The induction of a protective cell-mediated immune response also appears to depend on whether a live infection initiates the immunizing

response. In the guinea pig model of chlamydial genital infection, protection following parenteral immunization was observed. *Chlamydia*-specific IgG and IgA levels were comparable in the serum and genital secretions among vaginal, oral, and parenteral immunization routes when live EB were used. Moreover, guinea pigs could be protected from reinfection following a parenteral immunization with UV-inactivated *Chlamydia* which is most likely due to the production of a protective antibody response. In contrast, immunization of mice with UV-inactivated *Chlamydia* provided no protection against a genital infection.

These data show that to develop a protective vaccine many factors in addition to the antigen must be considered, such as route of immunization or form of antigen. A summary of different approaches to create a protective and safe vaccine against chlamydial infection is shown in Table 4.11.

4.3.3   Bacterial Vaginosis

Bacterial vaginosis (BV) is the most common adverse alteration of the vaginal flora, with a prevalence of about 10–60 % in different populations. For a normal vaginal flora after menarche, estrogen provides the conditions for survival of lactobacilli, the dominant vaginal flora in most adult females. There are various different species of lactobacilli with the dominant species being either *L. crispatus*, *L. gasseri*, *L. jensenii*, or *L. iners*. The healthy vaginal flora is characterized by high concentrations of this *Lactobacillus* spp. (10^8 colony forming units/ml) and a pH of less than 4.5. During menopause, there is a mixed flora with a considerable concentration of mycoplasmas and anaerobic bacteria. The roles of lactobacilli species are to produce lactate for acidification of the vaginal mucus; to produce bacteriocins, hydrogen peroxide, a bisurfactant, and organic acids; and furthermore to compete with pathogenic organisms for space, receptors, and nutrients.

The vaginal epithelium and its mucus layer helps to regulate the intrinsic bacterial and mucosal defense systems. The vagina is lined with squamous epithelium, whose thickness directly correlates with estrogen concentration. Glycogen supplied by the vaginal ECs supplies metabolic fuel for the generation of lactic acid by lactobacilli, thus enabling a low pH. This low pH helps to control potential overgrowth of other commensal flora such as Gardnerella vaginalis. Apparently, a low estrogenization of the vaginal mucous membrane will enhance the growth potential of flora that is normally encountered in small quantities in the vaginal mucus.

Some decades ago, Gardner and Duke reported aspects of the so-called Haemophilus vaginalis vaginitis which is now renamed BV. They proposed Haemophilus vaginalis, which is now Gardnerella vaginalis, as the single cause for BV.

Today it is generally known that BV significantly alters the vaginal ecosystem and a profuse mixed flora with anaerobic and facultative anaerobic bacteria besides depletion of *Lactobacillius* spp., especially those that produce hydrogen peroxide, is established. The vaginal flora in BV includes *Gardnerella vaginalis*, *Prevotella* spp., *Mobiluncus* spp., *Corynebacterium* spp., *Viridans* streptococci, coagulase-negative staphylococci, *Enterococcus faecalis*, *Atopobium vaginalis*, and *Mycoplasma hominis* (419, 874). There is not only a qualitative but also a quantitative change with bacterial concentrations about 100–1,000 times higher than normal. Production of fatty acids by these anaerobic bacteria leads to an elevated pH in the vagina which itself promotes anaerobic growth again.

Table 4.12   Amsel criteria for BV, of which at least three of four should be present

Vaginal pH greater than 4.5
Homogenous vaginal discharge on examination
Detection of fishy odor on addition of potassium hydroxide to vaginal fluid
Pretence of significant clue cells in vaginal smear (>20 % of total vaginal ECs)

M. Wirth 2006, Personal communication

BV is the most prevalent form of vaginal infection in women of reproductive age, affecting about 3 million women in the United States per year, and is the most common etiology of vaginal symptoms leading women to seek medical care. Symptomatic BV, which only accounts for 60 % of all cases, causes abnormal amounts of a malodorous vaginal discharge deriving from degraded vaginal mucus. Symptoms of a vaginitis including vaginal pruritus, burning, or dyspareunia, however, are rare and visible local inflammation signs are absent. BV is clinically diagnosed by the Nugent criteria which quantify the number of lactobacilli relative to BV-associated morphotypes or by the Amsel criteria (Table 4.12).

4.3.3.1 Pathogenesis and Implications of BV Infection

What influences susceptibility to BV in some women is currently not clear. Prepuberty and postmenopause are rarely associated with BV which has led to the proposal that vaginal microbial changes may be due to hormonal variations during the menstrual cycle. It is also considered that BV is a genetically determined miscolonization of the vagina or may be another example of an STD.

One virulence factor in bacteria associated with BV is a hemolytic toxin produced by *G. vaginalis*. Women who lack an adequate IgA immune response against this toxin are said to be at risk for BV. Another hypothesis respecting the pathogenesis is that hydrolytic enzymes degrade the mucin and thus damage the protective vaginal mucosa. In comparison with healthy women, women affected by BV are also known to have significantly higher vaginal concentrations of the hydrolytic enzymes sialidase and proline dipeptidase. Proline dipeptidase is produced by both *Mobiluncus* spp. and *G. vaginalis*. Sialidase, which is produced by, for instance, *Prevotella* spp., is thought to be an important virulence factor in BV pathogenesis, not only because it leads to lysis of the mucin, thus aiding the adherence of bacteria, but also through its ability to counteract a specific IgA defense against *G. vaginalis* toxin. It was furthermore suggested that a high sialidase activity in BV gives rise to a significant risk of prematurity.

A causal relationship between BV and the acquisition of HIV has been supported by studies evaluating HIV genital shedding in BV and from prospective studies examining the risk of HIV infection associated with abnormal vaginal flora. The presence of BV was associated with a sixfold increase in the quantity of HIV shed relative to normal flora. Relations between BV and the acquisition of HSV-2 have also been reported. It may be speculated that the increased risk of incurring infections such as HIV and HSV-2 in the presence of an abnormal vaginal microbiota is due in part to the fact that vaginal acidity falls as lactobacillus levels decline and this circumstance benefits the survival of other microorganisms. A further factor arising from the decrease of lactobacilli is a corresponding decline in production of H_2O_2, which has an antimicrobial effect. It is also to be noted that some anaerobes associated with BV augment expression of HIV in T cells in vitro, which might enhance the amount of HIV shedding or activate these T cells to further support viral transmission.

Studies have shown that genital mucosal fluids from women with BV are potent stimulators of leukocytes, eliciting secretion of TNF-α and expression of mRNA for both TLR4 and TLR2. Thus, findings suggest that TNF-α levels in genital mucosal fluids from women with BV would be higher than those in women with normal flora. Activation of cells through TLR2 and TLR4 with microbial products enhances HIV expression through stimulation of TNF-α secretion or direct activation of NF-κB and subsequent binding of

NF-κB to the HIV promoter. Therefore the secretion of TNF-α and mRNA expression of TLR2 and TLR4 by genital mucosal fluid of women with BV could play a role in mediating HIV transmission. Proinflammatory cytokines such as IL-1 and TNF-α were found to be elevated in BV patients. As these cytokines could upregulate local HIV replication by activating NF-κB in the LTR-promoter region of HIV, this could partly explain the mechanism by which this risk factor enhances HIV transmission.

Further data support the association between BV and adverse sequelae related to the upper genital tract. Studies have raised suspicion that there is a correlation between BV and CIN or cervical carcinoma.

During pregnancy, BV is associated with an increased risk of preterm delivery and low-birth-weight children, first-trimester miscarriage among women undergoing in vitro fertilization (IVF), chorioamnionitis, and other infections. Screening for BV and treatment has been considered a strategy to reduce the rate of preterm birth. But its effectiveness remains unproven. In nonpregnant women, BV increases the risk for posthysterectomy infections and PID as well as the risk for acquiring *Neisseria gonorrhoeae* or *Chlamydia*. The correlation between BV and infection in the upper genital tract is believed to be due to the fact that an abundant vaginal overgrowth of BV-associated bacteria makes ascending infections in the genital tract more likely. Considering the concept of vaginal inflammation, a balanced and appropriate immune response is thought to be crucial to clear infectious agents through the production of antimicrobial agents, phagocytosis, and clearance of microorganisms. Individuals differ in their ability to mount an inflammatory response; some are hyperresponders with an excessive local and systemic response and others are hyporesponders with the risk of an overwhelming infection. In this context, there is a hypothesis to understand the relationship between changes in the vaginal flora, inflammatory response, and clinical outcome. Hyporesponsive mothers may not be able to control microbial challenge which results in ascending intrauterine infection and clinical chorioamnionitis. Hyperresponders develop an excessive local immune response and clinical symptoms of vaginitis and be at risk for preterm delivery. To underline this hypothesis, Simhan reported that women with low concentrations of cytokines IL-1β, IL-6, and IL-8 in vaginal fluid in early pregnancy are more likely to develop chorioamnionitis than those without low concentration of these cytokines. Also, women with elevated vaginal cytokines may be at risk for preterm delivery. More data concerning the circumstances of preterm delivery associated with infections such as BV are discussed below in the chapter on disturbances in maternal–fetal interactions.

4.3.3.2 Innate and Specific Immune Responses in BV

BV is generally regarded as a noninflammatory vaginal condition, and inflammatory signs are rare in BV-positive women. Activation and recruitment of neutrophils is one of the main components of innate immunity in general against microbial and viral infections in the mucous membrane of the genitalia. However, the number of vaginal neutrophils in most BV-positive patients is not increased in comparison with healthy women, which is surprising, given the massive microbial colonization (192, 195). A subgroup of BV-positive patients actually shows high numbers of neutrophils together with a tenfold increase in proinflammatory cytokine concentrations when compared to the subgroup with low numbers of neutrophils. This implies that some women with BV do experience a strong activation of the innate immune response. Other innate immune factors, such as the anti-inflammatory and antimicrobial SLPI, which is produced by mucosal ECs, are present at lower levels in vaginal fluid in BV-positive women. Since SLPI has been shown to inhibit HIV infection in vitro, it has been suggested that low levels of SLPI in conjunction with a BV-positive status might contribute to the risk of contracting HIV. The concentration of neutrophil defensins is also not increased in BV.

Proinflammatory cytokines IL-1α and IL-1β are released by phagocytes which are stimulated by bacterial surface antigens and trigger an inflammatory reaction by activating T-helper cells. Production of local proinflammatory cytokines, which has been shown to be increased in genital tract infections with *Candida* or *T. vaginalis*, for example, has been investigated in BV. The levels of IL-1α and IL-1β in CVS are higher in BV-positive patients whether pregnant or not (37, 192, 890, 1494). Furthermore, there is a correlation between a gradual disruption of lactobacillus dominance and a gradual increase in IL-1α and IL-1β. This shows that the innate immune system is reacting strongly and trying to combat abnormal microbial colonization, although most BV-positive women do not show any inflammatory signs. However, increased levels of IL-1α seem to be associated with BV in pregnancy.

In a trial of the Munich study group on 45 symptomatic BV patients and 36 asymptomatic controls, the proinflammatory cytokines IL-6 and IL-10 and the anti-inflammatory IL-12 in vaginal secretions were measured. Results showed no significant difference in levels of all three cytokines between the two study groups. These findings are consistent with results from other studies. An association between IL-6 concentrations and BV has not been demonstrated yet, but significant increases in IL-1α and, to a lesser extent, IL-8 in BV-positive pregnant patients have been reported. In pregnant women, BV can probably result in the induction of a local immune response mediated by IL-1α and IL-8. A significant rise in concentrations of IL-6 and TNF-α in pregnant BV-positive women compared to controls could not be demonstrated, whereas vaginal levels of IL-1β were increased. As IL-6 is expressed in endometrial ECs, the absence of an IL-6 response in BV may be because the mucosal ECs are not triggered by BV-associated bacteria or their components to secrete IL-6 above the constitutive levels. Nonetheless, oral and vaginal metronidazole treatment of BV-positive pregnant patients has been shown to reduce cervical mucus levels of IL-6 as well as IL-1β and IL-8. In the group of patients with persistent BV, however, the metronidazole treatment did not result in a cytokine reduction. Another study by the Munich study group determined the levels of the proinflammatory cytokines IL-1α and IL-1β and the anti-inflammatory cytokines IL-5 and IL-10 in vaginal secretions of BV patients and healthy women. They found significantly increased levels of IL-1β and significantly decreased levels of IL-10 in BV patients compared to healthy women; however, levels of IL-1α were not elevated in nonpregnant BV patients. Thus, there may be a difference in the response of the local immune system during pregnancy.

IL-1β is a master cytokine inducing several cytokines, especially IL-8. IL-8 is a potent chemotactic and activating factor for neutrophils that has been detected in vaginal fluid of women with BV and other vaginal infections, including trichomoniasis. The numbers of neutrophils in BV-positive patients and in healthy women are associated with the levels of IL-8. Another study by the same authors showed that impairment of IL-8 induction in women with BV is associated with low levels of vaginal IgA against hemolysin produced by *G. vaginalis*, a low number of leukocytes, and high microbial hydrolytic enzyme activities. IL-8 does not, however, seem to be correlated with the presence of BV in the same distinct manner as IL-1β. The BV microbial flora appears to produce virulence factors that specifically inhibit IL-8 more than IL-1β. The resulting low IL-8 levels may be responsible for the low counts of vaginal leukocytes and for the clinically observed absence of inflammatory symptoms in most women with BV. Further findings indicate that microbial hydrolytic enzymes could be responsible for dampening the expected proinflammatory response cascade after IL-1β induction. The impairment of IL-8 induction may explain the absence of neutrophil increase in most women exposed to a massive anaerobic vaginal colonization.

Anti-inflammatory IL-10 inhibits activation of Th1 cells, thereby suppressing cell-mediated immunity. There are inconsistent results concerning this cytokine in BV. In a Munich study no significant difference in vaginal IL-10 levels of BV patients compared to healthy women could be demonstrated, whereas other studies showed higher IL-10 levels in CVS of BV patients compared to controls. They suggested that higher IL-10 levels in CVS of BV patients may be another mechanism to increase susceptibility to HIV infection. As mentioned above, in another study, vaginal levels of IL-10 were significantly higher in healthy controls than in BV patients. These differences may be caused by recruitment of different patients into the studies.

Some evidence points to microbial hydrolytic enzymes, sialidases and prolidases, and toxins as factors that degrade human Igs and thus impair the immune response. So far, the only characterized specific adaptive immune response in BV is IgA antibody against the hemolysin produced by *G. vaginalis*. Levels of these vaginal IgA antibodies are positively associated with IL-8 and IL-1β concentrations and are inversely related to microbial enzyme activity. An association between levels of IL-1β and anti-*G. vaginalis* hemolysin IgA in vaginal fluids has been also proposed, suggesting a necessary association between the innate and adaptive immune responses for protection from ascent of pathogens to the upper genital tract. High levels of anti-*G. vaginalis* hemotoxin IgA in BV-positive pregnant women appear to be protective against adverse pregnancy outcomes whereas BV with high prolidase and sialidase activity was associated with a higher risk for low birth weight. Increased IL-1β level during BV could upregulate local HIV replication through activation of the LTR-promoter region and therefore partly explain the mechanism how BV enhances HIV transmission.

All bacterial species associated with BV, with the possible exception of *Mobiluncus* spp., appear in small quantities in the flora of healthy vaginae, but they increase considerably in the vaginae of women with BV. BV might well be an endogenous infection since microorganisms associated with BV are shown to have their natural habitat in the gastrointestinal tract. The pathogenetic mechanisms that lead to BV among a subpopulation of women are still unknown. The consequences of any interaction between different species of bacteria are not clear. All in all, however, it seems that an increased level of proinflammatory cytokines in conjunction with a disruption of the vaginal flora does not evoke an inflammatory effect in the usual clinical sense, but that it nonetheless is a host response to a growing potential threat. One could propose that the condition of BV can be considered as a mucosal immunity disorder or genetically determined miscolonization of the vagina resulting in the lack of an adequate immune response against the intruding microorganisms. Another option would be that the prevalence of certain bacteria inhibits the local host response.

It seems to be important to clearly differentiate between the prevalence of BV with its typical clinical picture, on the one hand, and the state of bacterial dysbiosis, on the other hand, which is more precisely characterized as a dysbalance of the vaginal flora. Studies have generally investigated an abnormal vaginal flora but concentrated on BV instead of taking into account other forms of a dysbalanced vaginal flora. Such forms of abnormal flora have been termed "intermediate flora" in some studies or have been included with BV in other studies (334, 335). However, a distinction between the classic finding of BV and an "intermediate" vaginal fluid should be considered. Abnormal vaginal flora comprises a wide range of changes, which include not only BV but also other less well-characterized conditions. Novel aspects raised the question of whether inflammation really exists with BV or whether it is a separate entity. In opposition to BV with no signs of local inflammation, some women with abnormal vaginal flora showed signs of a vaginitis including redness, pruritus, and burning pain. This was referred to as a condition characterized by a decrease in lactobacilli, high vaginal pH, absence of clue cells, and the presence of leukocytes which Donders called "aerobic vaginitis." Women with "aerobic vaginitis" were reported to have decreased levels of lactic acid and a local inflammatory response with high concentrations of vaginal IL-1β, IL-6, and LIF.

This is consistent with work by the Munich study group, who investigated 102 patients with a symptomatic vaginal dysbiosis, similar to the picture of an aerobic vaginitis of the Donders study, and 50 healthy asymptomatic controls. In women with vaginal dysbiosis, the proinflammatory cytokines IL-1α and IL-1β were significantly increased, whereas IL-2 and IL-4 were significantly lower in this group compared to healthy controls. This could also be due to bacterial proteins and proteases, which have been shown to inhibit cytokine release. The production of prostaglandin E2 by monocytes also inhibits IL-2 production, which was proposed as one important factor in recurrent vaginitis by Witkin. An inhibition of the cytokine response results in incompetent effector functions of the immune response, stimulating further bacterial growth and the prevalence of symptoms. Possible therapeutic interventions in vaginal dysbiosis, such as immunostimulation through IL-2, are implicated but need further study. Whether bacterial dysbiosis can be considered a separate entity or a state of transition to BV remains unclear. There is as yet no consensus about the diagnostics and classifications of vaginal flora to better define different states of abnormal vaginal flora, which also has important implications for therapy. Further studies to differentiate the effects of BV and aerobic vaginitis on the outcome of pregnancy are needed as well. Some studies have found no association between BV and pregnancy outcome, whereas others have indicated an association.

An association of an abnormal vaginal flora with elevated cervical levels of IL-1β has been also demonstrated. Concentrations of proinflammatory cytokines in an abnormal vaginal flora could be higher due to bacterial release of LPS and endotoxins. Elevated IL-1β was also demonstrated in patients with cervical dysplasia, which was more frequent in women with an abnormal vaginal flora than in women with normal vaginal flora. IL-1β could be responsible for stimulation of HPV replication, similar to HIV. Also the concentration of neutrophil defensins is increased in patients with "intermediate" flora whereas in BV it is not elevated.

Finally, in a study on 193 women attending an outpatient clinic for vaginal discharge problems, vaginal swabs were investigated for pathogens, lactobacilli, and leukocytes, as well as vaginal secretions for IL-4, IL-10, and IL-12. Preliminary results proposed an association of high vaginal levels of IL-12 with high leukocyte numbers and a high total BV-related pathogen count, whereas low levels of IL-10 were correlated with high total BV-related pathogen counts. High vaginal IL-10 levels were therefore assumed to be associated with healthy women, whereas high levels of IL-12 were positively correlated with infection and inflammation.

4.4 Candidiasis

Vulvovaginal candidiasis (VVC) is a common mucosal fungal infection caused in about 80–90 % by the opportunistic pathogen *Candida albicans*, a commensal organism in the gastrointestinal and reproductive tracts. Other causative agents are *Candida glabrata*, *Candida krusei*, and others. VVC affects an estimated three out of four women at least once during their reproductive age, and a significant percentage of those women (5–10 %) experience recurrent VVC (RVVC). An overview of different clinical forms of vaginal *Candida* infection is presented in Table 4.13.

Several exogenous predisposing factors such as pregnancy, oral contraceptives, and uncontrolled diabetes mellitus are known to cause acute episodes of VVC. However, RVVC seems to be idiopathic. Chronic RVVC (CRVVC) is clinically defined as at least four episodes per year in the absence of any predisposing factors.

Table 4.13 Different clinical forms of vaginal candidiasis

Asymptomatic form	Colonization, lack of symptoms
Acute form	Burning, itching, vaginal discharge
	Vaginal erythema and edema
Persistent form	Persistence after antifungal therapy
Recurrent form	Recurrence after antifungal therapy
	CRVVC: ≥4 episodes/year, caused mainly by *C. albicans*, but increasing rate of *C. glabrata* and non-albicans strains

M. Wirth 2006, Personal communication

Unlike symptomatic oropharyngeal candidiasis of HIV-positive subjects, which seems to be closely dependent upon both the severity of cellular immunodeficiency and reduced CD4+ cell counts, symptomatic VVC is common in women, regardless of HIV serostatus and immunodeficiency. Recurrences seem to be caused by persistent yeast in the vagina, rather than by reinfections, as demonstrated by the isolation of the same karyotypically identical strains in relapses.

Acute VCC can be treated topically with nystatin, imidazole, or amphotericin B or systemically with fluconazole or itraconazole. Antifungal therapy is highly effective for individual attacks of VCC and RVCC but does not prevent recurrence. Thus, RVVC is presumed to result from some local innate and/or acquired dysfunction in the normal protective immune response most healthy individuals acquire from early exposure to *Candida albicans*.

4.4.1 Cell-Mediated Immunity in *Candida* Infection

Cell-mediated immunity by T cells and cytokines, specifically a Th1-type response, is considered to be the predominant host defense mechanism against mucosal candidiasis and is thought to play a role in maintaining the organism in its commensal state at those sites as well. This is evidenced not only by the high incidence of *Candida* infections in HIV-positive persons with reduced cell-mediated immunity but also by a similar prevalence under other conditions of T-cell immunosuppression, as, for example, corticosteroid therapy.

Several experimental studies show that Th1-type cell-mediated immune responses are associated with resistance against systemic and mucosal *C. albicans* infections, whereas Th2-type responses are associated with susceptibility to infection. A murine model of VCC has been used to study host immune responses against *C. albicans*. In this model, the most important requirement for a persistent infection is a state of pseudoestrus. In the absence of estrogen treatments, the infection is short-lived with a low fungal burden in the vagina. However, the local vaginal immune responses in *Candida* infection are not clearly understood so far. Clinical as well as experimental estrogen-dependent murine model studies examining *C. albicans* vaginitis show that although *Candida*-specific systemic Th1-type responses are clinically present or experimentally induced during a vaginal infection, these responses appear to have no effect on the infection (405, 407). Further experimental studies using the murine model show that partial protection against infection can be achieved, but without involvement of systemic Th1-type cell-mediated immunity. Through clinical and experimental studies, it has become apparent that the host response to a *C. albicans* vaginal infection is more dependent on local immunity than the response observed in the systemic circulation (404, 405).

Other studies evaluated the role of local vaginal-associated Th1 cell immunity. Data to assess vaginally associated T cells showed no changes in the percentage or composition of local phenotypically distinct T cells during primary or secondary *C. albicans* vaginal infection and also showed no evidence for systemic T-cell infiltration into the vaginal mucosa during infection. It can therefore be concluded that if T cells are responsible for any host defense in vaginal *Candida* infection, they exert their protective effect without significant changes in number and composition.

In the absence of any clear exogenous predisposing factor, the risk of clinical infection has been correlated with a partial T-cell dysregulation, which might be exacerbated by the hormonal balance present during the follicular phase. Indeed, a significant reduction in the proliferation of peripheral blood lymphocytes from women in the follicular phase with RVVC has been reported, following their in vitro stimulation with *Candida* cells. These women had a depleted T-cell pool and, in response to *Candida* stimulation, showed significantly reduced IFN-γ production which is normally a hallmark of anti-Candida protection. However, in at least partial contradiction with these data, clinical evidence has demonstrated that *Candida*-specific cell-mediated

immunity at the periphery is normal in women with RVVC and is also remarkably similar both in HIV-positive subjects with oral candidiasis and in HIV-negative subjects.

It is obvious that innate and adaptive humoral and cellular immune mechanisms are involved in the host defense against *C. albicans* infections, but they exert their functions in a site-specific manner. Innate immunity by PMNs and macrophages seems to dominate protection against systemic candidiasis, which accounts for the high incidence of systemic candidiasis in neutropenic patients. There is now evidence that human and animal vaginal ECs may represent an important innate anti-*Candida* host defense mechanism. Interestingly, a study in humans showed that while the vaginal EC anti-*Candida* activity was not different at the various stages of the menstrual cycle, it was significantly reduced in women with a history of RVVC. Thus, reduced EC anti-*Candida* activity may represent, in part, a local immune deficiency associated with RVVC.

Experimentally, both humoral and cellular protective anti-*Candida* responses at the vaginal level are totally uncoupled from those occurring at the periphery, suggesting either an immunological independence, or compartmentalization of the vaginal mucosa, or a differential regulation of T-cell recruitment between different regions of the genital tract. Interestingly, murine vaginal T cells are phenotypically distinct from T cells in the blood. However, *Candida*-specific cell-mediated immunity was expressed by vaginal T cells in rats immunized against *Candida* after healing a primary infection, and vaginal T cells, particularly the CD4+ subset, transferred protection to naïve rats (unpublished data). These apparently contradictory data raise the issue of whether the data from experimental models of vaginal infection can be extrapolated to human disease.

Mice given an experimental *C. trachomatis* genital tract infection exhibit a CD4+ T-cell infiltrate into the genital tract. This Th1-type response is critical for the resolution of infection and indicates that T cells can reach the genital mucosa and provide substantial protection. Interestingly the question has been addressed whether or not a dual infection with *C. albicans* and *C. trachomatis* could enhance the local recruitment of a cell-mediated host response against *C. albicans* and facilitate clearance of the infection. The result was that a concurrent *Candida* and *Chlamydia* infection could not accelerate or modulate the anti-*Candida* cell-mediated response. These results suggest that host responses to these two genital tract infections are independent and not influenced by the presence of each other.

There is experimental and clinical evidence that supports immunoregulation or tolerance against *Candida* at the vaginal mucosa. Mice deficient in δ-chain TCR are more resistant to experimental vaginitis than WT mice, suggesting a tolerance role for vaginal γ/δ T cells that are in higher numbers compared with the circulation. Vaginal tissue homogenates in mice showed high constitutive concentrations of the immunoregulatory cytokine TGF-β, which were increased further in vaginally infected mice together with low levels of other cytokines. Furthermore, *Candida-specific* T cells with appropriate homing receptors for infiltration into the vaginal mucosa are reduced during a vaginal *Candida* infection in mice despite the upregulation of reciprocal adhesion molecules on the vaginal epithelium. Moreover, PMNs, which have significant killing activity against *C. albicans* in vitro and are often observed in vaginal lavage fluid of infected animals, are not effective against Candida in the vaginal environment. One report using a live challenge model in humans revealed a possible paradigm shift for factors associated with susceptibility and resistance to candidal vaginitis. Among women with no history of vaginitis, only a few became symptomatic with vaginitis or were even colonized. In contrast, inclusion of women with documented infrequent episodes of VVC resulted in significantly higher rates of symptomatic infection, with the remaining women becoming asymptomatically colonized. Interestingly, protection occurred in the absence of any evidence of inflammation or an inflammatory response, whereas those with symptomatic infection had a heavy vaginal cellular infiltrate consisting entirely of neutrophils. Furthermore, a high neutrophil infiltration score correlated with higher fungal burden. Therefore, symptomatic

infection appeared to be associated with a hyper-response by neutrophils rather than a deficiency in adaptive immunity, whereas resistance to infection appears to be associated with a noninflammatory innate presence rather than an adaptive cell-mediated response. This would change the paradigm for host defense against VVC away from adaptive immune dysfunction and toward dichotomous roles for innate immunity in both resistance and susceptibility to VVC.

4.4.2   Cytokine Responses in Candidiasis

Concerning cytokines, clinical evaluation of Th1/Th2 cytokines in vaginal lavage fluid of women with RVVC showed no differences in comparison to control women without a history of vaginitis. Cytokine production was associated with the elicitation of Th1-type (IL-2, IL-12, IFN-γ) and Th2-type (IL-4, IL-10, TGF-β) responses in the vagina and draining lymph nodes during an experimental *C. albicans* vaginal infection in mice. It was found that in naïve animals TGF-β1 production was at least twofold higher at the protein level and tenfold higher at the mRNA level than the other cytokines evaluated, while most of the Th1 and Th2 cytokines were present at extremely low levels. These high levels of TGF-β1 were further increased as a result of pseudoestrus and/or infection, and furthermore, the levels of TGF-β in naïve or infected mice were significantly higher in the vagina compared to other areas of the genital tract. Finally, TGF-β1 predominated as well in the draining, but not in nondraining lymph nodes during infection. Of the evaluated Th1/Th2 cytokines, TGF-β1 had the greatest likelihood of impacting the vaginal microenvironment and the local immune response, which may be suggestive of the newly classified Th3-type response based on the predominance of TGF-β1 and the virtual absence of changes in other Th-type cytokines during infection.

Witkin reported that PBMCs from patients with CRVVC showed a decreased in vitro proliferative response to *Candida* as compared to controls. This was shown to be due to the amplified production of prostaglandin E2 by macrophages which inhibits production of IL-2 and, therefore, the proliferation of lymphocytes. Due to this impaired lymphocyte response, *C. albicans* can proliferate and initiate a clinical infection. Prostaglandin E2 production can arise as a consequence of a vaginal allergic response due to local release of histamine. The allergen could be a semen constituent, an environmental product or a component of *C. albicans*. The result of a vaginal allergy can thus result in a weakened immune response against vaginal infections. Epitopes of *C. albicans* enolase have been detected as binding sites for IgE antibodies. The role of *Candida* IgE in vaginal candidiasis is considered to be an important one. Earlier studies proposed the existence of allergic reactions to *Candida* in the sense of a local vaginal hypersensitive immune response and suggested an allergic cause for chronic and recurrent symptoms. In patients with CRVVC, *Candida*-specific IgE were detected in vaginal secretions, which further supports the presence of a local vaginal hypersensitivity.

One hundred and four women with clinical symptoms of a CRVVC and 44 healthy controls were analyzed regarding IgE expression. *Candida* was detected by cultures in about 30 % of all symptomatic patients and by PCR in 42 % of all symptomatic patients. Prostaglandin E2, whole IgE, and *Candida*-specific-IgE were investigated. Prostaglandin E2 and the *Candida* IgE were significantly higher in comparison with the control group. A further study concentrated on the comparison of 150 healthy women and 74 women with vaginal *Candida*-infection with respect to IL-8 and glucose in vaginal secretions. Healthy women showed not only higher concentrations of physiological lactobacilli, lower levels of neutrophils, and a significantly lower presence of gram-positive cocci but also higher titers of IL-8. With respect to glucose levels, there was no difference between these two groups. An explanation could be that higher vaginal levels of the proinflammatory IL-8 in healthy persons serve as expression of an activated immune state or that IL-8 may be inhibited in women with vaginal infection or downregulated in a kind of feedback mechanism.

4.4.3 Antibody Responses in Candidiasis

The efficacy of humoral immune mechanisms and the role of antibodies against *C. albicans* has been a controversial subject for decades. It is usually assumed that antibodies play little or no role in defense against this infection. This is based on the fact that the disease is not more common or more clinically serious in subjects with Ig disorders, and that subjects with candidiasis often have high titres of anti-*Candida* antibodies in their plasma, not different from that of uninfected subjects. Such *Candida*-specific antibodies have not been associated with protection against infection, while other reports indicated that antibodies against *C. albicans* might be protective against experimental disseminated candidiasis (310, 983).

Similar to other studies, higher levels of *Candida*-specific IgA, IgG1, and IgG4 have been found in those with symptomatic VVC. The authors suggested that the increase in antibodies may indicate a role in fungal clearance. However, similar to previous studies showing similar findings, the increase in antibodies correlated with increased rather than decreased fungal burden, and the study was not designed to examine an endpoint of clearance. Thus, it would appear that the antibodies are induced in response to the organism, but there is no evidence of any role in clearance or protection. Instead, it is equally possible that the antibodies actually contribute to the pathogenesis.

The fact that VVC and RVVC occur in normal antibodies responders does not mean that women with VVC produce identical antibodies at the same location. Protective antibodies with specificity to a limited number of yeast epitopes might not necessarily be produced at protective levels, and some relevant yeast epitopes might not be expressed constitutively. Several earlier studies reported that antibodies are not protective against candidiasis but in the 1960s; however, reports indicated that antibodies against *C. albicans* might be protective against experimental disseminated candidiasis. Evidence from experimental settings of rodent models suggests that antibodies against specific virulence factors of the fungus play an important role in protection. This indicates that antibodies and cell-mediated immune responses are both active in the host–fungus relationship and can contribute to the host protection against yeast.

Finally, it is important to consider the extracellular nature of the infectious agent and its possession of several virulence traits, many of which are in principle inhibitable by suitable antibodies. Indeed, protective antibodies against well-defined virulence factors of the fungus have been reported. Furthermore, anti-idiotypic killer antibodies (KAbs) have been described that carry the internal image of a yeast killer toxin (KT) from a selected strain of the yeast *Pichia anomala* (PaKT), thus functionally mimicking it. KTs are glycosylated proteins secreted by self-immune yeasts, which exert a microbicidal activity against sensitive microorganisms characterized by the presence of specific KT cell wall receptors (KTR). On the basis of previous observations, and through the exploitation of new molecular technologies, three different possible immunotherapeutic strategies have been developed based on protective antibodies, KAbs, and therapeutic vaccines, as discussed below.

4.4.4 Effect of Reproductive Hormones

The use of oral contraceptives and hormone replacement therapy was shown to predispose women to VCC. Clinical observations indicated that VVC most often occurred in women during the luteal phase of the menstrual cycle, when estrogen and progesterone levels were elevated. In contrast, premenarchal and postmenopausal women who do not receive hormone replacement therapy, rarely, suffer from VVC.

Estrogen and progesterone have been shown to inhibit aspects of both innate and acquired immunity at the systemic or local level, including *Candida*-specific human peripheral blood lymphocyte responses or neutrophil anti-*Candida* activity in vitro. Furthermore, in vitro *Candida-specific* lymphocyte responses were reduced in

women during the luteal phase of the menstrual cycle concomitant with increased serum-induced germination of *C. albicans*.

Although estrogen-dependent experimental rodent models of *C. albicans* vaginal infection are used for many applications, the role of reproductive hormones and their limits in the acquisition of vaginal candidiasis remain unclear. The effects of estrogen and progesterone on several aspects of an experimental infection together with cell-mediated immune responses were also evaluated. Results showed that near-physiological concentrations of estrogen were as capable as supraphysiological concentrations of sustaining experimental infections induced by a wide range of *C. albicans* inocula. Additionally, it was found that a persistent infection with high numbers of organisms could equally occur if estrogen treatments were initiated several days before or after inoculation. The requirement for a maintained state of pseudoestrus was confirmed by the rapid clearance of the infection when the estrogen treatments were removed. Finally, estrogen was found to reduce the ability of vaginal ECs to inhibit the growth of *C. albicans*. In contrast to estrogen, progesterone treatment alone could not support an experimental vaginal infection for any significant period of time. In fact, vaginal fungal burdens in progesterone-treated animals were lower than those in untreated animals. This may have been due to a lack of or reduced influence by endogenous estrogen. Interestingly, progesterone had no effect on the titers of *C. albicans* in the vagina, rates of infection, or chronicity of the vaginal infection in the presence of estrogen. Furthermore, estrogen and progesterone treatment of mice had no effect on *Candida*-specific systemic cell-mediated immunity, i.e., in vitro proliferation of lymph node cells in response to *Candida* antigens.

Taken together, estrogen is predicted to be the primary factor in susceptibility to vaginitis during the luteal phase of the menstrual cycle, despite higher concentrations of progesterone than estrogen during that time. This is also consistent with the lack of prevalence of *Candida* vaginitis in women taking progesterone contraceptives. On the other hand, one may speculate that it is the peak levels of estrogen during the short ovulatory phase of the menstrual cycle that precipitates the vaginal infection and that the symptomatic infection does not fully present itself until the luteal phase. Similarly, one would predict that despite high levels of progesterone during pregnancy, the high incidence of vaginitis in pregnant women is more likely due to estrogen.

4.4.5 Immunotherapeutic Strategies

The first immunotherapeutic strategy is based on protective antibodies against immunodominant candidal antigens. Many candidal virulence factors such as adhesins and the enzymes aspartyl proteinases can stimulate the immune system to generate an immune response. Several studies tested antibodies against specific candidal proteins which were protective against natural and experimental disseminated candidiasis. Protective antibodies against disseminated candidiasis and vaginal infection were elicited by a vaccine composed of liposome-encapsulated C. albicans surface mannan. An IgM monoclonal antibody (mAb) specific for β-1,2-mannotriose, an acid-labile component of the cell wall phosphomannoproteins acting as an adhesin, protected normal inbred, outbred, severe combined immunodeficient, and neutropenic mice against disseminated or vaginal experimental candidiasis. Passive transfer of vaginal fluids from animals clearing a primary C. albicans infection conferred significant protection against vaginitis in naïve rats. This protection was associated with the presence of both anti-mannan and anti-Sap antibodies, mostly of the IgG and IgA isotypes. However, the mechanisms of protection by these antibodies against Candida infection are still unclear.

The second immunotherapeutic approach is based on KAbs. KAbs exert a remarkable candidacidal activity in vitro and confer significant immunoprotection against infection in systemic and mucosal animal models of candidiasis. KAbs functionally mimic PaKT by interacting with a putative PaKT receptor expressed on the yeast cell wall. The mimicry of the yeast killer phenomenon through the Id network has allowed the development of exclusive models of Id vaccination and anti-Id therapy, which could represent new approaches to the control of systemic and mucosal candidiasis. Direct use of the toxic and instable PaKT is not possible but a marked systemic or mucosal immunoprotection mediated by KAbs has been induced by parenteral or vaginal Id vaccination using a PaKT-neutralizing mAb in mice and in rats. An active immunization with immunogenic and protective microbial antigens represents a hallmark strategy to prevent or fight infectious diseases. To date, no effective prophylactic or therapeutic vaccine has been developed against candidiasis, although studies are in progress in animal models. Because of the antigenic complexity of Candida, it has been difficult to define the putative protective antigens to be considered for an effective vaccine. Moreover, the human commensal nature of the fungus, and the consequent natural "immunization" against it, poses several obstacles for the feasibility of a prophylactic vaccine. More realistic might be the generation of therapeutic vaccines. Generally, one might question whether a vaccine against vaginal candidiasis will be useful, given that women with VVC or RVVC are not generally immunosuppressed.

Interestingly, immunization with the L-mannan vaccine in mice induced an increased resistance to VVC. A recombinant form of the mannoprotein which was identified as the major target of T-cell response in humans is investigated as an active immunogen in mice and rats. A therapeutic vaccine in a murine model of oral candidiasis was recently reported. They have used this model to identify regulatory and effector molecules of T-cell activation as parameters of induced immunity. Oral but not systemic immunization with the blastospore yeast form induced clinical immunity with a shift in parameters of cytokine response characterized by an early and sustained production of both IFN-γ and IL-4 from antigen-stimulated cervical node T lymphocytes. As studies have demonstrated the importance of the Th1 cytokine pattern in the anti-*Candida* immune response and in the vaginal mucosa, a role for some cytokines typical of a Th1 response has been considered. However, no evidence for a beneficial outcome of a pure cytokine or anti-cytokine treatment has yet been reported. Some antifungals, such as amphotericin B, have direct immunomodulatory properties, suggesting that a combination of chemotherapy with cytokines and antibodies might have greater potential for the treatment of RVVC.

4.5 Trichomoniasis

Vaginal infections caused by the parasitic protozoan *Trichomonas vaginalis* are among the most common conditions found in women attending reproductive health facilities. The prevalence of trichomoniasis in young women attending American STD clinics for routine care typically approaches 25–48 % in certain populations. The WHO has estimated that this infection with 170 million cases per year accounts for almost half of all curable STDs worldwide. Based on WHO estimates, it is one of the two most common STDs in the United States with approximately 7.4 million new cases in 2000. Symptoms of trichomoniasis in women include vaginal discharge, odor, irritation, and pruritus; however, about half of all women infected with *T. vaginalis* are asymptomatic, and in males the infection appears usually to be asymptomatic. The pathogenesis of *T. vaginalis* is not well understood, also in respect to factors causing symptomatic versus asymptomatic infections in women. The extent of the inflammatory response to the parasite may determine the severity of the symptoms.

Although survival on fomites is documented, the organism is thought to be transmitted almost exclusively by sexual activity. Epidemiologically, *T. vaginalis* infections are also commonly associated with other STDs, particularly BV (322, 613). Unlike other STDs, which have a higher prevalence among adolescents and young adults, the rates of trichomoniasis are more evenly distributed among sexually active women of all age groups, further strengthening its potential utility

as a sensitive marker for high-risk sexual behavior.

Acquisition of HIV has been associated with trichomoniasis in several African studies, possibly as a result of local inflammation caused by the parasite. A significant difference between the prevalence of trichomoniasis among a cohort of HIV-infected and noninfected pregnant women in Rwanda was recently demonstrated, with 20.2 % versus 10.9 %, respectively. In a prospective analysis an incident trichomoniasis was significantly associated with HIV seroconversion among a cohort of women in Zaire in multivariate analysis. Additionally, significantly higher rates of vaginal trichomoniasis among women residing in high HIV prevalence cities than in low HIV prevalence cities was reported, suggesting that trichomoniasis may be an important factor in determining rates of HIV. Moreover, trichomoniasis is associated with adverse pregnancy outcome, such as preterm birth and premature rupture of placental membranes; this is further elucidated in the chapter on infections and preterm birth.

The existing literature provides little information on the host and parasite factors leading to symptomatic or asymptomatic *T. vaginalis* infection in women. The existence of two types of *T. vaginalis* strains, each differing in its morphological characteristics and intrinsic virulence, has been suggested.

4.5.1 Innate Immune Responses in Trichomoniasis

Current understanding of immunity to *T. vaginalis* has come largely from observations of responses in human patients and experimentation using in vitro models and animal models of the related species, *T. foetus*. The host immune responses to *T. vaginalis* infection are reported to be usually low and variable. Moreover, natural infection seems to produce immunity that is only partially protective, since the reinfection rate of patients can be as high as 36 % on follow-up. Factors that influence the host inflammatory response are not well understood but may include hormone levels, the coexisting vaginal flora, and the strain and relative concentration of the organisms present in the vagina. Observations indicate that innate immunity involving chemotaxis and subsequent influx of neutrophils may be more important than acquired immunity in controlling infections with *T. vaginalis*, since neutrophils are the predominant inflammatory cells found in vaginal discharges in response to infection.

4.5.1.1 Toll-Like Receptors

While it is clear that *T. vaginalis* infection can induce an inflammatory response in the female genital tract, the types of receptors involved in host recognition of the pathogen have not yet been established. Additionally, *T. vaginalis* infection of women is associated with the presence in the genital tract of a substance produced either by *T. vaginalis* or by genital tract cells as an innate immune response to infection that interacts with TLR4. Genital tract secretions from infected women stimulated TNF-α production by cells with functional TLR4 but significantly less by cells that were unresponsive to TLR4 ligands. Secretions collected after clearance of infection also induced significantly lower responses in cells with functional TLR4. TNF-α responses were not reduced by polymyxin B and did not correlate with β2-defensin levels, indicating that stimulation of cells was not through LPS or β2-defensin. These studies show that *T. vaginalis* infection results in the appearance of substances in the genital tract that stimulate cells through TLR4, suggesting a mechanism for the inflammation caused by this infection.

Interestingly, however, ECs from normal human vagina, ectocervix, and endocervix do not appear to express TLR4 and consequently do not respond to LPS, but they do express mRNA for TLR1, TLR2, TLR3, TLR5, and TLR6. Findings therefore suggest that ECs in the genital tract would not be stimulated during infection with *T. vaginalis*, and a severe inflammatory response is initially avoided until the migration of leukocytes into the genital tract establishes an inflammatory response since neutrophils, monocytes, and macrophages express TLR4. It may be relevant that in many cases *T. vaginalis* infection is relatively

asymptomatic until menses although numbers of *T. vaginalis* organisms decrease at this time. Thus, the initiation of symptoms correlates with the introduction of leukocytes into the lower genital tract from the upper genital tract that likely come into contact with *T. vaginalis* organisms.

4.5.1.2 The Role of Neutrophils

Vaginal inflammatory leukocytes in urogenital trichomoniasis were almost exclusively PMNs, and their concentration was positively correlated with the number of trichomonads in the vaginal exudate. Also, patients with a clinical picture of severe mucosal inflammation had significantly higher vaginal exudate leukocyte concentrations and viability than those without inflammatory signs. Groups of PMNs surrounding large trichomonads are able to fragment them and phagocytose the pieces.

Little is known about the exact mechanism of how neutrophils accumulate or mediate the initial inflammatory response after acute *T. vaginalis* infection. The parasite has been shown to secrete proteins, for example, excretory–secretory product (ESP), that are chemotactic to PMNs. These neutrophils can be further stimulated by *T. vaginalis* to produce chemokines such as IL-8 and GRO-α, mediated through the NF-κB and MAP-kinase signaling pathways. IL-8 is found in high levels in vaginal discharges of symptomatic trichomoniasis patients. *T. vaginalis* membrane components have been shown to induce blood monocytes and neutrophils to produce IL-8, probably with the help of TNF-α. IL-8 has been shown to enhance antimicrobial activities of neutrophils by inducing neutrophil degranulation and respiratory burst. However, during prolonged *T. vaginalis* adhesion, later proinflammatory production of TNF-α and IL-12 was suppressed, accompanied by inhibition of NF-κB activity, suggesting that *T. vaginalis* may inhibit the NF-κB activity of macrophages. A further chemoattractant found in high levels in vaginal discharges of symptomatic patients is leukotriene B4, and its presence at such levels could be due to release from *T. vaginalis* or from neutrophils induced by the interaction of trichomonads and humoral immunity. Humoral immunity could further promote the interaction of neutrophils with *T. vaginalis* and augment the inflammatory response through the amplification of leukotriene B4 production.

In vitro experiments showed that *T. vaginalis* selectively adhered to human vaginal ECs and exerted their cytopathogenic effects. It is possible that IL-8 production is induced in vaginal ECs early in infection when vaginal ECs are activated with *T. vaginalis*. *Candida* and *N. gonorrhoeae* have been reported to induce IL-8 production by vaginal ECs early in infection as well. These may subsequently induce more infiltration and recruitment of neutrophils by chemotaxis at the reaction site.

4.5.1.3 Complement

Of the known chemoattractants involved in the inflammatory response of *T. vaginalis* infection, complement components have been documented to play a role in the activation of neutrophils as well. Human neutrophils in combination with serum were able to kill *T. vaginalis*. This serum was shown to have specific IgG antibodies for *T. vaginalis*, which facilitated neutrophil killing by an IgG-enhanced classical component pathway. However, also antibody-independent alternative complement pathway activation provided C3 for *T. vaginalis* to facilitate neutrophil killing. The importance of the alternative complement pathway in host defense against *T. vaginalis* was investigated in vitro. Kinetic studies using immunofixation following electrophoresis showed that both a strongly and weakly virulent strain of *T. vaginalis* activated murine serum C3. In vivo studies on mice showed that the presence of C5 is also a significant factor in innate host resistance to primary infection with a strongly, but not a weakly virulent trichomonad strain.

T. vaginalis seems to have taken advantage of a niche in which little complement is present as cervical mucus is surprisingly deficient in complement. However, a role for an alternative pathway activation of complement and the trichomonocidal effect of menstrual blood complement has suggested. Menstrual blood represents the only source of complement available to the vagina and has appreciable complement-mediated cytotoxicity toward *T. vaginalis*, and

although a reduction in parasite concentration is seen during menses, trichomonal infection persists even after menses.

It has also been found that iron is a contributing factor in complement resistance. Fresh isolates of *T. vaginalis* differ in their susceptibility or resistance to complement-mediated lysis in serum. It appears that complement-resistant fresh isolates become susceptible to complement after prolonged in vitro cultivation, which is consistent with the hypothesis that phenotypic variation allows the trichomonad to avoid lysis by complement. Resistance to complement is dependent upon a high concentration of iron, a nutrient which is indeed abundant during menses. It seems that iron upregulates the expression of proteases, which have been found to degrade the C3 portion of complement on the surface of the organism; this allows the organism to evade complement-mediated destruction.

4.5.1.4 Nitric Oxide and RNIs

It has become increasingly clear that the oxidant–antioxidant balance is essential for immune cell function. Neutrophil and macrophage phagocytosis can also stimulate other cellular processes, including the respiratory burst, whereby increased cellular oxygen uptake results in the production of antimicrobial compounds, *T. vaginalis* by O_2 dependent mechanisms. PMNs were able to eliminate *T. vaginalis* in vitro under aerobic conditions, which speaks for the importance of oxidative microbicidal systems.

Nitric oxide and other ROS/ROI produced by immune effector cells such as macrophages are important cytotoxic mediators in microbial infections. The synthesis of nitric oxide by macrophages also results in antimicrobial activity against another protozoan, *Leishmania major*, which was regulated by the cytokines TNF and TGF controlling parasite survival or killing via IFN-γ.

The mean concentration of RNI in vaginal tissue of mice infected with isolates from symptomatic women was significantly higher than that of vaginal tissue of mice infected with isolates from asymptomatic women while it was less than in the vaginal washes and plasma of mice infected with isolates from symptomatic women compared to those infected with isolates from asymptomatic women. This may have been due to different macrophage populations with different functional capabilities. However, this would suggest a possible role for RNI production in establishing the infection. Mean RNI concentration was significantly higher in leukocytes and vaginal washes of asymptomatic women as compared to symptomatic women and was also higher in samples of infected as compared to healthy women. This suggests that RNI may have a role in limiting *T. vaginalis* infection in asymptomatic women.

4.5.2 Specific Immunity in Trichomoniasis

4.5.2.1 Antibodies

T. vaginalis infection in humans results in parasite-specific antibodies that can be found in the serum and vaginal secretions of infected individuals. IgA antibodies in serum of infected patients correlate to their clinical status. The presence of systemic IgG antibodies of all subclasses may be related to a local response of IgG-secreting cells but may also represent a systemic response to released antigen. Moreover, IgG, IgM, and IgA antibodies have been found in serum of patients. Specific antibody responses to *T. vaginalis* antigens in serum and specific local antibodies, both IgG and IgA, have also been identified in women.

An experimental mouse model showed a significant increase in serum and vaginal IgA levels in mice infected with *T. vaginalis* isolates from asymptomatic women compared with mice infected with isolates from symptomatic women and control mice. A further significant response was also observed in group A and group B mice as compared with the control group. In another study, a significant increase in the specific IgA antibody response was detected in serum samples and vaginal washes of *T. vaginalis*-infected women. These results suggest that specific IgA antibodies might help to protect asymptomatic individuals from severe infection. IgA antibodies

may also act as a first line of defense for immune exclusion of the parasite at the mucosal surface. Nevertheless, although an association between the presence of local antibody and low parasite counts has been postulated, there is no conclusive evidence to suggest that the presence of IgA antibodies is specifically related to the immune response to *T. vaginalis*.

Several trichomonad antigens appear to be important for the above-mentioned responses, including α-actinin and adhesins, and the recently detected TV44 via an IgA mAb. Multiple signaling pathways seem to be functional for distinct surface proteins of *T. vaginalis*, and *T. vaginalis* responds during infection both to environmental cues like iron and to adherence to vaginal ECs by up- and downregulating expression of genes. Also *Candida albicans* undergoes both up- and downregulation of surface proteins after host cell contact. However, despite the first report describing IgA mAb reactivity to a surface protein of *T. vaginalis*, the protective role of IgA in recognition of surface protein immunogens in trichomoniasis is poorly understood. IgA has been associated with resistance to a number of other mucosal pathogens, such as *Chlamydia trachomatis* or mycobacteria.

Anti-*Trichomonas* IgG, IgM, IgA, and IgG subclass antibody responses on different postinfection days in serum and vaginal washes of mice infected intravaginally with *T. vaginalis* isolates from 15 symptomatic and 15 asymptomatic women. A significant increase in parasite load was observed on the 14th postinfection day (pid) in mice inoculated with *T. vaginalis* isolates from symptomatic women as compared to asymptomatic women, followed by reduction until the 28th pid. A significant increase in specific IgG and in particular IgG1 and IgM responses was observed on the 14th pid in serum and vaginal washes of mice infected with *T. vaginalis* isolates from symptomatic women as compared to asymptomatic women. Significant increases in specific IgG, IgM, and IgG1 responses were observed on the 14th pid in serum samples as compared with vaginal washes of mice infected with *T. vaginalis* isolates from symptomatic and asymptomatic women, whereas no significant difference was observed in IgA, IgG2a, IgG2b, and IgG3 antibody responses. The study indicates that specific IgG, particularly IgG1 and IgM, may be playing a role in establishing symptomatic infection. Provenzano and Alderete have reported that numerous proteases secreted by *T. vaginalis* degrade IgG, IgM, and IgA, which allows the organism to survive the antibody response.

Four antigenic surface molecules have also been implicated in the adhesion of *T. vaginalis* to vaginal ECs; their expression is upregulated during attachment to host cells. Antibodies to these molecules protected target cells from parasite-mediated cytotoxicity, suggesting that anti-adhesion immune responses could be important in in vivo protection against the pathogenic effects of *T. vaginalis*.

Alternatively, antibodies specific for soluble parasite molecules such as proteases, cytoactive molecules, or lytic factors such as phospholipases may also be protective. However, proof of the protective nature of antibodies in eliminating infection or limiting pathogenesis in vivo has been hampered by lack of an adequate experimental animal model for vaginal infection studies.

4.5.2.2 T Lymphocytes

The presence of parasite-specific IgG and IgA responses also indicates priming of T-helper cells, although the relevant antigens are largely unknown, as are the exact effects of antibodies on the parasites. A significant increase in the population of total T cells, as well as CD4+ T cells, was detected in mice infected with isolates from asymptomatic women compared with mice infected with symptomatic isolates. No significant difference was observed in CD8+ cells, whereas a significant difference between the two groups was noticed in the vital CD4+/CD8+ ratio. Also a significant increase in NK cells was observed in animals infected with isolates from asymptomatic women compared with mice infected with isolates from symptomatic women and control uninfected mice, indicating that NK cells might be playing a role in the pathogenesis of this disease. An increase in CD4+ T cells in mice infected with isolates from asymptomatic women appears to be beneficial; it suggests that these cells have a role in the elimination of *T. vaginalis* from their mucosal surface. Clearance of *T. vaginalis* in these animals correlated well with development of anti-IgA antibodies. These results on cytokine production also suggest that the Th1-type response might play a role in the elimination of *T. vaginalis*.

4.5.3 The Role of Cytokines

The cytokine profile in vaginal cervical tissues of mice infected intravaginally with *T. vaginalis* isolates from 15 symptomatic and 15 asymptomatic women was the subject of a bath further analysis, demonstrating that the concentrations of IFN-γ and TNF-α in vaginal washes of mice infected with isolates from symptomatic and asymptomatic women were significantly higher compared to uninfected mice. Between the two infected groups, IFN and TNF levels were higher in the group of mice infected with isolates of asymptomatic women. Significantly higher IL-2 production was observed in mice infected with isolates from asymptomatic women compared mice infected with isolates from symptomatic women or the uninfected control group. IL-4 levels were found to be significantly higher when results from both groups infected with isolates were compared with controls.

IL-8 is found in high levels in vaginal discharges of symptomatic trichomoniasis patients. This cytokine has been shown to enhance antimicrobial activities of neutrophils by inducing neutrophil degranulation and respiratory burst. The possible role of IL-8 was also analyzed, demonstrating that membrane components of *T. vaginalis* induced blood monocytes to produce large dose- and time-dependent amounts of this cytokine. Amounts of IL-8 were higher than those induced by live trichomonads or ESP. Neutrophil chemotaxis was inhibited by a neutralizing mAb directed against IL-8 itself or partly decreased by a mAb directed against TNF-α, suggesting also a role for TNF-α in the release of IL-8. Interestingly, *T. vaginalis* can induce IL-8 production in neutrophils which may be mediated through the NF-κB and mitogen-activated protein (MAP) kinase signaling pathways. Live *T. vaginalis* produced higher amounts of IL-8 than ESP or *T. vaginalis* lysate. Moreover, GRO-α, another chemoattractant for PMNs, was also produced by neutrophils in response to *T. vaginalis* activation. NF-κB is implicated in the regulation of inflammatory responses by inducing cytokines such as IL-12 and TNF-α and activating effector molecules of innate immunity including macrophages. *T. vaginalis* induced a rapid activation of NF-κB in RAW264.7 macrophage during the early stage of adhesion which was not maintained but led to inhibition of the production of the proinflammatory cytokines. Furthermore, *T. vaginalis* infection induced a state of nonresponsiveness to subsequent stimulation with bacterial LPS which suggests that *T. vaginalis* induces an inhibitory mechanism that prevents or delays the immune response of host cells, thereby leading to their apoptotic cell death.

4.5.4 Vaccination Strategies

Systemic immunization of cows with a purified surface antigen of *T. foetus* induced serum and vaginal IgG and IgA antibodies, and intravaginal boosting enhanced the genital IgA response to infectious challenge. IgG and IgA antibodies in vaginal secretions were associated with protection or faster clearance of infection. Interestingly, lymphoid aggregates in the vagina and uterus in response to infectious challenge were demonstrated in control and intravaginally immunized animals, which suggests development of mucosal inductive sites for local IgA responses. Immunity has been difficult to produce in vivo, since in humans, repeated infections with *T. vaginalis* do not confer immune protection. Despite this, antibodies can be found in the serum and vaginal secretions of infected individuals and a cell-mediated immune response is also invoked. Older experimental work using subcutaneous or intraperitoneal injections in mice suggested that antibodies could be protective, and more recent experiments with immunized mice challenged by

intravaginal inoculation indeed indicate some protection.

Interestingly an induction of immunity to *T. vaginalis* was demonstrated in a mouse model, which may lead to the development of a vaccine. Whole, live trichomonads at different concentrations were injected subcutaneously into mice, first with Freund's complete adjuvant and then in a booster dose with the trichomonads and Freund's incomplete adjuvant. The mice were given estrogen and inoculated intravaginally with *Lactobacillus acidophilus* to simulate the conditions in the human vagina; they were then inoculated intravaginally with *T. vaginalis*. Immunized mice had significantly less intravaginal infection and had elevated antibody levels in the serum and vagina compared with naïve control groups. Mice that had been infected vaginally, treated, and reinfected vaginally were not protected and did not mount an immune response which suggests that antigen presentation may be crucial for developing protective immunity. To date, only one vaccine, the Solco Trichovac vaccine, had been produced against *T. vaginalis*. It was prepared from inactive lactobacilli and was thought to work by inducing antibodies to abnormal lactobacilli and *T. vaginalis* without adversely affecting the growth of normal lactobacilli in the vagina. However, a lack of antigenic similarity between this vaccine and *T. vaginalis* was shown, which makes this cross-reaction hypothesis unlikely. It is also to be noted that antiserum to *L. acidophilus* failed to inhibit trichomonad cytoadherence or host cell killing.

4.5.5 Summary

In conclusion, the findings suggest that both humoral and cellular immune responses might contribute to the varied symptomatology in trichomoniasis-infected patients, thereby reducing symptoms to asymptomatic levels. Periodic changes in immune competence, perhaps induced by parasite-derived products, might be responsible for an increase in parasite numbers, leading to increased epithelial damage and inflammatory response. However, the current understanding of immunity to *T. vaginalis* remains unsatisfactory, and it is not clear whether acquired immune responses are required for protection and, if so, what role is played by acquired immunity in containing or eliminating infections. Although there is some evidence that protection may be achieved by immunization of laboratory animals, strong protective immunity does not seem to follow natural infection in humans. A study of patients infected with *T. vaginalis* and HIV indicated no evidence of increased levels or longevity of parasite infection in these patients compared to those in patients infected with *T. vaginalis* but not HIV positive. These observations may indicate that innate immunity involving chemotaxis and the subsequent influx of neutrophils is much more important than acquired immunity in controlling infections with *T. vaginalis*.

Further Reading

Introduction

Donovan B. Sexually transmissible infections other than HIV. Lancet. 2004;363:545–56.

Weinstock H, Berman S, Cates Jr W. Sexually transmitted diseases among American youth: incidence and prevalence estimates, 2000. Perspect Sex Reprod Health. 2004;36:6–10.

World Health Organisation. Global prevalence and incidence of selected curable sexually transmitted infections: overview and estimates. Geneva: WHO; 2001.

Herpes Simplex Virus

Alsallaq RA, Schiffer JT, Longini Jr IM, Wald A, Corey L, Abu-Raddad LJ. Population level impact of an imperfect prophylactic vaccine for herpes simplex virus-2. Sex Transm Dis. 2010;37:290–7.

Ashkar AA, Rosenthal KL. Interleukin-15 and natural killer and NKT cells play a critical role in innate protection against genital herpes simplex virus type 2 infection. J Virol. 2003;77:10168–71.

Ashkar AA, Bauer S, Mitchell WJ, Vieira J, Rosenthal KL. Local delivery of CpG oligodeoxynucleotides induces rapid changes in the genital mucosa and inhibits replication, but not entry, of herpes simplex virus type 2. J Virol. 2003;77:8948–56.

Ashley RL, Corey L, Dalessio J, Wilson P, Remington M, Barnum G, Trethewey P. Protein- specific antibody responses to primary genital herpes simplex virus type 2 infections. J Infect Dis. 1994a;170:20–6.

Ashley RL, Wald A, Corey L. Cervical antibodies in patients with oral herpes simplex virus type 1 (HSV-1) infection: local anamnestic responses after genital HSV-2 infection. J Virol. 1994b;68:5284–6.

Aurelian L. Herpes simplex virus type 2 vaccines: new ground for optimism? Clin Diagn Lab Immunol. 2004; 11:437–45.

Bernstein DI, Harrison CJ, Tomai MA, Miller RL. Daily or weekly therapy with resiquimod (R- 848) reduces genital recurrences in herpes simplex virus-infected guinea pigs during and after treatment. J Infect Dis. 2001;183:844–9.

Bernstein DI, Cardin RD, Bravo FJ, et al. Potent adjuvant activity of cationic liposome-DNA complexes for genital herpes vaccines. Clin Vaccine Immunol. 2009;16: 699–705.

Cassatella MA. The production of cytokines by polymorphonuclear neutrophils. Immunol Today. 1995;16:21–6.

Chentoufi AA, Dasgupta G, Christensen ND, et al. A novel HLA (HLA-A*0201) transgenic rabbit model for preclinical evaluation of human CD8+ T cell epitope-based vaccines against ocular herpes. J Immunol. 2010;184:2561–71.

Cheshenko N, Herold BC. Glycoprotein B plays a predominant role in mediating herpes simplex virus type 2 attachment and is required for entry and cell-to-cell spread. J Gen Virol. 2002;83:2247–55.

Clinical Effectiveness Group. National guideline for the management of genital herpes. Sex Transm Infect. 1999;75:524–8.

Corwin E, Bozoky I, Pugh L, Johnston N. Interleukin-1beta elevation during the postpartum period. Ann Behav Med. 2003;25:41–7.

Cunningham AL, Mikloska Z. The Holy Grail: immune control of human herpes simplex virus infection and disease. Herpes. 2001;8 Suppl 1:6A–10.

Cunningham AL, Turner RR, Miller AC, Para MF, Merigan TC. Evolution of recurrent herpes simplex virus lesions: a immunohistologic study. J Clin Invest. 1985;75:226–33.

Duerst RJ, Morrison LA. Innate immunity to herpes simplex virus type 2. Viral Immunol. 2003;16:475–90.

Fleming DT, McQillan GM, Johnson RE, Nahmias AJ, Aral SO, Lee FK, St. Louis ME. Herpes simplex virus type 2 in the United States, 1976 to 1994. N Engl J Med. 1997;337:1105–11.

Fries LF, Friedman HM, Cohen GH, Eisenberg EJ, Hammer CH, Frank MM. Glycoprotein C of herpes simplex virus 1 is an inhibitor of the complement cascade. J Immunol. 1986;137:1636–41.

Gadjeva M, Paludan SR, Thiel S, Slavov V, Ruseva M, Eriksson K, Lowhagen GB, Shi L, Takahashi K, Ezekowitz A, Jensenius JC. Mannan-binding lectin modulates the response to HSV-2 infection. Clin Exp Immunol. 2004;138:304–11.

Gallichan WS, Woolstencroft RN, Guarasci T, McCluskie MJ, Davis HL, Rosenthal KL. Intranasal immunization with CpG oligodeoxynucleotides as an adjuvant dramatically increases IgA and protection against herpes simplex virus-2 in the genital tract. J Immunol. 2001;166:3451–7.

Garg S, Anderson RA, Chany 2nd CJ, Waller DP, Diao XH, Vermani K, Zaneveld LJ. Properties of a new acid-buffering bioadhesive vaginal formulation (ACIDFORM). Contraception. 2001;64:67–75.

Garred P, Madsen HO, Balsley U, Hofmann B, Pedersen C, Gerstoft J, Svejgaard A. Susceptibility to HIV infection and progression of AIDS in relation to variant alleles of mannose-binding lectin. Lancet. 1997; 349:236–40.

Gill N, Rosenthal KL, Ashkar AA. NK and NKT cell-independent contribution of interleukin-15 to innate protection against mucosal viral infection. J Virol. 2005;79:4470–8.

Gutzeit C, Raftery MJ, Peiser M, et al. Identification of an important immunological difference between virulent varicella-zoster virus and its avirulent vaccine: viral disruption of dendritic cell instruction. J Immunol. 2010;185:488–97.

Halford WP, Maender JL, Gebhardt BM. Re-evaluating the role of natural killer cells in innate resistance to herpes simplex type 1. Virol J. 2005;17:56.

Harandi AM, Svennerholm B, Holmgren J, Eriksson K. Differential roles of B cells and IFN- gamma-secreting CD4(+) T cells in innate and adaptive immune control of genital herpes simplex virus type 2 infection in mice. J Gen Virol. 2001;82:845–53.

Hashemi H, Bamdad T, Jamali A, Pouyanfard S, Mohammadi MG. Evaluation of humoral and cellular immune responses against HSV-1 using genetic immunization by filamentous phage particles: a comparative approach to conventional DNA vaccine. J Virol Methods. 2010;163:440–4.

Hashido M, Kawana T. Herpes simplex virus-specific IgM, IgA and IgG subclass antibody responses in primary and nonprimary genital herpes patients. Microbiol Immunol. 1997;41:415–20.

Hill A, Jugovic P, York I, Russ G, Bennink J, Yewdell J, Ploegh H, Johnson D. Herpes simplex virus turns off TAP to evade host immunity. Nature. 1995;375:411–5.

Iwasaki A. The role of dendritic cells in immune responses against vaginal infection by herpes simplex virus type 2. Microbes Infect. 2003;5:1221–30.

John M, Keller MJ, Fam EH, Cheshenko N, Hogarty K, Kasowitz A, Wallenstein S, Carlucci MJ, Tuyama AC, Lu W, Klotman ME, Lehrer RI, Herold BC. Cervicovaginal secretions contribute to innate resistance to herpes simplex virus infection. J Infect Dis. 2005;192:1731–40.

Kaushic C, Ashkar AA, Reid LA, Rosenthal KL. Progesterone increases susceptibility and decreases immune responses to genital herpes infection. J Virol. 2003;77:4558–65.

Keller MJ, Madan RP, Shust G, Carpenter CA, Torres NM, Cho S, Khine H, Huang ML, Corey L, Kim M, Herold BC. Changes in the soluble mucosal immune environment during genital herpes outbreaks. J Acquir Immune Defic Syndr. 2012;61(2):194–202.

King NJ, Parr EL, Parr MB. Migration of lymphoid cells from vaginal epithelium to iliac lymph nodes in relation to vaginal infection by herpes simplex virus type 2. J Immunol. 1998;160:1173–80.

Koelle DM, Tigges MA, Burke RL, Symington FW, Riddell SR, Abbo H, Corey L. Herpes simplex virus infection of human fibroblasts and keratinocytes inhibits recognition by cloned CD8+ cytotoxic T lymphocytes. J Clin Invest. 1993;91:961–8.

Koelle DM, Abbo H, Peck A, Ziegweid K, Corey L. Direct recovery of herpes simplex virus (HSV)-specific T lymphocyte clones from recurrent genital HSV-2 lesions. J Infect Dis. 1994;169:956–61.

Koelle DM, Frank JM, Johnson ML, Kwok WW. Recognition of herpes simplex virus type 2 tegument proteins by CD4 T cells infiltrating human genital herpes lesions. J Virol. 1998a;72:7476–83.

Koelle DM, Posavad CM, Barnum GR, Johnson ML, Frank JM, Corey L. Clearance of HSV-2 from recurrent genital lesions correlates with infiltration of HSV-specific cytotoxic T lymphocytes. J Clin Invest. 1998b; 101:1500–8.

Koelle DM, Chen HB, Gavin MA, Wald A, Kwok WW, Corey L. CD8 CTL from genital herpes lesions: recognition of viral tegument and immediate early proteins and lysis of infected cutaneous cells. J Immunol. 2001;166:4049–58.

Krieg AM. CpG motifs in bacterial DNA and their immune effects. Annu Rev Immunol. 2002;20:709–60.

Kuklin NA, Daheshia M, Chun S, Rouse BT. Role of mucosal immunity in Herpes simplex virus infection. J Immunol. 1998;160:5998–6003.

Kurt-Jones EA, Chan M, Zhou S, Wang J, Reed G, Bronson R, Arnold MM, Knipe DM, Finberg RW. Herpes simplex virus 1 interaction with toll-like receptor 2 contributes to lethal encephalitis. Proc Natl Acad Sci USA. 2004;101:1315–20.

Kwant A, Rosenthal KL. Intravaginal immunization with viral subunit protein plus CpG oligodeoxynucleotides induces protective immunity against HSV-2. Vaccine. 2004;22:3098–104.

Linehan MM, Richman S, Krummenacher C, Eisenberg RJ, Cohen GH, Iwasaki A. In vivo role of nectin-1 in entry of herpes simplex virus type 1 (HSV-1) and HSV-2 through the vaginal mucosa. J Virol. 2004;78: 2530–6.

Lubinski JM, Jiang M, Hook L, Chang Y, Sarver C, Mastellos D, Lambris JD, Cohen GH, Eisenberg RJ, Friedman HM. Herpes simplex virus type 1 evades the effects of antibody and complement in vivo. J Virol. 2002;76:9232–41.

Lund J, Sato A, Akira S, Medzhitov R, Iwasaki A. Toll-like receptor 9-mediated recognition of herpes simplex virus-2 by plasmacytoid dendritic cells. J Exp Med. 2003;198:513–20.

Marchetti M, Trybala E, Superti F, Johansson M, Bergstrom T. Inhibition of herpes simplex virus infection by lactoferrin is dependent on interference with the virus binding to glycosaminoglycans. Virology. 2004;318:405–13.

Martin Jr HL, Nyange PM, Richardson BA, Lavreys L, Mandaliya K, Jackson DJ, Ndinya-Achola JO, Kreiss J. Hormonal contraception, sexually transmitted diseases, and risk of heterosexual transmission of human immunodeficiency virus type 1. J Infect Dis. 1998;178: 1053–9.

MasCasullo V, Fam E, Keller MJ, Herold BC. Role of mucosal immunity in preventing genital herpes infection. Viral Immunol. 2005;18:595–606.

Mastrolorenzo A, Tiradritti L, Salimbeni L, Zuccati G. Multicentre clinical trial with herpes simplex virus vaccine in recurrent herpes infection. Int J STD AIDS. 1995;6:431–5.

Mbopi-Keou FX, Belec L, Dalessio J, Legoff J, Gresenguet G, Mayaud P, Brown DWG, Morrow RA. Cervicovaginal neutralizing antibodies to herpes simplex virus (HSV) in women seropositive for HSV types 1 and 2. Clin Diagn Lab Immunol. 2003;10:388–93.

McCluskie MJ, Cartier JLM, Patrick AJ, Sajic D, Weeratna RD, Rosenthal KL, Davis H. Treatment of intravaginal HSV-2 infection in mice. A comparison of CpG oligodeoxynucleotides and resiquimod (R-848). Antiviral Res. 2006;69:77–85.

McDermott MR, Brais IJ, Evelegh MJ. Mucosal and systemic antiviral antibodies in mice inoculated intravaginally with herpes simplex virus type 2. J Gen Virol. 1990;71:1497–504.

McLean CS, Erturk M, Jennings R, Ni Challanain D, Minson AC, Duncan I, Boursnell MEG, Inglis SC. Protective vaccination against primary and recurrent disease caused by herpes simplex virus (HSV) type 2 using a genetically disabled HSV-1. J Infect Dis. 1994; 170:1100–9.

McNeely TB, Dealy M, Dripps DJ, Orenstein JM, Eisenberg SP, Wahl SM. Secretory leukocyte protease inhibitor: a human saliva protein exhibiting antihuman immunodeficiency virus 1 activity in vitro. J Clin Invest. 1995;96:456–64.

Meignier B, Longnecker R, Roizman B. In vivo behavior of genetically engineered herpes simplex viruses R7017 and R7020: construction and evaluation in rodents. J Infect Dis. 1988;158:602–14.

Meschi J, Crouch EC, Skolnik P, Yahya K, Holmskov U, Leth-Larsen R, Tornoe I, Tecle T, White MR, Hartshorn KL. Surfactant protein D binds to human immunodeficiency virus (HIV) envelope protein gp120 and inhibits HIV replication. J Gen Virol. 2005;86:3097–107.

Mikloska Z, Danis VA, Adams S, Lloyd AR, Adrian DL, Cunningham AL. In vivo production of cytokines and β (C-C) chemokines in human recurrent herpes simplex virus lesions-do herpes simplex virus infected keratinocytes contribute to their production? J Infect Dis. 1998;177:827–38.

Mikloska Z, Sanna PP, Cunningham AL. Neutralizing antibodies inhibit axonal spread of herpes simplex virus type 1 to epidermal cell in vitro. J Virol. 1999;73: 5933–44.

Mikloska Z, Bosnjak L, Cunningham AL. Immature monocyte-derived dendritic cells are productively infected with herpes simplex virus type 1. J Virol. 2001;75:5958–64.

Milligan GN, Bernstein DI. Analysis of herpes simplex virus-specific T cells in the murine female genital tract following genital infection with herpes simplex virus type 2. Virology. 1995;212:481–9.

Milligan GN, Bernstein DI, Bourne N. T lymphocytes are required for protection of the vaginal mucosae and sensory ganglia of immune mice against reinfection with herpes simplex virus type 2. J Immunol. 1998; 160:6093–100.

Mohamedi SA, Heath AW, Jennings R. A comparison of oral and parenteral routes for therapeutic vaccination with HSV-2 ISCOMs in mice; cytokine profiles, antibody responses and protection. Antiviral Res. 2001;49: 83–99.

Nagashunmugam T, Lubinski J, Wang L, Goldstein LT, Weeks BS, Sundaresan P, Kang EH, Dubin G, Friedman HM. In vivo immune evasion mediated by the herpes simplex virus type 1 immunoglobulin G Fc receptor. J Virol. 1998;72:5351–9.

Nordström I, Nurkkala M, Collinns V, Eriksson K. CD8+ T-cells suppress antigen-specific and allogeneic CD4+ T-cell responses to herpes simplex virus type 2-infected human dendritic cells. Viral Immunol. 2005;18:616–26.

Orange JS, Geha RS. Finding NEMO: genetic disorders of NF-[kappa]B activation. J Clin Invest. 2003;112: 983–5.

Parr EL, Parr MB. Immunoglobulin G is the main protective antibody in mouse vaginal secretions after vaginal immunization with attenuated herpes simplex virus type 2. J Virol. 1997;71:8109–15.

Parr EL, Parr MB. Immunoglobulin G, plasma cells, and lymphocytes in the murine vagina after vaginal or parenteral immunization with attenuated herpes simplex virus type 2. J Virol. 1998a;72:5137–45.

Parr MB, Parr EL. Mucosal immunity to herpes simplex virus type 2 infection in the mouse vagina is impaired by in vivo depletion of T lymphocytes. J Virol. 1998b;72:2677–85.

Parr MB, Parr EL. Immunity to vaginal herpes simplex virus-2 infection in B-cell knockout mice. Immunology. 2000a;101:126–31.

Parr MB, Parr EL. Interferon-gamma up-regulates intercellular molecule-1 and vascular cell adhesion molecule-1 and recruits lymphocytes into the vagina of immune mice challenged with herpes simplex virus-2. Immunology. 2000b;99:540–5.

Parr MB, Parr EL. Vaginal immunity in the HSV-2 mouse model. Int Rev Immunol. 2003;22:43–63.

Parr EL, Parr MB. Female genital tract infections and immunity in animal models. In: Mestecky J, Lamm ME, Strober W, Bienenstock J, McGhee JR, Mayer L, editors. Handbook of mucosal immunology. 3rd ed. Oxford: Elsevier Academic Press; 2005. p. 1613–30.

Parr MB, Kepple L, McDermott MR, Drew MD, Bozzola JJ, Parr EL. A mouse model for studies of mucosal immunity to vaginal infection by herpes simplex virus type 2. Lab Invest. 1994;70:369–80.

Parr EL, Bozzola JJ, Parr MB. Immunity to vaginal infection by herpes simplex virus type 2 in adult mice: characterization of the antibody in vaginal mucus. J Reprod Immunol. 1998a;38:15–30.

Parr MB, Harriman GR, Parr EL. Immunity to vaginal HSV-2 infection in immunoglobulin A knockout mice. Immunology. 1998b;95:208–13.

Parsania M, Bamdad T, Hassan ZM, et al. Evaluation of apoptotic and anti-apoptotic genes on efficacy of DNA vaccine encoding glycoprotein B of Herpes Simplex Virus type 1. Immunol Lett. 2010;128:137–42.

Pellis V, De Seta F, Crovella S, Bossi F, Bulla R, Guaschino S, Radillo O, Garred P, Tedesco F. Mannose binding lectin and C3 act as recognition molecules for infectious agents in the vagina. Clin Exp Immunol. 2005;139:120–6.

Peretti S, Shaw A, Blanchard J, Bohm R, Morrow G, Lifson JD, Gettie A, Pope M. Immunomodulatory effects of HSV-2 infection on immature macaque dendritic cells modify innate and adaptive responses. Blood. 2005;106:1305–13.

Posavad CM, Koelle DM, Corey L. High frequency of CD8+ cytotoxic T-lymphocyte precursors specific for herpes simplex viruses in persons with genital herpes. J Virol. 1996;70:8165–8.

Prechtel AT, Turza NM, Kobelt DJ, Eisemann JI, Coffin RS, McGrath Y, Hacker C, Ju X, Zenke M, Steinkasser A. Infection of mature dendritic cells with herpes simplex virus type 1 dramatically reduces lymphoid chemokine-mediated migration. J Gen Virol. 2005;86:1645–57.

Pyles RB, Higgins D, Chalk C, Zalar A, Eiden J, Brown C, Van Nest G, Stanberry LR. Use of immunostimulatory sequence-containing oligonucleotides as topical therapy for genital herpes simplex virus type 2 infection. J Virol. 2002;76:11387–96.

Reszka NJ, Dudek T, Knipe DM. Construction and properties of a herpes simplex virus 2 dl5-29 vaccine candidate strain encoding an HSV-1 virion host shutoff protein. Vaccine. 2010;28:2754–62.

Rosenthal KS, Killius J, Hodnichak CM, Venetta TM, Gyurgyik L, Janiga K. Mild acidic pH inhibition of the major pathway of herpes simplex virus entry into HEp-2 cells. J Gen Virol. 1989;70:857–67.

Siegal FP, Lopez C, Hammer GS, Brown AE, Kornfeld SJ, Gold J, Hassett J, Hirschman SZ, Cunningham-Rundles C, Adlsberg BR. Severe acquired immunodeficiency in male homosexuals, manifested by chronic perianal ulcerative herpes simplex lesions. N Engl J Med. 1981;305:1439–44.

Singh M, Carlson JR, Briones M, Ugozzoli M, Kazzaz J, Barackman J, Ott G, O'Hagan D. A comparison of biodegradable microparticles and MF59 as systemic adjuvants for recombinant gD from HSV-2. Vaccine. 1998;16:1822–7.

Smith CC, Peng T, Kulka M, Aurelian L. The PK domain of the large subunit of herpes simplex virus type 2 ribonucleotide reductase (ICP10) is involved in immediate-early gene transcription and virus growth. J Virol. 1998;72:9131–41.

Spruance S, Tyring S, Smith M, Meng TC. Application of a topically applied immune response modifier, resiquimod gel, to modify the recurrence rate of recurrent genital herpes: a pilot study. J Infect Dis. 2001;84:196–200.

Stanberry LR. Clinical trials of prophylactic and therapeutic herpes simplex virus vaccines. Herpes. 2004;11:A161–70.

Stanberry LR, Bernstein DI, Burke RL, Pachl C, Myers MG. Vaccination with recombinant herpes simplex virus glycoproteins: protection against initial and recurrent genital herpes. J Infect Dis. 1987;155:914–20.

Stanberry LR, Cunningham AL, Mindel A, Scott LL, Spruance SL, Aoki FY, Lacey CJ. Prospects for control of herpes simplex virus disease through immunization. Clin Infect Dis. 2000;30:549–66.

Torseth JW, Merigan TC. Significance of local γ-interferon in recurrent herpes simplex infection. J Infect Dis. 1986;153:979–84.

Wald A, Link K. Risk of human immunodeficiency virus infection in herpes simplex virus type 2-seropositive persons: a meta-analysis. J Infect Dis. 2002;185:45–52.

Wald A, Zeh J, Selke S, Warren T, Ryncarz AJ, Ashley R, Krieger JN, Corey L. Reactivation of genital herpes simplex virus type 2 infection in asymptomatic seropositive persons. N Engl J Med. 2000;342:844–50.

Whitley RJ, Kimberlin DW, Roizman B. Herpes simplex viruses. Clin Infect Dis. 1998;26:541–53.

Wilson M, Seymour R, Henderson B. Bacterial perturbation of cytokine networks. Infect Immun. 1998;66:2401–9.

Yasin B, Wang W, Pang M, Cheshenko N, Hong T, Waring AJ, Herold BC, Wagar EA, Lehrer RI. Theta defensins protect cells from infection by herpes simplex virus by inhibiting viral adhesion and entry. J Virol. 2004;78:5147–56.

Zhao X, Deak E, Soderberg S, Linehan M, Spezzano D, Zhu J, Knipe DM, Iwasaki A. Vaginal submucosal dendritic cells, but not Langerhans cells, induce protective Th1 responses to herpes simplex virus-2. J Exp Med. 2003;197:153–62.

Human Immunodeficiency Virus

Agostini C, Semenzato G. Immunologic effects of HIV in the lung. Clin Chest Med. 1996;17:633–45.

Ahmed SM, Al-Doujaily H, Johnson MA, Kitchen V, Reid WM, Poulter LW. Immunity in the female lower genital tract and the impact of HIV infection. Scand J Immunol. 2001;54:225–38.

Ahn WS, Bae SM, Kim TY, Kim TG, Lee JM, Namkoong SE, Kim CK, Sin JI. A therapy modality using recombinant IL-12 adenovirus plus E7 protein in a human papillomavirus 16 E6/E7-associated cervical cancer animal model. Hum Gene Ther. 2003;14:1389–99.

Al-Harthi L, Landay A. HIV in the female genital tract: viral shedding and mucosal immunity. Clin Obstet Gynecol. 2001;44:144–53.

Al-Harthi L, Spear GT, Hashemi FB, Landay A, Sha BE, Roebuck KA. A human immunodeficiency virus (HIV)-inducing factor from the female genital tract activates HIV-1 gene expression through the kappaB enhancer. J Infect Dis. 1998;178:1343–51.

Al-Harthi L, Roebuck KA, Olinger GG, Landay A, Sha BE, Hashemi FB, Spear GT. Bacterial vaginosis-associated microflora isolated from the female genital tract activates HIV-1 expression. J Acquir Immune Defic Syndr. 1999;22:194–202.

Al-Harthi L, Kovacs A, Coombs RW, Reichelderfer PS, Wright DJ, Cohen MH, Cohn J, Cu-Uvin S, Watts H, Lewis S, Beckner S, Landay A, WHS 001 study team. A menstrual cycle pattern for cytokine levels exists in HIV-positive women: implication for HIV vaginal and plasma shedding. AIDS. 2001;15: 1535–43.

Anderson DJ, Politch JA, Tucker LD, Fichorova R, Haimovici F, Tuomala RE, Mayer KH. Quantitation of mediators of inflammation and immunity in genital tract secretions and their relevance to HIV type 1 transmission. AIDS Res Hum Retroviruses. 1998;14 Suppl 1:S43–9.

Asin S, Fanger M, Wildt-Perinic D, Ware P, Wira C, Howell A. HIV-1 transmission by primary human uterine epithelial and stromal cells. J Infect Dis. 2004; 190:236–45.

Bélec L, Meillet D, Hernvann A, Grésenguet G, Gherardi R. Differential elevation of circulating interleukin-1β, tumor necrosis factor alpha, and interleukin-6 in AIDS-associated cachectic states. Clin Diagnos Lab Immunol. 1994;1:177–20.

Belec L, Dupre T, Prazuck T, Tevi-Benissan C, Kanga JM, Pathey O, Lü XS, Pillot J. Cervicovaginal overproduction of specific IgG to human immunodeficiency virus (HIV) contrasts with normal or impaired IgA local response in HIV infection. J Infect Dis. 1995a;172: 691–7.

Belec L, Gherardi R, Payan C, Prazuck T, Malkin JE, Tevi-Benissan C, Pillot J. Proinflammatory cytokine expression in cervicovaginal secretions of normal and HIV-infected women. Cytokine. 1995b;7: 568–74.

Berger EA, Murphy PM, Farber JM. Chemokine receptors as HIV-1 coreceptors: roles in viral entry, tropism and disease. Annu Rev Immunol. 1999;17:657–700.

Bienzle D, MacDonald K, Smaill F, Kovacs C, Baqi M, Courssaris B, Luscher MA, Walmsley SL, Rosenthal KL. Factors contributing to the lack of human immunodeficiency virus type 1 (HIV-1) transmission in HIV-1-discordant partners. J Infect Dis. 2000;182: 123–32.

Braida L, Boniotto M, Pontillo A, Tovo PA, Amoroso A, Crovella S. A single-nucleotide polymorphism in the human beta-defensin 1 gene is associated with HIV-1 infection in Italian children. AIDS. 2004;18: 1598–600.

Coombs RW, Reichelderfer PS, Landay AL. Recent observations on HIV type-1 infection in the genital tract of men and women. AIDS. 2003;17:455–80.

Diaz-Mitoma F, Kumar A, Karimi S, Kryworuchko M, Daftarian MP, Creery WD, Filion LG, Cameron W. Expression of IL-10, IL-4 and interferon-gamma in unstimulated and mitogen- stimulated peripheral blood lymphocytes from HIV-seropositive patients. Clin Exp Immunol. 1995;102:31–9.

Donaghy H, Stebbing J, Patterson S. Antigen presentation and the role of dendritic cells in HIV. Curr Opin Infect Dis. 2004;17:1–6.

Dorrell L, Hessell AJ, Wang M, Whittle H, Sabally S, Rowand-Jones S, Burton DR, Parren PW. Absence of specific mucosal antibody responses in HIV-exposed uninfected sex workers from the Gambia. AIDS. 2000;14:1117–22.

Dreyfus M, Baldauf JJ, Ritter J, Obert G. Seric and local antibodies against a synthetic peptide of HPV16. Eur J Obstet Gynecol Reprod Biol. 1995;59:187–91.

Farrar DJ, Cu-Uvin S, Caliendo AM, Costello SF, Murphy DM, Flanigan TP, Mayer KH, Carpenter CC. Detection of HIV-1 RNA in vaginal secretions of HIV-1-seropositive women who have undergone hysterectomy. AIDS. 1997;11:1296–7.

Fauci AS. Host factors and the pathogenesis of HIV-induced disease. Nature. 1996;384:529–34.

Fortis C, Polis G. Dendritic cells and natural killer cells in the pathogenesis of HIV infection. Immunol Res. 2005;33:1–21.

Geijtenbeek TB, Kwon DS, Torensma R, van Vliet SJ, van Duijnhoven GCF, Mddel J, Cornelissen ILMHA, Nottet HSLM, KewalRamani VN, Littman DR, Figdor CG, van Kooyk Y. DC-SIGN, a dendritic cell-specific HIV-1-binding protein that enhances transinfection of T cells. Cell. 2000;100:587–97.

Ghosh D. Glucocorticoid receptor-binding site in the human immunodeficiency virus long terminal repeat. J Virol. 1992;66:586–90.

Gray RH, Waver MJ, Brookmeyer R, Sewankambo NK, Serwadda D, Wabwire-Mangen F, Lutalo T, Li X, van Cott T, Quinn TC, Rakai Project Team. Probability of HIV-1 transmission per coital act in monogamous, heterosexual, HIV-1 discordant couples in Rakai, Uganda. Lancet. 2001;357:1149–53.

Gupta P, Collins KB, Ratner D, Watkins S, Naus GJ, Landers DV, Patterson BK. Memory CD4+ T cells are the earliest detectable human immunodeficiency virus type 1 (HIV-1)- infected cells in the female genital mucosal tissue during HIV-1 transmission in an organ culture system. J Virol. 2002;76:9868–76.

Harlow SD, Schuman P, Cohen M, Ohmit SE, Cu-Uvin S, Lin X, Anastos K, Burns D, Greenblatt R, Minkoff H, Muderspach L, Rompalo A, Warren D, Young MA, Klein RS. Effect of HIV infection on menstrual cycle length. J Acquir Immune Defic Syndr Hum Retrovirol. 2000;24:68–75.

Hocini H, Bomsel M. Infectious human immunodeficiency virus can rapidly penetrate a tight human epithelial barrier by transcytosis in a process impaired by mucosal immunoglobulins. J Infect Dis. 1999;179 Suppl 3:S448–53.

Howell AL, Edkins RD, Rier SE, Yeaman GR, Stern JE, Fanger MW, Wira CR. Human immunodeficiency virus type 1 infection of cells and tissues from the upper and lower human female reproductive tract. J Virol. 1997;71:3498–506.

Howell AL, Asin SN, Yeaman GR, Wira CR. HIV-1 infection in the female reproductive tract. Curr HIV/AIDS Rep. 2005;2:35–8.

Hu J, Gardner MB, Miller CJ. Simian immunodeficiency virus rapidly penetrates the cervicovaginal mucosa after intravaginal inoculation and infects intraepithelial dendritic cells. J Virol. 2000;74:6087–95.

Jameson BA, Rao PE, Kong LI, Hahn BH, Shaw GM, Hood LE, Kent SB. Location and chemical synthesis of a binding site for HIV-1 on the CD4 receptor. Science. 1988;240:1335–9.

Janoff EN, Jackson S, Wahl SM, Thomas K, Peterman JH, Smith PD. Intestinal mucosal immunoglobulins during human immunodeficiency virus type 1 infection. J Infect Dis. 1994;170:299–307.

Kaul R, Plummer FA, Kimani J, Dong T, Kiama P, Rostron T, Njagi E, MacDonald KS, Bwayo JJ, McMichael AJ, Rowland-Jones SL. HIV-1 specific mucosal CD8+ lymphocyte responses in the cervix of HIV-1 resistant prostitutes in Nairobi. J Immunol. 2000;164:1602–11.

Kaul R, Thottingal P, Kimani J, Kiama P, Waigwa CW, Bwayo JJ, Plummer FA, Rowland-Jones SL. Quantitative ex vivo analysis of functional virus-specific CD8 T lymphocytes in the blood and genital tract of HIV-infected women. AIDS. 2003;17: 1139–44.

Kemal KS, Foley B, Burger H, Anastos K, Minkoff H, Kitchen C, Philpott SM, Gao W, Robison E, Holman S, Dehner C, Beck S, Meyer III WA, Landay A, Kovacs A, Bremer J, Weiser B. HIV-1 in genital tract and plasma of women: Compartmentalization of viral sequences, coreceptor usage, and glycosylation. Proc Natl Acad Sci USA. 2003;100:12972–7.

Kostense S, Ogg GS, Manting EH, Gillespie G, Joling J, Vandenberghe K, Veenhof EZ, van Baarle D, Juriaans S, Klein MR, Miedema F. High viral burden in the presence of major HIV- specific CD8+ T cell expansions: evidence for impaired CTL effector function. Eur J Immunol. 2001;31:677–86.

Kwon DS, Gregorio G, Bitton N, Hendrickson WA, Littman DR. DC-SIGN-mediated internalization of HIV is required for trans-enhancement of T cell infection. Immunity. 2002;16:135–44.

Lervin NL, Barouch DH, Montefiori DC. Prospects for vaccine protection against HIV-1 infection and AIDS. Annu Rev Immunol. 2002;20:73–99.

Lohman BL, Miller CJ, McChesney MB. Antiviral cytotoxic T lymphocytes in vaginal mucosa of simian immunodeficiency virus-infected rhesus macaques. J Immunol. 1995;155:5855–60.

Lü FX. Predominate HIV1-specific IgG activity in various mucosal compartments of HIV1- infected individuals. Clin Immunol. 2000;97:59–68.

Ma G, Greenwell-Wild T, Lei K, Jin W, Swisher J, Hardegen N, Wild CT, Wahl SM. Secretory leukocyte protease inhibitor binds to annexin II, a cofactor for macrophage HIV-1 infection. J Exp Med. 2004; 200:1337–46.

Marx PA, Spira AI, Gettie A, Dailey PJ, Veazey RS, Lackner AA, Mahoney CJ, Miller CJ, Claypool LE, Ho DD, Alexander NJ. Progesterone implants enhance SIV vaginal transmission and early virus load. Nat Med. 1996;2:1084–9.

McMichael AJ, Rowland-Jones SL. Cellular immune responses to HIV. Nature. 2001;410:980–7.

McNeely TB, Dealy M, Dripps DJ, Orenstein JM, Eisenberg SP, Wahl SM. Secretory leukocyte protease inhibitor: a human saliva protein exhibiting anti-human immunodeficiency virus 1 activity in vitro. J Clin Invest. 1995;96:456–64.

Miller CJ, Lü FX. Anti-HIV and -SIV immunity in the vagina. Int Rev Immunol. 2003;22:65–76.

Miller CJ, Alexander NJ, Sutjipto S, Lackner AA, Gettie A, Hendrickx AG, Lowenstine LJ, Jennings M, Marx PA. Genital mucosal transmission of simian immunodeficiency virus: animal model for heterosexual transmission of human immunodeficiency virus. J Virol. 1989;63:4277–84.

Mostad SB. Prevalence and correlates of HV type 1 shedding in the female genital tract. AIDS Res Hum Retroviruses. 1998;14 Suppl 1:11–5.

Musey L, Hu Y, Eckert L, Christensen M, Karchmer T, McElrath MJ. HIV-1 induces cytotoxic T lymphocytes in the cervix of infected women. J Exp Med. 1997; 185:293–303.

Ogg GS, Jin X, Bonhoeffer S, Dunbar PR, Nowak MA, Monard S, Segal JP, Cao Y, Rowland-Jones SL, Cerundolo V, Hurley A, Markowitz M, Ho DD, Nixon DF, McMichael AJ. Quantitation of HIV-1 specific cytotoxic T lymphocytes and plasma load of viral RNA. Science. 1998;279:2103–6.

Olaitan A, Johnson MA, Reid WM, Poulter LW. Changes to the cytokine microenvironment in the genital tract mucosa of HIV1 women. Clin Exp Immunol. 1998; 112:100–4.

Olinger GG, Hashemi FB, Sha BE, Spear GT. Association of indicators of bacterial vaginosis with a female genital tract factor that induces expression of HIV-1. AIDS. 1999;13:1905–12.

Pearce-Pratt R, Phillips DM. Studies of adhesion of lymphocytic cells: implications for sexual transmission of human immunodeficiency virus. Biol Reprod. 1993; 48:431–45.

Pett SL, Zaunders J, Bailey M, et al. A novel chemokine-receptor-5 (CCR5) blocker, SCH532706, has differential effects on CCR5 + CD4+ and CCR5 + CD8+ T cell numbers in chronic HIV infection. AIDS Res Hum Retroviruses. 2010;26:653–61.

Pillay K, Coutsoudis A, Agadzi-Naqvi AK, Kuhn L, Coovadia HM, Janoff EN. Secretory leukocyte protease inhibitor in vaginal fluids and perinatal human immunodeficiency virus type 1 transmission. J Infect Dis. 2001;183:653–6.

Poli G, Fauci AS. The effect of cytokines and pharmacologic agents on chronic HIV infection. AIDS Res Hum Retroviruses. 1992;8:191–7.

Politch JA, Mayer KH, Anderson DJ. Depletion of CD4+ T cells in semen during HIV infection and their restoration following antiretroviral therapy. J Acquir Immune Defic Syndr. 2009;50:283–9.

Poppe W, Drijkoningen M, Ide P, Lauweryns J, Van Assche F. Lymphocytes and dendritic cells in the normal uterine cervix. An immunohistochemical study. Reprod Biol. 1998;81:277–82.

Pudney J, Quayle AJ, Anderson DJ. Immunological microenvironments in the human vagina and cervix: mediators of cellular immunity are concentrated in the cervical transformation zone. Biol Reprod. 2005;73:1253–63.

Qiu JT, Chang TC, Lin CT, et al. Novel codon-optimized GM-CSF gene as an adjuvant to enhance the immunity of a DNA vaccine against HIV-1 Gag. Vaccine. 2007;25:253–63.

Quinones-Mateu ME, Lederman MM, Feng Z, Chakraborty B, Weber J, Rangel HR, Marotta ML, Mirza M, Jiang B, Kiser P, Medvik K, Sieg SF, Weinberg A. Human epithelial beta- defensins 2 and 3 inhibit HIV-1 replication. AIDS. 2003;17:F39–48.

Rabot M, Tabiasco J, Polgar B, Aguerre-Girr M, Berrebi A, Bensussan A, Strbo N, Rukavina D, Le Bouteiller P. HLA class I/NK cell receptor interaction in early human decidua basalis: possible functional consequences. Chem Immunol Allergy. 2005;89:72–83.

Raghupathy R, Mutawa EA, Makhseed M, Azizieh F, Szekeres-Bartho J. Modulation of cytokine production by dehydrogesterone in lymphocytes from women with recurrent miscarriage. BJOG. 2005;112:1096–101.

Reichelderfer PS, Coombs RW, Wright DJ, Cohn J, Burns DN, Cu-Uvin S, Baron PA, Coheng MH, Landay AL, Beckner SK, Lewis SR, Kovacs AA. Effect of menstrual cycle on human immunodeficiency virus type 1 levels in the peripheral blood and genital tract. WHS 001 study team. AIDS. 2000;14:2101–7.

Reka S, Kotler DP. Detection and localisation of HIV RNA and TNF mRNA in rectal biopsies from patients with AIDS. Cytokine. 1993;5:305–8.

Shaheen F, Sison AV, McIntosh L, Mukhtar M, Pomerantz RJ. Analysis of HIV-1 in the cervicovaginal secretions and blood of pregnant and nonpregnant women. J Hum Virol. 1999;2:154–66.

Smith S, Charkraborty P, Baskin G. Estrogen protects against vaginal transmission of SIV. In: Program and abstracts (abstract 119) of the 7th Conference on Retroviruses and Opportunistic Infections, Chicago, 30 Jan–2 Feb 2000.

Smith BA, Gartner S, Liu Y, Perelson AS, Stilianakis NI, Keele BF, Kerkering TM, Ferreira-Gonzalez A, Szakal AK, Tew JG, Burton GF. Persistence of infectious HIV on follicular dendritic cells. J Immunol. 2001;166:690–6.

Terry VH, Johnston IC, Spina CA. CD44 microbeads accelerate HIV-1 infection in T cells. Virology. 2009;388:294–304.

Thurman AR, Doncel GF. Innate immunity and inflammatory response to Trichomonas vaginalis and bacterial vaginosis: relationship to HIV acquisition. Am J Reprod Immunol. 2011;65:89–98.

Turville SG, Cameron PU, Handley A, Lin G, Pohlmann S, Doms RW, Cunningham AL. Diversity of receptors binding HIV on dendritic cell subsets. Nat Immunol. 2002;3:975–83.

Vassiliadou N, Tucker L, Anderson DJ. Progesterone-induced inhibition of chemokine receptor expression on peripheral blood mononuclear cells correlates with reduced HIV-1 infectability in vitro. J Immunol. 1999;162:7510–8.

Vatakis DN, Nixon CC, Bristol G, Zack JA. Differentially stimulated CD4+ T cells display altered human immunodeficiency virus infection kinetics: implications for the efficacy of antiviral agents. J Virol. 2009;83:3374–8.

Wang CC, McClelland RS, Overbaugh J, Reilly M, Panteleeff DD, Mandaliya K, Chohan B, Lavreys L, Ndinya-Achola J, Kreiss JK. The effect of hormonal contraception on genital tract shedding of HIV-1. AIDS. 2004;18:205–9.

Wang X, Xu H, Gill AF, et al. Monitoring alpha4beta7 integrin expression on circulating CD4+ T cells as a surrogate marker for tracking intestinal CD4+ T-cell loss in SIV infection. Mucosal Immunol. 2009;2(6):518–26.

Wijewardana V, Brown KN, Barratt-Boyes SM. Studies of plasmacytoid dendritic cell dynamics in simian immunodeficiency virus infection of nonhuman primates provide insights into HIV pathogenesis. Curr HIV Res. 2009;7:23–9.

WHO/UNAIDS AIDS epidemic update 2004 WHO and UNAIDS, Geneva, December 2004

Wu Z, Cocchi F, Gentles D, Ericksen B, Lubkowski J, Devico A, Lehrer RI, Lu W. Human neutrophil alpha-defensin 4 inhibits HIV-1 infection in vitro. FEBS Lett. 2005;579:162–6.

Yeaman GR, Howell AL, Weldon S, Demian DJ, Collins JE, O'Connell DM, Asin SN, Wira CR, Fanger MF. Human immunodeficiency virus receptor and coreceptor expression on human uterine ECs: regulation of expression during the menstrual cycle and implications for human immunodeficiency virus infection. Immunology. 2003;109:137–46.

Yeaman GR, Asin S, Weldon S, Demian DJ, Collins JE, Gonzalez JL, Wira CR, Fanger MW, Howell AL. Chemokine receptor expression in human ectocervix: implications for infection by the human immunodeficiency virus-type 1. Immunology. 2004;113:524–33.

Zhang Z, Schuler T, Zupancic M, Wietgrefe S, Staskus KA, Reimann KA, Reinhart TA, Rogan M, Cavert W, Miller CJ, Veazey RS, Notermans D, Little S, Danner SA, Richmann DD, Havlir D, Wong J, Jordan HL, Schacker TW, Racz P, Tenner-Racz K, Letvin L, Wolinsky S, Haase AT. Sexual transmission and propagation of SIV and HIV in resting and activated CD4+ T cells. Science. 1999;286:1353–7.

Zhang SY, Zhang Z, Fu JL, et al. Progressive CD127 down-regulation correlates with increased apoptosis of CD8 T cells during chronic HIV-1 infection. Eur J Immunol. 2009;39:1425–34.

Zhu T, Wang N, Carr A, Nam DS, Moor-Jankowski R, Cooper DA, Ho DD. Genetic characterization of human immunodeficiency virus type 1 in blood and genital secretions: evidence for viral compartmentalization and selection during sexual transmission. J Virol. 1996;70:3098–107.

Zhu J, Hladik F, Woodward A, et al. Persistence of HIV-1 receptor-positive cells after HSV-2 reactivation is a potential mechanism for increased HIV-1 acquisition. Nat Med. 2009;15:886–92.

Human Papillomavirus

Alexander M, Salgaller ML, Celis E, Sette A, Barnes WA, Rosenberg SA, Steller MA. Generation of tumor specific cytolytic T-lymphocytes from peripheral blood of cervical cancer patients by in vitro stimulation with a synthetic HPV-16 E7 epitope. Am J Obstet Gynecol. 1996;175:1586–93.

Ault KA, Giuliano AR, Edwards RP, Tamms G, Kim LL, Smith JF, Jansen KU, Allende M, Taddeo FJ, Skulsky D, Barr E. A phase I study to evaluate a human papillomavirus (HPV) type 18 L1 VLP vaccine. Vaccine. 2004;22:3004–7.

Bard E, Riethmüller D, Meillet D, Pretet JL, Schaal JP, Mougin C, Seilles E. High-risk papillomavirus infection is associated with altered antibody responses in genital tract: non- specific responses in HPV infection. Viral Immunol. 2004;17:381–9.

Bontkes HJ, de Gruijl TD, Walboomers JM, Coursaget P, Stukart MJ, Dupuy C, Kueter E, Verheijen RH, Helmerhorst TJ, Duggan-Keen MF, Stern PL, Meijer CJ, Scheper RJ. Immune responses against human papillomavirus (HPV) type 16 virus-like particles in a cohort study of women with cervical intraepithelial neoplasia: II. Systemic but not local IgA responses correlate with clearance of HPV-16. J Gen Virol. 1999;80:409–17.

Bornstein J. The HPV vaccines–which to prefer? Obstet Gynecol Surv. 2009;64:345–50.

Bubenik J. Animal models for development of therapeutic HPV16 vaccines (review). Int J Oncol. 2002;20:207–12.

Campo MS. Animal models of papillomavirus pathogenesis. Virus Res. 2002;89:249–61.

Chellappan S, Kraus VB, Kroger B, Munger K, Howley PM, Phelps PM, Nevins JR. Adenovirus E1A, simian virus 40 tumor antigen, and human papillomavirus E7 protein share the capacity to disrupt the interaction between transcription factor E2F and the retinoblastoma gene product. Proc Natl Acad Sci U S A. 1992;89:4549–53.

Cho YS, Kang JW, Cho M, Cho CW, Lee S, Choe YK, Kim Y, Choi I, Park SN, Kim S, Dinarello CA, Yoon DY. Downmodulation of IL-18 expression by human papillomavirus type 16 E6 oncogene via binding to IL-18. FEBS Lett. 2001;501:139–45.

Clerici M, Merola M, Ferrario E, Trabattoni D, Villa ML, Stefanon B, Venzon DJ, Shearer GM, De Palo G, Cerici E. Cytokine production patterns in cervical intraepithelial neoplasia: association with human papillomavirus infection. J Natl Cancer Inst. 1997;89:245–50.

Daayana S, Elkord E, Winters U, et al. Phase II trial of imiquimod and HPV therapeutic vaccination in patients with vulval intraepithelial neoplasia. Br J Cancer. 2010;102:1129–36.

Dillner J. The serological response to papillomaviruses. Sem Cancer Biol. 1999;9:423–30.

Dreyfus M, Baldauf JJ, Ritter J, Obert G. Seric and local antibodies against a synthetic peptide of HPV16. Eur J Obstet Gynecol Reprod Biol. 1995;59:187–91.

Dupuy C, Buzoni-Gatel D, Touze A, Bout D, Coursaget P. Nasal immunization of mice with human papillomavirus type 16 (HPV-16) virus-like particles or with the HPV-16 L1 gene elicits specific cytotoxic T lymphocytes in vaginal draining lymph nodes. J Virol. 1999;73:9063–71.

Einstein MH, Baron M, Levin MJ, et al. Comparison of the immunogenicity and safety of Cervarix and Gardasil human papillomavirus (HPV) cervical cancer vaccines in healthy women aged 18–45 years. Hum Vaccin. 2009;5:705–19.

Einstein MH, Baron M, Levin MJ, et al. Comparison of the immunogenicity of the human papillomavirus (HPV)-16/18 vaccine and the HPV-6/11/16/18 vaccine for oncogenic non-vaccine types HPV-31 and HPV-45 in healthy women aged 18–45 years. Hum Vaccin. 2011;7:1359–73.

Fattorossi A, Battaglia A, Ferrandina G, Buzzonetti A, Legge F, Salutari V, Scambia G. Lymphocyte composition of tumor draining lymph nodes from cervical and endometrial cancer patients. Gynecol Oncol. 2004;92:106–15.

Frazer IH, Thomas R, Zhou J, Leggatt GR, Dunn L, McMillan N, Tindle RW, Filgueira L, Manders P, Barnard P, Sharkey M. Potential strategies utilised by papillomavirus to evade host immunity. Immunol Rev. 1999;168:131–42.

Govind CK, Gupta SK. Failure of female baboons (Papio anubis) to conceive following immunization with recombinant non-human primate zona pellucida glycoprotein-B expressed in Escherichia coli. Vaccine. 2000;18:2970–8.

Hagensee ME, Koutsky LA, Lee SK. Detection of cervical antibodies to human papillomavirus type 16 (HPV-16) antigens in relation to detection of HPV-16 DNA and cervical lesions. J Infect Dis. 2000;181:1234–9.

Harper DM, Franco EL, Wheeler C, Ferris DG, Jenkins D, Schuind A, Zahaf T, Innis B, Naud P, De Carvalho NS, Roteli-Martins CM, Teixeira J, Blatter MM, Korn AP, Quint W, Dubin G, GlaxoSmithKline HPV Vaccine Study Group. Efficacy of a bivalent L1 virus-like particle vaccine in prevention of infection of human papillomavirus types 16 and 18 in young women: a randomised controlled trial. Lancet. 2004;364:1731–2.

Hildesheim A, Wang SS. Host and viral genetics and risk of cervical cancer: a review. Virus Res. 2002;89: 229–40.

Hinchliffe SA, Van Velzen D, Korporaal H, Kok PL, Boon ME. Transience of cervical HPV infection in sexually active, young women with normal cervicovaginal cytology. Br J Cancer. 1995;72:943–5.

Hoffmann C, Stanke J, Kaufmann AM, Loddenkemper C, Schneider A, Cichon G. Combining T-cell vaccination and application of agonistic anti-GITR mAb (DTA-1) induces complete eradication of HPV oncogene expressing tumors in mice. J Immunother. 2010;33: 136–45.

Hopfl R, Heim K, Christensen N, Zumbach K, Wieland U, Volgger B, Widschwendter A, Haimbuchner S, Müller-Holzner E, Pawlita M, Pfister H, Fritsch P. Spontaneous regression of CIN and delayed-type hypersensitivity to HPV-16 oncoprotein E7. Lancet. 2000;356: 1985–6.

Howley PM. Role of the human papillomaviruses in human cancer. Cancer Res. 1991;51(Suppl):S5019–22.

Huang CY, Chen CA, Lee CN, et al. DNA vaccine encoding heat shock protein 60 co-linked to HPV16 E6 and E7 tumor antigens generates more potent immunotherapeutic effects than respective E6 or E7 tumor antigens. Gynecol Oncol. 2007;107:404–12.

Jemal A, Siegel R, Ward E, Murray T, Xu J, Smigal C, Thun MJ. Cancer statistics, 2006. CA Cancer J Clin. 2006;56:106–30.

Kadish AS, Ho GYF, Burk BD, Wang Y, Romney SL, Ledwidge R, Angeletti RH. Lymphoproliferative responses to human papillomavirus (HPV) type 16 proteins E6 and E7: outcome of HPV infection and associated neoplasia. J Natl Cancer Inst. 1997;89:1285–93.

Kase H, Aoki Y, Tanaka K. Fas ligand expression in cervical adenocarcinoma: relevance to lymph node metastasis and tumor progression. Gynecol Oncol. 2003;90:70–4.

Kaufmann AM, Nieland J, Schinz M, et al. HPV16 L1E7 chimeric virus-like particles induce specific HLA-restricted T cells in humans after in vitro vaccination. Int J Cancer. 2001;92:285–93.

Kaufmann AM, Stern PL, Rankin EM, Sommer H, Nuessler V, Schneider A, Adams M, Onon TS, Bauknecht T, Wagner U, Kroon K, Hickling J, Boswell CM, Stacey SN, Kitchener HC, Gillard J, Wanders J, Roberts JS, Zwierzina H. Safety and immunogenicity of TA-HPV, a recombinant vaccinia virus expressing modified human papillomavirus (HPV)-16 and HPV-18 E6 and E7 genes, in women with progressive cervical cancer. Clin Cancer Res. 2002;8:3676–85.

Kessis TD, Slebos RJ, Nelson WG, Kastan MB, Plunkett BS, Han SM, Lorincz AT, Hedrick L, Cho KR. Human papillomavirus 16 E6 expression disrupts the p53-mediated cellular response to DNA damage. Proc Natl Acad Sci U S A. 1993;90:3988–92.

Kim YJ, Kim KT, Kim JH, et al. Vaccination with a human papillomavirus (HPV)-16/18 AS04-adjuvanted cervical cancer vaccine in Korean girls aged 10–14 years. J Korean Med Sci. 2010;25:1197–204.

Kleine-Lowinski K, Rheinwald JG, Fichorova RN, Anderson DJ, Basile J, Munger K, Daly CM, Rosl F, Rollins BJ. Selective suppression of monocyte chemoattractant protein-1 expression by human papillomavirus E6 and E7 oncoproteins in human cervical epithelial and epidermal cells. Int J Cancer. 2003;107: 407–15.

Kupper TS, Fuhlbrigge RC. Immune surveillance in the skin: mechanisms and clinical consequences. Nat Rev Immunol. 2004;4:211–22.

Lamikanra A, Pan ZK, Isaacs SN, Wu TC, Paterson Y. Regression of established human papillomavirus type 16 (HPV-16) immortalized tumors in vivo by vaccinia viruses expressing different forms of HPV-16 E7 correlates with enhanced CD8+ T cell responses that home to the tumor site. J Virol. 2001;75:9654–64.

Li S, Labrecque S, Gauzzi MC, Cuddihy AR, Wong AH, Pellegrini S, Matlashewski GJ, Koromilas AE. The human papilloma virus (HPV)-18 E6 oncoprotein physically associates with Tyk2 and impairs Jak-STAT activation by interferon alpha. Oncogene. 1999;18: 5727–37.

Lin CT, Tsai YC, He L, et al. DNA vaccines encoding IL-2 linked to HPV-16 E7 antigen generate enhanced E7-specific CTL responses and antitumor activity. Immunol Lett. 2007;114:86–93.

Lin K, Doolan K, Hung CF, Wu TC. Perspectives for preventive and therapeutic HPV vaccines. J Formos Med Assoc. 2010a;109:4–24.

Lin K, Roosinovich E, Ma B, Hung CF, Wu TC. Therapeutic HPV DNA vaccines. Immunol Res. 2010b;47:86–112.

Lorincz AT, Reid R, Jenson AB, Greenberg MD, Lancaster W, Kurman RJ. Human papillomavirus infection of the cervix: relative risk associations of 15 common anogenital types. Obstet Gynecol. 1992;79:328–37.

Man S, Fiander A. Immunology of human papillomavirus infection in lower genital tract neoplasia. Best Pract Res Clin Obstet Gynecol. 2001;15:701–14.

McKenzie J, King A, Hare J, Fulford T, Wilson B, Stanley M. Immunocytochemical characterization of large granular lymphocytes in normal cervix and HPV-associated disease. J Pathol. 1991;165:75–80.

Mota F, Rayment N, Chong S, Singer A, Chain B. The antigen-presenting environment in normal and human papillomavirus (HPV)-related premalignant cervical epithelium. Clin Exp Immunol. 1999;116:33–40.

Muderspach L, Wilczynski S, Roman L, Bade L, Felix J, Small LA, Kast WM, Fascio G, Marty V, Weber J. A phase I trial of a human papillomavirus (HPV) peptide vaccine for women with high-grade cervical and vulvar intraepithelial neoplasia who are HPV 16 positive. Clin Cancer Res. 2000;6:3406–16.

Munoz N, Castellsague X, de Gonzalez AB, Gissmann L. Chapter 1: HPV in the etiology of human cancer. Vaccine. 2006;24 Suppl 3:S3/1–10.

Nees M, Geoghegan JM, Hyman T, Frank S, Miller L, Woodworth CD. Papillomavirus type 16 oncogenes downregulate expression of interferon-responsive genes and upregulate proliferation-associated and

NF-κB-responsive genes in cervical keratinocytes. J Virol. 2001;75:4283–96.

Nonn M, Schinz M, Zumbach K, Pawlita M, Schneider A, Durst M, Kaufmann AM. Dendritic cell-based tumor vaccine for cervical cancer I: in vitro stimulation with recombinant protein- pulsed dendritic cells induces specific T cells to HPV16 E7 or HPV18 E7. J Cancer Res Clin Oncol. 2003;129:511–20.

Orth G, Favre M. Human papillomaviruses. Biochemical and biologic properties. Clin Dermatol. 1985;3: 27–42.

Padilla-Paz LA. Human papillomavirus vaccine: history, immunology, current status, and future prospects. Clin Obstet Gynecol. 2005;48:226–40.

Palmroth J, Namujju P, Simen-Kapeu A, et al. Natural seroconversion to high-risk human papillomaviruses (hrHPVs) is not protective against related HPV genotypes. Scand J Infect Dis. 2010;42:379–84.

Pecoraro G, Morgan D, Defendi V. Differential effects of human papillomavirus type 6, 16, and 18 DNAs on immortalization and transformation of human cervical ECs. Proc Natl Acad Sci U S A. 1989;86:563–7.

Pilch H, Hoehn H, Schmidt M, et al. CD8 + CD45RA + CD27-CD28-T-cell subset in PBL of cervical cancer patients representing CD8 + T-cells being able to recognize cervical cancer associated antigens provided by HPV 16 E7. Zentralbl Gynakol. 2002;124:406–12.

Pinto LA, Edwards J, Castle PE, Harro CD, Lowy DR, Schiller JT, Wallace D, Kopp W, Adelsberger JW, Baseler MW, Berzofsky JA, Hildesheim A. Cellular immune responses to human papillomavirus (HPV)-16 L1 in healthy volunteers immunized with recombinant HPV- 16 L1 virus-like particles. J Infect Dis. 2003;188:327–38.

Pinto LA, Castle PE, Boden RB, Harro CD, Lowy DR, Schiller JT, Wallace D, Williams M, Kopp W, Frazer IH, Berzofsky JA, Hildesheim A. HPV-16 L1 VLP vaccine elicits a broad-spectrum of cytokine responses in whole blood. Vaccine. 2005;23:3555–64.

Santin AD, Bellone S, Palmieri M, et al. HPV16/18 E7-pulsed dendritic cell vaccination in cervical cancer patients with recurrent disease refractory to standard treatment modalities. Gynecol Oncol. 2006;100: 469–78.

Sewell DA, Douven D, Pan ZK, Rodriguez A, Paterson Y. Regression of HPV-positive tumors treated with a new Listeria monocytogenes vaccine. Arch Otolaryngol Head Neck Surg. 2004;130:92–7.

Sheu BC, Lin HC, Lien HC, Ho HN, Hsu SM, Huang SC. Predominant Th2/Tc2 polarity of tumor infiltrating lymphocytes in human cervical cancer. J Immunol. 2001;167:2972–8.

Sigstad E, Lie A, Luostarinen T, Dillner J, Jellum E, Lehtinen M, Thoresen S, Abeler V. A prospective study of the relationship between prediagnostic human papillomavirus seropositivity and HPV DNA in subsequent cervical carcinomas. Br J Cancer. 2002;87:175–80.

Simon P, Buxant F, Hallez S, et al. Cervical response to vaccination against HPV16 E7 in case of severe dysplasia. Eur J Obstet Gynecol Reprod Biol. 2003; 109:219–23.

Smith G. Virus proteins that bind cytokines, chemokines or interferons. Curr Opin Immunol. 1996;8:467–71.

Stanley MA. Immunobiology of papillomavirus infection. J Reprod Immunol. 2001;52:45–59.

Stanley MA. Immune interventions in HPV infections: current progress and future developments. Expert Rev Vaccines. 2003a;2:615–7.

Stanley MA. Progress in prophylactic and therapeutic vaccines for human papillomavirus infection. Expert Rev Vaccines. 2003b;2:381–9.

Stanley MA. Human papillomavirus (HPV) vaccines: prospects for eradicating cervical cancer. J Fam Plann Reprod Health Care. 2004;30:213215.

Stanley MA. Immune responses to human papillomavirus. Vaccine. 2006;24 Suppl 1:S16–22.

Stern PL. Immune control of human papillomavirus (HPV) associated anogenital disease and potential for vaccination. J Clin Virol. 2005;32:S72–81.

Stoler MH. A brief synopsis of the role of human papillomaviruses in cervical carcinogenesis. Am J Obstet Gynecol. 1996;175:1091–8.

Tjalma WAA, Arbyn M, Paavonen J, Van Waes TR, Bogers JJ. Prophylactic human papillomavirus vaccines: the beginning of the end of cervical cancer. Int J Gynecol Cancer. 2004;14:751–61.

Trimble CL, Peng S, Kos F, et al. A phase I trial of a human papillomavirus DNA vaccine for HPV16+ cervical intraepithelial neoplasia 2/3. Clin Cancer Res. 2009;15:361–7.

Van Poelgeest MI, Nijhuis ER, Kwappenberg KMC, Hamming IE, Drijfhout JW, Fleuren GJ, van der Zee AGJ, Melief CJ, Kenter GG, Nijman HW, Offringa R, van der Burg SH. Distinct regulation and impact of type 1 T-cell immunity against HPV16 L1, E2 and E6 antigens during HPV16-induced cervical infection and neoplasia. Int J Cancer. 2006;118:675–83.

Veress G, Konya J, Csiky-Meszaros T, Czegledy J, Gergely L. Human papillomavirus DNA and anti-HPV S-IgA antibodies in cytologically normal cervical specimens. J Med Virol. 1994;43:201–7.

Viac J, Guerin-Reverchon I, Chardonnet Y, Bremond A. Langerhans cells and EC modifications in cervical intraepithelial neoplasia: correlation with human papillomavirus infection. Immunobiology. 1990;180:328–38.

Villa LL, Costa RLR, Petta CA, Andrade RP, Ault KA, Giuliano AR, Wheeler CM, Koutsky LA, Malm C, Lehtinen M, Skjeldestad FE, Olsson SE, Steinwall M, Brown DR, Kurman RJ, Ronnett BM, Stoler MH, Ferenczy A, Harper DM, Tamms GM, Yu J, Lupinacci L, Railkar R, Taddeo FJ, Jansen KU, Esser MT, Sings HL, Saah AJ, Barr E. Prophylactic quadrivalent human papillomavirus (types 6, 11, 16, and 18) L1 virus-like particle vaccine in young women a randomised double-blind placebo-controlled multicentre phase II efficacy trial. Lancet Oncol. 2005;6:271–8.

Youde SJ, Dunbar PR, Evans EM, Fiander AN, Borysiewicz LK, Cerundolo V, Man S. Use of fluorogenic histocompatibility leukocyte antigen-A*201/

HPV16 E7 peptide complexes to isolate rare human cytotoxic T-lymphocyte-recognising endogenous human papillomavirus antigens. Cancer Res. 2000; 60:365–71.

Zaks TZ, Chappell DB, Rosenberg SA, Restifo NP. Fas-mediated suicide of tumor-reactive T cells following activation by specific tumor: selective rescue by caspase inhibition. J Immunol. 1999;162:3273–9.

Zeng Q, Peng S, Monie A, et al. Control of cervicovaginal HPV-16 E7-expressing tumors by the combination of therapeutic HPV vaccination and vascular disrupting agents. Hum Gene Ther. 2011;22:809–19.

Zhang B, Li P, Wang E, Brahmi Z, Dunn KW, Blum JS, Roman A. The E5 protein of human papillomavirus type 16 perturbs MHC class II antigen maturation in human foreskin keratinocytes treated with interferon-gamma. Virology. 2003;310:100–8.

Gonorrhea

Apicella MA, Ketterer M, Lee FK, Zhou D, Rice PA, Blake MS. The pathogenesis of gonococcal urethritis in men: confocal and immunoelectron microscopic analysis of urethral exudates from men infected with Neisseria gonorrhoeae. J Infect Dis. 1996;173:636–46.

Batteiger BE, Fraiz J, Newhall WJ, Katz BP, Jones RB. Association of recurrent chlamydial infection with gonorrhea. J Infect Dis. 1989;159:661–9.

Binnicker MJ, Williams RD, Apicella MA. Infection of human urethral epithelium with Neisseria gonorrhoeae elicits an upregulation of host anti-apoptotic factors and protects cells from staurosporine-induced apoptosis. Cell Microbiol. 2003;5:549–60.

Blake M, Holmes KK, Swanson J. Studies on gonococcus infection. XVII. IgA1-cleaving protease in vaginal washings from women with gonorrhea. J Infect Dis. 1979;139:89–92.

Bohmer JT, Schemmer G, Harrison Jr FN, Kreft W, Elliot M. Cervical wet mount as a negative predictor for gonococci- and Chlamydia trachomatis-induced cervicitis in a gravid population. Am J Obstet Gynecol. 1999;181:283–7.

Boslego JW, Tramont EC, Chung RC, McChesney DG, Ciak J, Sadoff JC, Piziak MV, Brown JD, Brinton CC, Wood SW, Bryan JR. Efficacy trial of a parenteral gonococcal pilus vaccine in men. Vaccine. 1991;9:154–62.

Burch CL, Danaher RJ, Stein DC. Antigenic variation in Neisseria gonorrhoeae: production of multiple lipooligosaccharides. J Bacteriol. 1997;179:982–6.

Buve A, Weiss H, Laga M, Van Dyck E, Musonda R, Zekeng L, Kahindo M, Anagonou S, Morison L, Robinson NJ, Hayes RJ, The Study Group on Heterogeneity of HIV Epidemics in African Cities. The epidemiology of trichomoniasis in women in four African cities. AIDS. 2001;15 Suppl 4:S89–96.

Cahoon LA, Seifert HS. An alternative DNA structure is necessary for pilin antigenic variation in Neisseria gonorrhoeae. Science. 2009;325:764–7.

Chen A, Boulton IC, Pongoski J, Cochrane A, Gray-Owen SD. Induction of HIV-1 long terminal repeat-mediated transcription by Neisseria gonorrhoeae. AIDS. 2003;17:625–8.

Cohen MS, Cannon JG. Human experimentation with Neisseria gonorrhoeae: progress and goals. J Infect Dis. 1999;179 Suppl 2:S375–9.

Duffin PM, Seifert HS. ksgA mutations confer resistance to kasugamycin in Neisseria gonorrhoeae. Int J Antimicrob Agents. 2009;33:321–7.

Duncan JA, Gao X, Huang MT, et al. Neisseria gonorrhoeae activates the proteinase cathepsin B to mediate the signaling activities of the NLRP3 and ASC-containing inflammasome. J Immunol. 2009;182: 6460–9.

Edwards JL, Apicella MA. The molecular mechanisms used by Neisseria gonorrhoeae to initiate infection differ between men and women. Clin Microbiol Rev. 2004;17:965–81.

Edwards JL, Brown EJ, Ault KA, Apicella MA. The role of complement receptor 3 (CR3) in Neisseria gonorrhoeae infection of human cervical epithelia. Cell Microbiol. 2001;3:611–22.

Edwards JL, Brown EJ, Uk-Nham S, Cannon JG, Blake MS, Apicella MA. A co-operative interaction between Neisseria gonorrhoeae and complement receptor 3 mediates infection of primary cervical ECs. Cell Microbiol. 2002;4:571–84.

Eley A, Pacey AA, Galdiero M, Galdiero M, Galdiero F. Can Chlamydia trachomatis directly damage your sperm? Lancet Infect Dis. 2005;5:53–7.

Fichorova RN, Desai PJ, Gibson III FC, Genco CA. Distinct proinflammatory host responses to Neisseria gonorrhoeae infection in immortalized human cervical and vaginal ECs. Infect Immun. 2001;69:5840–8.

Fichorova RN, Cronin AO, Lien E, Anderson DJ, Ingalls RR. Response to Neisseria gonorrhoeae by cervicovaginal ECs occurs in the absence of toll-like receptor 4-mediated signaling. J Immunol. 2002;168:2424–32.

Follows SA, Murlidharan J, Massari P, Wetzler LM, Genco CA. Neisseria gonorrhoeae infection protects human endocervical epithelial cells from apoptosis via expression of host antiapoptotic proteins. Infect Immun. 2009;77:3602–10.

Geisler WM, Wang C, Tang J, Wilson CM, Crowley-Nowick PA, Kaslow RA. Immunogenetic correlates of Neisseria gonorrhoeae infection in adolescents. Sex Transm Dis. 2008;35:656–61.

Harvey HA, Porat N, Campbell CA, Jennings MP, Gibson BW, Phillips NJ, Apicella MA, Blake MS. Gonococcal lipooligosaccharide is a ligand for the asialoglycoprotein receptor on human sperm. Mol Microbiol. 2000;36:1059–70.

Harvey HA, Jennings MP, Campbell CA, Williams R, Apicella MA. Receptor-mediated endocytosis of Neisseria gonorrhoeae into primary human urethral ECs: the role of the asialoglycoprotein receptor. Mol Microbiol. 2001;42:659–72.

Harvey HA, Post DMB, Apicella MA. Immortalization of human urethral ECs: a model for the study of the pathogenesis of and the inflammatory cytokine response to Neisseria gonorrhoeae infection. Infect Immun. 2002;70:5808–15.

Hedger MP. Testicular leukocytes: what are they doing? Rev Reprod. 1997;2:38–47.

Hedger MP. Macrophages and the immune responsiveness of the testis. J Reprod Imunol. 2002;57:19–34.

Hedger MP, Meinhardt A. Cytokines and the immune-testicular axis. J Reprod Immunol. 2003;58:1–26.

Hedges SR, Mayo MS, Kallmann L, Mestecky J, Hook 3rd EW, Russell MW. Evaluation of immunoglobulin A1 (IgA1) protease and IgA1 protease-inhibitory activity in human female genital infection with Neisseria gonorrhea. Infect Immun. 1998a;66: 5826–32.

Hedges SR, Sibley D, Mayo MS, Hook 3rd EW, Russell MW. Cytokine and antibody responses in women infected with Neisseria gonorrhoeae: effects of concomitant infections. J Infect Dis. 1998b;178:742–51.

Hedges SR, Mayo MS, Mestecky J, Hook 3rd EW, Russell MW. Limited local and systemic antibody responses to Neisseria gonorrhoeae during uncomplicated genital infections. Infect Immun. 1999;67:3937–46.

Hill SA, Davies JK. Pilin gene variation in Neisseria gonorrhoeae: reassessing the old paradigms. FEMS Microbiol Rev. 2009;33:521–30.

Ison CA, Hadfield SG, Bellinger CM, Dawson SG, Glynn AA. The specificity of serum and local antibodies in female gonorrhea. Clin Exp Immunol. 1986;65: 198–205.

Jerse AE. Experimental gonococcal genital tract infection and opacity protein expression in estradiol-treated mice. Infect Immun. 1999;182:848–55.

Källström HD, Blackmer G, Albiger B, Liszewski MK, Atkinson JP, Jonsson AB. Attachment of Neisseria gonorrhoeae to the cellular pilus receptor CD46: identification of domains important for bacterial adherence. Cell Microbiol. 2001;3:133–43.

Klotman ME, Rapista A, Teleshova N, et al. Neisseria gonorrhoeae-induced human defensins 5 and 6 increase HIV infectivity: role in enhanced transmission. J Immunol. 2008;180:6176–85.

Lee HS, Ostrowski MA, Gray-Owen SD. CEACAM1 dynamics during neisseria gonorrhoeae suppression of CD4+ T lymphocyte activation. J Immunol. 2008;180: 6827–35.

Lis-Tonder J, Cybulski Z. Antimicrobial susceptibility and biochemical patterns of Neisseria gonorrhoeae strains in Vejle area, Denmark. J Eur Acad Dermatol Venereol. 2009;23:1193–6.

Makepeace BL, Watt PJ, Heckels JE, Christodoulides M. Interactions of Neisseria gonorrhoeae with mature human macrophage opacity proteins influence production of proinflammatory cytokines. Infect Immun. 2001;69:1909–13.

Miettinen A, Hakkarainen K, Grönroos P, Heinonen P, Teisala K, Aine R, Sillantaka I, Saarenmaa K, Lehtinen M, Punnonen R, Paavonen J. Class specific antibody response to gonococcal infection. J Clin Pathol. 1989; 42:72–6.

Müller A, Günther D, Brinkmann V, Hurwitz R, Meyer TF, Rudel T. Targeting of the pro- apoptotic VDAC-like porin (PorB) of Neisseria gonorrhoeae to mitochondria of infected cells. EBMO J. 2000;19:5332–43.

Pantelic M, Kim YJ, Bolland S, Chen I, Shively J, Che T. Neisseria gonorrhoeae kills carcinoembryonic antigen-related cellular adhesion molecule 1 (CD66a)-expressing human B cells and inhibits antibody production. Infect Immun. 2005;73:4171–9.

Plante M, Jerse A, Hamel J, Couture F, Rioux CR, Brodeur BR, Martin D. Intranasal immunization with gonococcal outer membrane preparations reduces duration of vaginal colonization of mice by Neisseria gonorrhoeae. J Infect Dis. 2000;182:848–55.

Price GA, Russell MW, Cornelissen CN. Intranasal administration of recombinant Neisseria gonorrhoeae transferring binding proteins A and B conjugated to the cholera toxin B subunit induces systemic and vaginal antibodies in mice. Infect Immun. 2005;73:3945–53.

Quan DN, Cooper MD, Potter JL, Roberts MH, Cheng H, Jarvis GA. TREM-2 binds to lipooligosaccharides of Neisseria gonorrhoeae and is expressed on reproductive tract epithelial cells. Mucosal Immunol. 2008;1:229–38.

Ramsey KH, Schneider H, Cross AS, Boslego JW, Hoover DL, Staley TL, Kuschner RA, Deal CD. Inflammatory cytokines produced in response to experimental human gonorrhea. J Infect Dis. 1995;172:186–91.

Rest RF, Fischer SH, Ingham ZZ, Jones JF. Interactions of Neisseria gonorrhoeae with human neutrophils: effects of serum and gonococcal opacity on phagocyte killing and chemiluminescence. Infect Immun. 1982;36: 737.744.

Shaughnessy J, Lewis LA, Jarva H, Ram S. Functional comparison of the binding of factor H short consensus repeat 6 (SCR 6) to factor H binding protein from Neisseria meningitidis and the binding of factor H SCR 18 to 20 to Neisseria gonorrhoeae porin. Infect Immun. 2009;77:2094–103.

Sheung A, Rebbapragada A, Shin LY, et al. Mucosal Neisseria gonorrhoeae coinfection during HIV acquisition is associated with enhanced systemic HIV-specific CD8 T-cell responses. AIDS. 2008;22:1729–37.

Soler-Garcia AA, Jerse AE. Neisseria gonorrhoeae catalase is not required for experimental genital tract infection despite the induction of a localized neutrophil response. Infect Immun. 2007;75:2225–33.

Sparling PF. Biology of Neisseria gonorrhoeae. In: Holmes KK, Mardh PA, Sparling PF, Lemon SM, Stamm WE, Piot P, Wasserheit JN, editors. Sexually transmitted diseases. 3rd ed. New York: McGraw-Hill; 1999. p. 433–49.

Spence JM, Chen JCR, Clark VL. A proposed role for the lutropin receptor in contact-inducible gonococcal invasion of Hec1B cells. Infect Immun. 1997;65: 3736–42.

Spencer SE, Valentin-Bon IE, Whaley K, Jerse AE. Inhibition of Neisseria gonorrhoea genital tract infection by leading candidate topical microbicides in a mouse model. J Infect Dis. 2004;189:410–9.

Swanson J. Studies on gonococcus infection. IV. Pili: their role in attachment of gonococci to tissue culture cells. J Exp Med. 1973;137:571–89.

Tramont EC. Inhibition of adherence of Neisseria gonorrhoeae by human genital secretions. J Clin Invest. 1977;59:117–24.

Tramont EC, Sadoff JC, Boslego JW, Ciak J, McChesney D, Brinton CC, Wood S, Takafuji E. Gonococcal pilus vaccine. Studies on antigenicity and inhibition of attachment. J Clin Invest. 1981;68:881–8.

Vonck RA, Darville T, O'Connell CM, Jerse AE. Chlamydial Infection Increases Gonococcal Colonization in a Novel Murine Coinfection Model. Infect Immun. 2011;79(4):1566–77.

Weel JFL, van Putten JPM. Fate of the major outer membrane protein P.IA in early and late events of gonococcal infection of ECs. Res Microbiol. 1991;142:985–93.

Wen KK, Giardina PC, Blake MS, Edwards JL, Apicella MA, Rubenstein PA. Interaction of the gonococcal porin P.IB with G and F-actin. Biochemistry. 2000;39:8638–47.

Wiesenfeld H, Hillier S, Krohn M, Landers DV, Sweet RL. Bacterial vaginosis is a strong predictor of Neisseria gonorrhoeae and Chlamydia trachomatis infection. Clin Infect Dis. 2003;36:663–8.

Wu H, Soler-Garcia AA, Jerse AE. A strain-specific catalase mutation and mutation of the metal-binding transporter gene mntC attenuate Neisseria gonorrhoeae in vivo but not by increasing susceptibility to oxidative killing by phagocytes. Infect Immun. 2009;77:1091–102.

Chlamydia trachomatis

Ajonuma LC, Fok KL, Ho LS, et al. CFTR is required for cellular entry and internalization of Chlamydia trachomatis. Cell Biol Int. 2010;34:593–600.

Andrews WW, Goldenberg RL, Mercer B, Iams J, Meis P, Moawad A, Das A, Vandorsten JP, Caritis SN, Thurnau G, Miodovnik M, Roberts J, McNellis D. The Preterm Prediction Study: association of second-trimester genitourinary Chlamydia infection with subsequent spontaneous preterm birth. Am J Obstet Gynecol. 2000;183:662–8.

Arno JN, Ricker VA, Batteiger BE, Katz BP, Caine VA, Jones RB. Interferon-gamma in endocervical secretions of women infected with Chlamydia trachomatis. J Infect Dis. 1990;162:1385–9.

Arno JN, Katz BP, McBride R, Carty GA, Batteiger BE, Caine VA, Jones RB. Age and clinical immunity to infections with Chlamydia trachomatis. Sex Transm Dis. 1994;21:47–52.

Ault KA, Tawfik OW, Smith-King MM, Gunter J, Terranova PT. Tumor necrosis factor-alpha response to infection with Chlamydia trachomatis in human fallopian tube organ culture. Am J Obstet Gynecol. 1996;175:1242–5.

Barteneva N, Theodor I, Peterson EM, de la Maza LM. Role of neutrophils in controlling early stages of a Chlamydia trachomatis infection. Infect Immun. 1996;64:4830–3.

Bashmakov YK, Zigangirova NA, Pashko YP, Kapotina LN, Petyaev IM. Chlamydia trachomatis growth inhibition and restoration of LDL-receptor level in HepG2 cells treated with mevastatin. Comp Hepatol. 2010;9:3.

Batteiger BE, Rank RG. Analysis of the humoral immune response to chlamydial genital infection in guinea pigs. Infect Immun. 1987;55:1767–73.

Batteiger BE, Fraiz J, Newhall WJ, Katz BP, Jones RB. Association of recurrent chlamydial infection with gonorrhea. J Infect Dis. 1989;159:661–9.

Batteiger BE, Xu F, Johnson RE, Rekart ML. Protective immunity to Chlamydia trachomatis genital infection: evidence from human studies. J Infect Dis. 2010;201 Suppl 2:S178–89.

Bauer S, Pollheimer J, Hartmann J, Husslein P, Aplin JD, Knofler M. Tumor necrosis factor- alpha inhibits trophoblast migration through elevation of plasminogen activator inhibitor-1 in first-trimester villous explant cultures. J Clin Endocrinol Metab. 2004;89:812–22.

Bavoil PM, Hsia RC, Rank RG. Prospects for a vaccine against Chlamydia genital disease I. – Microbiology and pathogenesis. Bull Inst Pasteur. 1996;94:5–54.

Beatty PR, Stephens RS. CD8+ T lymphocyte-mediated lysis of Chlamydia-infected L cells using an endogenous antigen pathway. J Immunol. 1994;153:4588–95.

Beatty WL, Morrison RP, Byrne GI. Immunoelectron-microscopic quantitation of different levels of chlamydial proteins in a cell culture model of persistent Chlamydia trachomatis infection. Infect Immun. 1994;62:4059–62.

Beer AE. Immunopathologic factors contributing to recurrent spontaneous abortions in humans. Am J Reprod Immunol. 1983;4:182–4.

Beer AE. New horizons in the diagnosis, evaluation and therapy of recurrent spontaneous abortions. Clin Obstet Gyn. 1986;13:115–24.

Beer AE, Semprini AE, Zhu XY, Quebbeman JF. Pregnancy outcome in human couples with recurrent spontaneous abortions: HLA antigen profiles; HLA antigen sharing; female serum MLR blocking factors; and paternal leukocyte immunization. Exp Clin Immunogenet. 1985;2:137–53.

Beer AE, Kwak JYH, Ruiz JE. Immunophenotypic profiles of peripheral blood lymphocytes in women with recurrent pregnancy losses and infertile women with multiple failed in vitro fertilization cycles. Am J Reprod Immunol. 1996;35:376–82.

Behbakht K, Friedman J, Heimler I, Aroutcheva A, Simoes J, Faro S. Role of the vaginal microbiological ecosystem and cytokine profile in the promotion of cervical dysplasia: a case- control study. Infect Dis Obstet Gynecol. 2002;10:181–6.

Belardelli F. Role of interferons and other cytokines in the regulation of the immune response. APMIS. 1995;103:161–79.

Belay T, Eko FO, Ananaba GA, Bowers S, Moore T, Igietseme JU. Chemokine and chemokine receptor dynamics during genital chlamydial infection. Infect Immun. 2002;70:844–50.

Bélec L, Meillet D, Hernvann A, Grésenguet G, Gherardi R. Differential elevation of circulating interleukin-1β, tumor necrosis factor alpha, and interleukin-6 in AIDS-associated cachectic states. Clin Diag Lab Immunol. 1994;1:177–20.

Belec L, Dupre T, Prazuck T, Tevi-Benissan C, Kanga JM, Pathey O, Lü XS, Pillot J. Cervicovaginal overproduction of specific IgG to human immunodeficiency virus (HIV) contrasts with normal or impaired IgA local response in HIV infection. J Infect Dis. 1995a; 172:691–7.

Belec L, Gherardi R, Payan C, Prazuck T, Malkin JE, Tevi-Benissan C, Pillot J. Proinflammatory cytokine expression in cervicovaginal secretions of normal and HIV-infected women. Cytokine. 1995b;7:568–74.

Bell SC, Billington WD. Antifetal alloantibody in the pregnant female. Immunol Rev. 1983;75:5–30.

Ben-Baruch A, Michiel DF, Oppenheim JJ. Signals and receptors involved in recruitment of inflammatory cells. J Biol Chem. 1995;270:11703–6.

Bengtsson AK, Ryan EJ, Giordano D, Magaletti DM, Clark EA. 17beta-estradiol (E2) modulates cytokine and chemokine expression in human monocyte-derived dendritic cells. Blood. 2004;104:1404–10.

Ben-Hur H, Gurevich P, Berman V, Tchanyshev R, Gurevich E, Zusman I. The secretory immune system as part of the placental barrier in the second trimester of pregnancy in humans. In Vivo. 2001;15:429–35.

Benki S, Mostad SB, Richardson BA, Mandaliya K, Kreiss JK, Overbaugh J. Cyclic shedding of HIV-1 RNA in cervical secretions during the menstrual cycle. J Infect Dis. 2004;189:2192–201.

Benoff S, Cooper GW, Hurley I, Mandel FS, Rosenfeld DL. Antisperm antibody binding to human sperm inhibits capacitation induced changes in the levels of plasma membrane sterols. Am J Reprod Immunol. 1993;30:113–30.

Berger EA, Murphy PM, Farber JM. Chemokine receptors as HIV-1 coreceptors: roles in viral entry, tropism and disease. Annu Rev Immunol. 1999;17:657–700.

Bergquist C, Johansson EL, Lagergård T, Holmgren J, Rudin A. Intranasal vaccination of humans with recombinant Cholera Toxin B subunit induces systemic and local antibody responses in the upper respiratory tract and the vagina. Infect Immun. 1997;65: 2676–84.

Bernstein DI, Harrison CJ, Tomai MA, Miller RL. Daily or weekly therapy with resiquimod (R- 848) reduces genital recurrences in herpes simplex virus-infected guinea pigs during and after treatment. J Infect Dis. 2001;183:844–9.

Betterle C, Rossi A, Dalla Pria S, Artifoni A, Pedini B, Gavasso S, Caretto A. Premature ovarian failure: autoimmunity and natural history. Clin Endocrinol. 1993;39:35–43.

Bianchi A, Dosquet C, Henry S, Couderc MC, Ferchal F, Scieux C. Chlamydia trachomatis growth stimulates interleukin-8 production by human monocytic U-937 cells. Infect Immun. 1997;65:2434–6.

Bohmer JT, Schemmer G, Harrison Jr FN, Kreft W, Elliot M. Cervical wet mount as a negative predictor for gonococci- and Chlamydia trachomatis-induced cervicitis in a gravid population. Am J Obstet Gynecol. 1999;181:283–7.

Brunham RC, Peeling RW. Chlamydia trachomatis antigens: role in immunity and pathogenesis. Infect Agents Dis. 1994;3:218–33.

Brunham RC, Kuo CC, Cles L, Holmes KK. Correlation of host immune response with quantitative recovery from Chlamydia trachomatis from the human ectocervix. Infect Immun. 1983;39:1491–4.

Brunham RC, Kimani J, Bwayo J, Maitha G, Maclean I, Yang C, Shen C, Roman S, Nagelkerke NJD, Cheang M, Plummer FA. The epidemiology of Chlamydia trachomatis within a sexually transmitted diseases core group. J Infect Dis. 1996;173:950–6.

Burstein GR, Gaydos CA, Diener-West M, Howell MR, Zenilman JM, Quinn TC. Incident Chlamydia trachomatis infections among inner-city adolescent women. JAMA. 1998;280:521–6.

Bussen SS, Steck T. Thyroid antibodies and their relation to antithrombin antibodies, anticardiolipin antibodies and lupus anticoagulant in women with recurrent spontaneous abortions (antithyroid, anticardiolipin and antithrombin autoantibodies and lupus anticoagulant in habitual aborters). Eur J Obstet Gynecol Reprod Biol. 1997;74:139–43.

Cain TK, Rank RG. Local Th1-like responses are induced by intravaginal infection of mice with the mouse pneumonitis biovar of Chlamydia trachomatis. Infect Immun. 1995;63:1784–9.

Caldwell HD, Schachter J. Antigenic analysis of the major outer membrane protein of Chlamydia spp. Infect Immun. 1982;35:1024–31.

Cotter TW, Ramsey KH, Miranpuri GS, Poulsen CE, Byrne GI. Dissemination of Chlamydia trachomatis chronic genital infection in gamma interferon gene knockout mice. Infect Immun. 1997;65: 2145–52.

Cunningham DS. Immune response characteristics in women with chlamydial genital tract infection. Gynecol Obstet Invest. 1995;39:54–9.

Darville T, Andrews Jr CW, Lafoon KK, Shymasani W, Kishen LR, Rank RG. Mouse strain- dependent variation in the course and outcome of chlamydial genital tract infection is associated with differences in host response. Infect Immun. 1997;65:3065–73.

Darville T, Andrews Jr CW, Rank RG. Does inhibition of tumor necrosis factor alpha affect chlamydial genital tract infection in mice and guinea pigs? Infect Immun. 2000;68:5299–305.

Dean D, Suchland RJ, Stamm WE. Evidence for long-term cervical persistence of Chlamydia trachomatis by omp1 genotyping. J Infect Dis. 2000;182:909–16.

den Hartog JE, Lyons JM, Ouburg S, et al. TLR4 in Chlamydia trachomatis infections: knockout mice, STD patients and women with tubal factor subfertility. Drugs Today (Barc). 2009;45(Suppl B):75–82.

Donati M, Di Francesco A, Delucca F, et al. Antibody-neutralizing activity against all urogenital Chlamydia trachomatis serovars in Chlamydia suis-infected pigs. FEMS Immunol Med Microbiol. 2011;61:125–8.

Du K, Wang F, Huo Z, et al. Localization and characterization of GTP-binding protein CT703 in the Chlamydia trachomatis-Infected cells. Curr Microbiol. 2011;62:465–71.

Eckert LO, Hawes SE, Wolner-Hanssen P, Money DM, Peeling RW, Brunham RC, Stevens CE, Eschenbach DA, Stamm WE. Prevalence and correlates of antibody to chlamydial heat shock protein in women attending sexually transmitted disease clinics and women with confirmed pelvic inflammatory disease. J Infect Dis. 1997;175:1453–8.

Eko FO, Ekong E, He Q, Black CM, Igietseme JU. Induction of immune memory by a multisubunit chlamydial vaccine. Vaccine. 2011;29:1472–80.

Eley A, Pacey AA, Galdiero M, Galdiero M, Galdiero F. Can Chlamydia trachomatis directly damage your sperm? Lancet Infect Dis. 2005;5:53–7.

Fan T, Lu H, Hu H, Shi LF, McClarty GA, Nance DM, Greenberg AH, Zhong GM. Inhibition of apoptosis in chlamydia-infected cells: blockade of mitochondrial cytochrome c release and caspase activation. J Exp Med. 1998;187:487–96.

Farris CM, Morrison RP. Vaccination against Chlamydia Genital Infection Utilizing the Murine C. muridarum Model. Infect Immun. 2011;79:986–96.

Fling SP, Sutherland RA, Steele LN, Hess B, D'Orazio SEF, Maissonneuve JF, Lampe MF, Probst P, Starnbach MN. CD8+ T cells recognize an inclusion membrane-associated protein from the vacuolar pathogen Chlamydia trachomatis. Proc Natl Acad Sci USA. 2001;98:1160–5.

Geisler WM. Approaches to the management of uncomplicated genital Chlamydia trachomatis infections. Expert Rev Anti Infect Ther. 2004;2:771–85.

Ghaem-Maghami S, Ratti G, Ghaem-Maghami M, Comanducci M, Hay PE, Bailey RL, Mabey DCW, Whittle HC, Ward ME, Lewis DJM. Mucosal and systemic immune responses to the plasmid protein pgp3 in patients with genital and ocular Chlamydia trachomatis infection. Clin Exp Immunol. 2003;132:436–42.

Gondek DC, Roan NR, Starnbach MN. T cell responses in the absence of IFN-gamma exacerbate uterine infection with Chlamydia trachomatis. J Immunol. 2009; 183:1313–9.

Gonzales GF, Muñoz G, Sánchez R, Henkel R, Gallegos-Avila G, Diaz-Gutierrez O, Vigil P, Vásquez F, Kortebani G, Mazzolli A, Bustos-Obregon B. Update on the impact of Chlamydia trachomatis infection on male infertility. Andrologia. 2004;36:1–23.

Hawkins RA, Rank RG, Kelly KA. Expression of mucosal homing receptor alpha4beta7 is associated with enhanced migration to the Chlamydia-infected murine genital mucosa in vivo. Infect Immun. 2000; 68:5587–94.

Hawkins RA, Rank RG, Kelly KA. A Chlamydia trachomatis-specific Th2 clone does not provide protection against a genital infection and displays reduced trafficking to the infected genital mucosa. Infect Immun. 2002;70:5132–9.

Hickey JM, Weldon L, Hefty PS. The atypical OmpR/PhoB response regulator ChxR from Chlamydia trachomatis forms homodimers in vivo and binds a direct repeat of nucleotide sequences. J Bacteriol. 2011; 193:389–98.

Hook CE, Matyszak MK, Hill Gaston JS. Infection of epithelial and dendritic cells by Chlamydia trachomatis results in IL-12 and IL-18 production, leading to interferon-γ production by human natural killer cells. FEMS Immunol Med Microbiol. 2005;45:113–20.

Huang J, Wang MD, Lenz S, Gao D, Kaltenboeck B. IL-12 administered during Chlamydia psittaci lung infection in mice confers immediate and long-term protection and reduces macrophage inflammatory protein-2 level and neutrophil infiltration in lung tissue. J Immunol. 1999;162:2217–26.

Igietseme JU, Ramsey KH, Magee DM, Williams DM, Kincy TJ, Rank RG. Resolution of murine chlamydial genital infection by the adoptive transfer of a biovar-specific, Th1 lymphocyte clone. Regional Immunol. 1993;5:317–24.

Igietseme JU, Perry LL, Ananaba GA, Uriri IM, Ojior OO, Kumar SN, Caldwell HD. Chlamydial infection in inducible nitric oxide synthase knockout mice. Infect Immun. 1998a;66:1282–6.

Igietseme JU, Uriri IM, Kumar SN, Ananaba GA, Ojior OO, Momodu IA, Candal DH, Black CM. Route of infection that induces a high intensity of gamma interferon-secreting T cells in the genital tract produces optimal protection against Chlamydia trachomatis infection in mice. Infect Immun. 1998b;66:4030–5.

Igietseme JU, Ananaba GA, Bolier J, Bowers S, Moore T, Belay T, Eko FO, Lyn D, Black CM. Suppression of endogenous IL-10 gene expression in dendritic cells enhances antigen presentation for specific Th1 induction: potential for cellular vaccine development. J Immunol. 2000;164:4212–9.

Igietseme JU, Eko FO, Black CM. Contemporary approaches to designing and evaluating vaccines against Chlamydia. Expert Rev Vaccines. 2003;2: 129–46.

Igietseme JU, He Q, Joseph K, et al. Role of T lymphocytes in the pathogenesis of Chlamydia disease. J Infect Dis. 2009;200:926–34.

Igietsieme JU, Murdin A. Induction of protective immunity against Chlamydia trachomatis genital infection by a vaccine based on major outer membrane protein-lipophilic immune response-stimulating complexes. Infect Immun. 2000;68:6798–806.

Ingalls RR, Rice PA, Qureshi N, Takayama K, Lin JS, Golenbock DT. The inflammatory cytokine response to Chlamydia trachomatis infection is endotoxin mediated. Infect Immun. 1995;63:3125–30.

Jayarapu K, Kerr MS, Katschke A, Johnson RM. Chlamydia muridarum-specific CD4 T-cell clones recognize infected reproductive tract epithelial cells in an interferon-dependent fashion. Infect Immun. 2009;77:4469–79.

Johansson M, Lycke NJ. Immunological memory in B cell-deficient mice conveys long-lasting protection against genital tract infection with Chlamydia trachomatis by rapid recruitment of T cells. Immunology. 2001;102:199–208.

Johansson M, Schön K, Ward M, Lycke NJ. Genital tract infection Chlamydia trachomatis fails to induce protective immunity in gamma interferon receptor-deficient mice despite a strong local immunoglobulin A response. Infect Immun. 1997a;65:1032–44.

Johansson M, Ward M, Lycke N. B-cell-deficient mice develop complete immune protection against genital tract infection with Chlamydia trachomatis. Immunol. 1997b;92:422–8.

Jones HM, Schachter J, Stephens RS. Evaluation of the humoral immune response in trachoma to Chlamydia trachomatis major outer membrane proteins by sequence-defined immunoassay. J Infect Dis. 1992; 166:915–9.

Karimi O, Ouburg S, de Vries HJ, et al. TLR2 haplotypes in the susceptibility to and severity of Chlamydia trachomatis infections in Dutch women. Drugs Today (Barc). 2009;45(Suppl B):67–74.

Karunakaran KP, Yu H, Foster LJ, Brunham RC. Development of a Chlamydia trachomatis T cell Vaccine. Hum Vaccine. 2011;6:676–80.

Katz BP, Batteiger BE, Jones RB. Effect of prior sexually transmitted disease on the isolation of Chlamydia trachomatis. Sex Transm Dis. 1987;14:160–4.

Kaushic C, Grant K, Crane M, Wira CR. Infection of polarized primary ECs from rat uterus with Chlamydia trachomatis: cell-cell interaction and cytokine secretion. Am J Reprod Immunol. 2000a;44:73–9.

Kaushic C, Zhou F, Murdin AD, Wira CR. Effects of estradiol and progesterone on susceptibility and early immune responses to Chlamydia trachomatis infection in the female reproductive tract. Infect Immunol. 2000b;68:4207–16.

Kelly KA. Cellular immunity and Chlamydia genital infection: induction, recruitment, and effector mechanisms. Int Rev Immunol. 2003;22:3–41.

Kelly KA, Rank RG. Identification of homing receptors that mediate the recruitment of CD4 T cells to the genital tract following intravaginal infection with Chlamydia trachomatis. Infect Immun. 1997;65: 5198–208.

Kelly KA, Robinson EA, Rank RG. Initial route of antigen administration alters the T cell cytokine profile produced in response to the mouse pneumonitis biovar of Chlamydia trachomatis following genital infection. Infect Immun. 1996;64:4976–83.

Kelly KA, Walker JC, Jameel SH, Gray HL, Rank RG. Differential regulation of CD4 lymphocyte recruitment between the upper and lower regions of the genital tract during Chlamydia infection. Infect Immun. 2000;68:1519–28.

Kelly KA, Gray HL, Walker JC, Rank RG, Wormley FL, Fidel Jr PL. Chlamydia trachomatis infection does not enhance local cellular immunity against concurrent Candida vaginal infection. Infec Immun. 2001;69: 3451–4.

Kimani J, MacLean IW, Bwayo JJ, MacDonald K, Oyugi J, Maitha GM, Peeling RW, Cheang M, Nagelkerke NJD, Plummer FA, Brunham RC. Risk factors for Chlamydia trachomatis pelvic inflammatory disease among sex workers in Nairobi, Kenya. J Infect Dis. 1996;173:1437–44.

King M, Poya H, Rao J, et al. CXCL13 expression in Chlamydia trachomatis infection of the female reproductive tract. Drugs Today (Barc). 2009;45(Suppl B):125–34.

Kinnunen A, Molander P, Laurila A, Rantala I, Morrison R, Lehtinen M, Karttunen R, Tiitinen A, Paavonen J, Surcel HM. Chlamydia trachomatis reactive T lymphocytes from upper genital tract tissue specimens. Hum Reprod. 2000;15:1484–9.

Krause W, Bohring C. Male infertility and genital chlamydial infection: victim or perpetrator? Andrologia. 2003;35:209–16.

Lampe MF, Wong KG, Kuehl LM, Stamm WE. Chlamydia trachomatis major outer membrane protein variants escape neutralization by both monoclonal antibodies and human immune sera. Infect Immun. 1997;65:317–9.

Lu H, Yang X, Takeda K, Zhang D, Fan Y, Luo M, Shen C, Wang S, Akira S, Brunham RC. Chlamydia trachomatis mouse pneumonitis lung infection in IL-18 and IL-12 knockout mice: IL-12 is dominant over IL-18 for protective immunity. Mol Med. 2000;7:604–12.

Martin DH, Eschenbach DA, Cotch MF, Nugent RP, Rao AV, Klebanoff MA, Lou Y, Rettig PJ, Gibbs RS, Pastorek 2nd JG, Regan JA, Kaslow RA. Double-blind placebo-controlled treatment trial of Chlamydia trachomatis endocervical infections in pregnant women. Infect Dis Obstet Gynecol. 1997;5:10–7.

Maxion HK, Kelly KA. Chemokine expression patterns differ within anatomically distinct regions of the genital tract during Chlamydia trachomatis infection. Infect Immun. 2002;70:1538–46.

Mayer J, Woods ML, Vavrin Z, Hibbs JB. Gamma interferon-induced nitric oxide production reduces Chlamydia trachomatis infectivity in McCoy cells. Infect Immun. 1993;61:491–7.

Meoni E, Faenzi E, Frigimelica E, et al. CT043, a protective antigen that induces a CD4+ Th1 response during Chlamydia trachomatis infection in mice and humans. Infect Immun. 2009;77:4168–76.

Morrison RP, Lyng K, Caldwell HD. Chlamydial disease pathogenesis. Ocular hypersensitivity elicited by a genus-specific 57kD protein. J Exp Med. 1989;169: 663–75.

Morrison RP, Feilzer K, Tumas DB. Gene knockout mice establish a primary protective role for major histocompatibility complex class II-restricted responses in Chlamydia trachomatis genital tract infection. Infect Immun. 1995;63:4661–8.

Ojcius DM, Hellio R, Dautry-Varsat A. Distribution of endosomal, lysosomal, and major histocompatibility complex markers in a monocytic cell line infected with Chlamydia psittaci. Infect Immun. 1997;65: 2437–42.

Olive AJ, Gondek DC, Starnbach MN. CXCR3 and CCR5 are both required for T cell-mediated protection against C. trachomatis infection in the murine genital mucosa. Mucosal Immunol. 2011;4:208–16.

Paavonen J. Chlamydia trachomatis infections of the female genital tract: state of the art. Ann Med. 2012; 44:18–28.

Pal S, Theodor I, Peterson EM, de la Maza LM. Monoclonal immunoglobulin A antibody to the major outer membrane protein of Chlamydia trachomatis mouse pneumonitis biovar protects mice against a chlamydial genital challenge. Vaccine 1997; 15:575–582 Patton DL, Kuo CC. Histopathology of Chlamydia trachomatis salpingitis after primary and repeated reinfections in the monkey subcutaneous pocket model. J Reprod Fertil. 1989;85:647–65.

Pal S, Peterson EM, de la Maza LM. Intranasal immunization induces long-term protection in mice against a Chlamydia trachomatis genital challenge. Infect Immun. 1996;64:5341–8.

Pal S, Hui W, Peterson EM, de la Maza LM. Factors influencing the induction of infertility in a mouse model of Chlamydia trachomatis ascending genital tract infection. J Med Microbiol. 1998;47:599–605.

Parks KS, Dixon PB, Richey CM, Hook EW. Spontaneous clearance of Chlamydia trachomatis infection in untreated patients. Sex Transm Dis. 1997;24:229–35.

Patton DL, Kuo CC. Histopathology of Chlamydia trachomatis salpingitis after primary and repeated reinfections in the monkey subcutaneous pocket model. J Reprod Fertil. 1989;85:647–65.

Perry LL, Feilzer K, Caldwell HD. Immunity to Chlamydia trachomatis is mediated by T helper 1 cells through IFN-γ-dependent and -independent pathways. J Immunol. 1997;158:3344–52.

Ramsey KH, Rank RG. Resolution of chlamydial genital infection with antigen-specific T- lymphocyte lines. Infect Immun. 1991;59:925–31.

Ramsey KH, Cotter TW, Salyer RD, Miranpuri GS, Yanez MA, Poulsen CE, DeWolfe JL, Byrne GI. Prior genital tract infection with a murine or human biovar of Chlamydia trachomatis protects mice against heterotypic challenge infection. Infect Immun. 1999; 67:3019–25.

Rank RG, Bavoil PM. Prospects for a vaccine against Chlamydia genital disease II. Immunity and vaccine development. Bull Inst Pasteur. 1996;94:55–82.

Rank RG, Sanders MM. Pathogenesis of endometritis and salpingitis in a guinea pig model of chlamydial genital infection. Am J Pathol. 1992;140:927–36.

Rank RG, Soderberg LSF, Barron AL. Chronic chlamydial genital infection in congenitally athymic nude mice. Infect Immun. 1985;48:847–9.

Rank RG, Batteiger BE, Soderberg LSF. Susceptibility to reinfection after a primary chlamydial genital infection. Infect Immun. 1988;56:2243–9.

Rank RG, Batteiger BE, Soderberg LSF. Immunization against chlamydial genital infection in guinea pigs with UV-inactivated and viable chlamydiae administered by different routes. Infect Immun. 1990;58: 2599–605.

Rank G, Ramsey KH, Pack EA, Williams DN. Effect of gamma interferon on resolution of murine chlamydial genital infection. Infect Immun. 1992;60:4427–9.

Rasmussen S, Eckmann L, Quayle AJ, Shen L, Zhang Y, Anderson DJ, Fierer J, Stephens RS, Kagnoff MF. Secretion of proinflammatory cytokines by ECs in response to Chlamydia infection suggests a central role for ECs in chlamydial pathogenesis. J Clin Invest. 1997;99:77–87.

Reddy BS, Rastogi S, Das B, Salhan S, Verma S, Mittal A. Cytokine expression pattern in the genital tract of Chlamydia trachomatis-positive infertile women-implications for T cell responses. Clin Exp Immunol. 2004;137:552–8.

Register KB, Morgan PA, Wyrick PB. Interaction between Chlamydia spp. and human polymorphonuclear leukocytes in vitro. Infect Immun. 1986;52:664–70.

Schautteet K, Stuyven E, Cox E, Vanrompay D. Validation of the Chlamydia trachomatis genital challenge pig model for testing recombinant protein vaccines. J Med Microbiol. 2011;60:117–27.

Shavlakadze N, Gorgoshidze B. IL-17/il-23 and Chlamydia trachomatis. Georgian Med News. 2010 (45–51).

Shemer-Avni Y, Wallach D, Sarov I. Inhibition of Chlamydia trachomatis growth by recombinant tumor necrosis factor. Infect Immun. 1988;56:2503–6.

Starnbach MN, Bevan MJ, Lampe MF. Protective cytotoxic T lymphocytes are induced during murine infection with Chlamydia trachomatis. J Immunol. 1994;153:5183–9.

Sweet RL, Blankfort-Doyle M, Robbie MO, Schachter J. The occurrence of chlamydial and gonococcal salpingitis during the menstrual cycle. JAMA. 1986;255:2062–4.

Tseng CK, Rank RG. Role of NK cells in early host response to chlamydial genital infection. Infect Immun. 1998;66:5867–75.

Van Voorhis WC, Barrett LK, Sweeney YT, Kuo CC, Patton DL. Repeated Chlamydia trachomatis infection of Macaca nemestrina fallopian tubes produces a Th1-like cytokine response associated with fibrosis and scarring. Infect Immun. 1997;65:2175–82.

Vardhan H, Dutta R, Vats V, et al. Persistently elevated level of IL-8 in Chlamydia trachomatis infected HeLa 229 cells is dependent on intracellular available iron. Mediators Inflamm. 2009;2009:417658.

Vignola MJ, Kashatus DF, Taylor GA, Counter CM, Valdivia RH. cPLA2 regulates the expression of type I interferons and intracellular immunity to Chlamydia trachomatis. J Biol Chem. 2010;285:21625–35.

Wang SP, Grayston JT. Three new serovars of Chlamydia trachomatis: Da, Ia, and L2a. J Infect Dis. 1991;163:403–5.

Wiesenfeld H, Hillier S, Krohn M, Landers DV, Sweet RL. Bacterial vaginosis is a strong predictor of

Neisseria gonorrhoeae and Chlamydia trachomatis infection. Clin Infect Dis. 2003;36:663–8.

Williams DM, Grubbs BG, Kelly KA, Rank RG. Humoral and cellular immunity in secondary infection due to murine Chlamydia trachomatis. Infect Immun. 1997;65:2876–82.

Williams DM, Grubbs BG, Darville T, Kelly KA, Rank RG. A role for interleukin-6 in host defense against murine Chlamydia trachomatis infection. Infect Immun. 1998;66:4564–7.

Witkin SS. Circulating antibodies to Chlamydia trachomatis in women: relationship to antisperm and antichlamydial antibodies in semen of male partners. Hum Reprod. 1996;11:1635–7.

Witkin SS. Immunological aspects of genital chlamydia infections. Best Pract Res Clin Obstet Gynaecol. 2002;16:865–74.

Witkin SS, Linhares IM. Chlamydia trachomatis in subfertile women undergoing uterine instrumentation: an alternative to direct microbial testing or prophylactic antibiotic treatment. Hum Reprod. 2002;17:1938–41.

Yang X, Gartner J, Zhu L, Wang S, Brunham RC. IL-10 gene knockout mice show enhanced Th1-like protective immunity and absent granuloma formation following Chlamydia trachomatis lung infection. J Immunol. 1999;162:1010–7.

Zhong G, Liu L, Fan T, Fan P, Ji H. Degradation of transcription factor RFX5 during the inhibition of both constitutive and interferon-γ-inducible major histocompatibility complex class I expression in Chlamydia-infected cells. J Exp Med. 2000;191:1525–34.

Bacterial Vaginosis

Aboul Enien WM, El Metwally HA. Association of abnormal vaginal flora with increased cervical tumour necrosis factor–alpha and interferon–gamma levels in idiopathic infertility. Egypt J Immunol. 2005;12:53–9.

Anton G, Rid J, Mylonas I, Weissenbacher ER. Proinflammatory and antiinflammatory cytokines in the vagina of healthy women and during bacterial vaginosis. In: 10th annual meeting of the International Infectious Disease Society for Obstetrics & Gynecology, San Francisco, 2005.

Balu RB, Savitz DA, Ananth CV, Hartmann KE, Miller WC, Thorp JM, Heine RP. Bacterial vaginosis and vaginal fluid defensins during pregnancy. Am J Obstet Gynecol. 2002;187:1267–71.

Cauci S. Vaginal immunity in bacterial vaginosis. Curr Infect Dis Rep. 2004;6:450–6.

Cauci S, Driussi S, Monte R, Lanzafame P, Pitzus E, Quadrifoglio F. Immunoglobulin A response against Gardnerella vaginalis hemolysin and sialidase activity in bacterial vaginosis. Am J Obstet Gynecol. 1998;178:511–5.

Cauci S, Driussi S, Guaschino S, Isola M, Quadrifoglio F. Correlation of local interleukin-1beta levels with

specific IgA response against Gardnerella vaginalis cytolysin in women with bacterial vaginosis. Am J Reprod Immunol. 2002a;47:257–64.

Cauci S, Guaschino S, Driussi S, De Santo D, Lanzafame P, Quadrifoglio F. Correlation of local interleukin-8 with immunoglobulin A against Gardnerella vaginalis hemolysin and with prolidase and sialidase levels in women with bacterial vaginosis. J Infect Dis. 2002b;185:1614–20.

Cauci S, Hitti J, Noonan C, Agnew K, Quadrifoglio F, Hillier SL, Eschenbach DA. Vaginal hydrolytic enzymes, immunoglobulin A against Gardnerella vaginalis toxin, and risk of early preterm birth among women in preterm labor with bacterial vaginosis or intermediate flora. Am J Obstet Gynecol. 2002c;187:877–81.

Cauci S, Guaschino S, de Aloysio D, Driussi S, De Santo D, Penacchioni P, Quadrifoglio F. Interrelationships of interleukin-8 with interleukin-1β and neutrophils in vaginal fluid of healthy and bacterial vaginosis positive women. Mol Hum Reprod. 2003a;9:53–8.

Cauci S, Thorsen P, Schendel DE, Brmmelgaard A, Quadrifoglio F, Guaschino S. Determination of immunoglobulin A against Gardnerella vaginalis hemolysin, sialidase, and prolidase activities in vaginal fluid: Implications for adverse pregnancy outcomes. J Clin Microbiol. 2003b;41:435–8.

Cherpes TL, Meyn LA, Krohn MA, Lurie JG, Hillier SL. Association between acquisition of herpes simplex virus type 2 in women and bacterial vaginosis. Clin Infect Dis. 2003;37:319–25.

Cherpes TL, Hillier SL, Meyn LA, Busch JL, Krohn MA. A delicate balance: risk factors for acquisition of bacterial vaginosis include sexual activity, absence of hydrogen peroxide-producing lactobacilli, black race, and positive herpes simplex virus type 2 serology. Sex Transm Dis. 2008;35:78–83.

Cohen CR, Plummer FA, Mugo N, et al. Increased interleukin-10 in the endocervical secretions of women with non-ulcerative sexually transmitted diseases: a mechanism for enhanced HIV-1 transmission? AIDS. 1999;13:327–32.

Culhane JF, Nyirjesy P, McCollum K, Goldenberg RL, Gelber SE, Cauci S. Variation in vaginal immune parameters and microbial hydrolytic enzymes in bacterial vaginosis positive pregnant women with and without Mobiluncus species. Am J Obstet Gynecol. 2006;195:516–21.

Demirezen S, Korkmaz E, Beksac MS. Association between trichomoniasis and bacterial vaginosis: examination of 600 cervicovaginal smears. Cent Eur J Public Health. 2005;13:96–8.

Devi KM, Devi Kh S, Singh NB, Singh NN, Singh ID. Co-infection of herpes simplex virus (HSV) with human immunodeficiency virus (HIV) in women with reproductive tract infections (RTI). J Commun Dis. 2008;40:193–7.

Discacciati MG, Simoes JA, Lopes ES, Silva SM, Montemor EB, Rabelo-Santos SH, Westin MC. Is bacterial vaginosis associated with squamous intraepithelial lesion of the uterine cervix? Diagn Cytopathol. 2006;34:323–5.

Discacciati MG, Simoes JA, Silva MG, et al. Microbiological characteristics and inflammatory cytokines associated with preterm labor. Arch Gynecol Obstet. 2011;283:501–8.

Donders GG, Vereecken A, Bosmans E, Dekeersmaecker A, Salembier G, Spitz B. Definition of a type of abnormal vaginal flora that is distinct from bacterial vaginosis: aerobic vaginitis. BJOG. 2002;109:34–43.

Fan SR, Liu XP, Liao QP. Human defensins and cytokines in vaginal lavage fluid of women with bacterial vaginosis. Int J Gynaecol Obstet. 2008;103:50–4.

Fichorova RN. Impact of T. vaginalis infection on innate immune responses and reproductive outcome. J Reprod Immunol. 2009;83:185–9.

Fichorova RN, Onderdonk AB, Yamamoto H, et al. Maternal microbe-specific modulation of inflammatory response in extremely low-gestational-age newborns. MBio. 2011a;2:e00280–00210.

Fichorova RN, Yamamoto HS, Delaney ML, Onderdonk AB, Doncel GF. Novel vaginal microflora colonization model providing new insight into microbicide mechanism of action. MBio. 2011b;2:e00168–00111.

Forsum U, Holst E, Larsson PG, Vasquez A, Jakobsson T, Mattsby-Baltzer I. Bacterial vaginosis-a microbiological and immunological enigma. APMIS. 2005;113: 81–90.

Genc MR, Karasahin E, Onderdonk AB, Bongiovanni AM, Delaney ML, Witkin SS. Association between vaginal 70-kd heat shock protein, interleukin-1 receptor antagonist, and microbial flora in mid trimester pregnant women. Am J Obstet Gynecol. 2005;192:916–21.

Genc MR, Vardhana S, Delaney ML, Witkin SS, Onderdonk AB. TNFA-308G > A polymorphism influences the TNF-alpha response to altered vaginal flora. Eur J Obstet Gynecol Reprod Biol. 2007;134:188–91.

Goepfert AR, Varner M, Ward K, et al. Differences in inflammatory cytokine and Toll-like receptor genes and bacterial vaginosis in pregnancy. Am J Obstet Gynecol. 2005;193:1478–85.

Gomez LM, Sammel MD, Appleby DH, et al. Evidence of a gene-environment interaction that predisposes to spontaneous preterm birth: a role for asymptomatic bacterial vaginosis and DNA variants in genes that control the inflammatory response. Am J Obstet Gynecol. 2010;202:386.e1–6.

Hashemi FB, Ghassemi M, Faro S, Aroutcheva A, Spear GT. Induction of human immunodeficiency virus type 1 expression by anaerobes associated with bacterial vaginosis. J Infect Dis. 2000;181:1574–80.

Hillier SL, Nugent RP, Eschenbach DA, Krohn MA, Gibbs RS, Martin DH, Cotch MF, Edelman R, Pastorek JG, Rao AV, McNellis D, Regan JA, Carey JC, Klebanoff MA. Association between bacterial vaginosis and preterm delivery of a low-birth-weight infant. N Engl J Med. 1995;333:1737–42.

Holst E. Reservoir of four organisms associated with bacterial vaginosis suggests lack of sexual transmission. J Clin Microbiol. 1990;28:2035–9.

James JA, Thomason JL, Gelbart SM, Osypowski P, Kaiser P, Hanson L. Is trichomoniasis often associated with bacterial vaginosis in pregnant adolescents? Am J Obstet Gynecol. 1992;166:859–62.

Klebanoff MA, Schwebke JR, Zhang J, Nansel TR, Yu KF, Andrews WW. Vulvovaginal symptoms in women with bacterial vaginosis. Obstet Gynecol. 2004;104: 267–72.

Lehtovirta P, Paavonen J, Heikinheimo O. Risk factors, diagnosis and prognosis of cervical intraepithelial neoplasia among HIV-infected women. Int J STD AIDS. 2008;19:37–41.

Leitich H, Bodner-Adler B, Brunbauer M, Kaider A, Egarter C, Husslein P. Bacterial vaginosis as a risk factor for preterm delivery: a meta-analysis. Am J Obstet Gynecol. 2003a;189:139–47.

Leitich H, Brunbauer M, Bodner-Adler B, Kaider A, Egarter C, Husslein P. Antibiotic treatment of bacterial vaginosis in pregnancy: a meta-analysis. Am J Obstet Gynecol. 2003b;188:752–8.

Macones GA, Parry S, Elkousy M, Clothier B, Ural SH, Strauss JF. A polymorphism in the promoter region of TNF and bacterial vaginosis: preliminary evidence of gene-environment interaction in the etiology of spontaneous preterm birth. Am J Obstet Gynecol. 2004; 190:1504–8.

Mardh PA. The definition and epidemiology of bacterial vaginosis. Rev Fr Gynecol Obstet. 1993;88:195–7.

Marrazzo JM. Evolving issues in understanding and treating bacterial vaginosis. Expert Rev Anti Infect Ther. 2004;2:913–22.

Mattsby-Baltzer I, Hosseini N. The IL-6 response in human cervix epithelial and monocytic cell lines stimulated by bacteria associated with bacterial vaginosis and Escherichia coli. Int J STD AIDS. 1997;8 Suppl 1:34.

Mattsby-Baltzer I, Platz-Christensen JJ, Hosseini N, Rosen P. IL-1beta, IL-6, TNFalpha, fetal fibronectin, and endotoxin in the lower genital tract of pregnant women with bacterial vaginosis. Acta Obstet Gynecol Scand. 1998;77:701–6.

McDonald H, Brocklehurst P, Parsons J. Antibiotics for treating bacterial vaginosis in pregnancy. Cochrane Database Syst Rev. 2005;1, CD000262.

Mitchell CM, Balkus J, Agnew KJ, et al. Bacterial vaginosis, not HIV, is primarily responsible for increased vaginal concentrations of proinflammatory cytokines. AIDS Res Hum Retroviruses. 2008;24:667–71.

Morris M, Nicoll A, Simms I, Wilson J, Catchpole M. Bacterial vaginosis: a public health review. BJOG. 2001a;108:439–50.

Morris MC, Rogers PA, Kinghorn GR. Is bacterial vaginosis a sexually transmitted disease? Sex Transm Infect. 2001b;77:63–8.

Nugent RP, Krohn MA, Hillier SL. Reliability of diagnosing bacterial vaginosis is improved by a standardized method of Gram stain interpretation. J Clin Microbiol. 1991;29:297–301.

Olinger GG, Hashemi FB, Sha BE, Spear GT. Association of indicators of bacterial vaginosis with a female genital tract factor that induces expression of HIV-1. AIDS. 1999;13:1905–12.

Ralph SG, Rutherford AJ, Wilson JD. Influence of bacterial vaginosis on conception and miscarriage in the first trimester: cohort study. Br Med J. 1999;319: 220–3.

Romero R, Chaiworapongsa T, Kuivaniemi H, Tromp G. Bacterial vaginosis, the inflammatory response and the risk of preterm birth: a role for genetic epidemiology in the prevention of preterm birth. Am J Obstet Gynecol. 2004;190:1509–19.

Schmid G, Markowitz L, Joesoef R, Koumans E. Bacterial vaginosis and HIV infection. Sex Transm Infect. 2000; 76:3–4.

Sewankambo N, Gray RH, Wawer MJ, Paxton L, McNaim D, Wabwire-Mangen F, Serwadda D, Li C, Kiwanuka N, Hillier SL, Rabe L, Gaydos CA, Quinn TC, Konde-Lule J. HIV-1 infection associated with abnormal vaginal flora morphology and bacterial vaginosis. Lancet. 1997;23(350):546–50.

Simhan HN, Caritis SN, Hillier SL, Krohn MA. Cervical anti-inflammatory cytokine concentrations among first-trimester pregnant smokers. Am J Obstet Gynecol. 2005;193:1999–2003.

Spandorfer SD, Neuer A, Giraldo PC, Rosenwaks Z, Witkin SS. Relationship of abnormal vaginal flora, proinflammatory cytokines and idiopathic infertility in women undergoing IVF. J Reprod Med. 2001;46: 806–10.

Sturm-Ramirez K, Gaye-Diallo A, Eisen G, Mboup S, Kanki PJ. High levels of tumor necrosis factor-alpha and interleukin-1 beta in bacterial vaginosis may increase susceptibility to human immunodeficiency virus. J Infect Dis. 2000;182:467–73.

Taylor-Robinson D, Morgan DJ, Sheehan M, Rosenstein IJ, Lamont RF. Relation between Gram-stain and clinical criteria for diagnosing bacterial vaginosis with special reference to Gram grade II evaluation. Int J STD AIDS. 2003;14:6–10.

Thurman AR, Doncel GF. Innate immunity and inflammatory response to Trichomonas vaginalis and bacterial vaginosis: relationship to HIV acquisition. Am J Reprod Immunol. 2011;65:89–98.

Ugwumadu A, Manyonda I, Reid F, Hay P. Effect of early oral clindamycin on late miscarriage and preterm delivery in asymptomatic women with abnormal vaginal flora and bacterial vaginosis: a randomised controlled trial. Lancet. 2003;361:983–8.

Verstraelen H, Verhelst R, Nuytinck L, et al. Gene polymorphisms of Toll-like and related recognition receptors in relation to the vaginal carriage of Gardnerella vaginalis and Atopobium vaginae. J Reprod Immunol. 2009;79:163–73.

Wiesenfeld H, Hillier S, Krohn M, Landers DV, Sweet RL. Bacterial vaginosis is a strong predictor of Neisseria gonorrhoeae and Chlamydia trachomatis infection. Clin Infect Dis. 2003;36:663–8.

Yudin MH, Landers DV, Meyn L, Hillier SL. Clinical and cervical cytokine response to treatment with oral or vaginal metronidazole for bacterial vaginosis during pregnancy: a randomized trial. Obstet Gynecol. 2003; 102:527–34.

Candidiasis

Babula O, Lazdane G, Kroica J, Linhares IM, Ledger WJ, Witkin SS. Frequency of interleukin-4 (IL-4) -589 gene polymorphism and vaginal concentrations of IL-4, nitric oxide, and mannose-binding lectin in women with recurrent vulvovaginal candidiasis. Clin Infect Dis. 2005;40:1258–62.

Barousse MM, Steele C, Dunlap K, Espinosa T, Boikov D, Sobel JD, Fidel Jr PL. Growth inhibition of Candida albicans by human vaginal epithelial cells. J Infect Dis. 2001;184:1489–93.

Black CA, Eyers FM, Dunkley ML, Clancy RL, Beagley KW. Major histocompatibility haplotype does not impact the course of experimentally induced murine vaginal candidiasis. Lab Anim Sci. 1999a;49: 668–72.

Black CA, Eyers FM, Russell A, Dunkley ML, Clancy RL, Beagley KW. Increased severity of Candida vaginitis in BALB/c nu/nu mice versus the parent strain is not abrogated by adoptive transfer of T cell enriched lymphocytes. J Reprod Immunol. 1999b;45:1–18.

Calderone RA, Fonzi WA. Virulence factors of Candida albicans. Trends Microbiol. 2001;9:327–33.

Cassone A, Boccanera M, Adriani D, Santoni G, De Bernardis F. Rats clearing a vaginal infection by Candida albicans acquire specific, antibody-mediated resistance to vaginal reinfection. Infect Immun. 1995; 65:2619–25.

Cheng G, Wozniak K, Wallig MA, Fid Jr PL, Trupin SR, Hoyer LL. Comparison between Candida albicans agglutinin-like sequence gene expression patterns in human clinical specimens and models of vaginal candidiasis. Infect Immun. 2005;73:1656–63.

Corrigan EM, Clancy RL, Dunkley ML, Eyers FM, Beagley KW. Cellular immunity in recurrent vulvovaginal candidiasis. Clin Exp Immunol. 1998;111: 574–8.

Cotch MF, Hillier SL, Gibbs RS, Eschenbach DA. Epidemiology and outcomes associated with moderate to heavy Candida colonization during pregnancy. Vaginal Infections and Prematurity Study Group. Am J Obstet Gynecol. 1998;178:374–80.

De Carvalho R, Cunha C, Silva D, Sopelete MC, Urzedo JE, Moreira TA, Moraes Pde S, Taketomi EA. IgA, IgE, and IgG subclasses to Candida albicans in serum and vaginal fluid from patients with vulvovaginal candidiasis. Rev Assoc Med Bras. 2003;49:434–8.

DeBernardis F, Santoni G, Boccanera M, Spreghini E, Adriani D, Morelli L, Cassone A. Local anticandidal immune responses in a rat model of vaginal infection by and protection against Candida albicans. Infect Immun. 2000;68:3297–304.

Elahi S, Clancy R, Pang G. A therapeutic vaccine for mucosal candidiasis. Vaccine. 2001;19:2516–21.

Fan SR, Liao QP, Liu XP, Liu ZH, Zhang D. Vaginal allergic response in women with vulvovaginal candidiasis. Int J Gynaecol Obstet. 2008;101:27–30.

Ferrer J. Vaginal candidosis: epidemiological and etiological factors. Int J Gynaecol Obstet. 2000;71 Suppl 1:S21–7.

Fichtenbaum CJ, Powderly W. Refractory mucosal candidiasis in patients with human immunodeficiency virus infection. Clin Infect Dis. 1998;26:556–65.

Fidel Jr PL. Immunity in vaginal candidiasis. Curr Opin Infect Dis. 2005;18:107–11.

Fidel Jr PL, Sobel JD. Immunopathogenesis of recurrent vulvovaginal candidiasis. Clin Microbiol Rev. 1996;9:335–48.

Fidel Jr PL, Lynch ME, Redondo-Lopez V, Sobel JD, Robinson R. Systemic cell-mediated immune reactivity in women with recurrent vulvovaginal candidiasis (RVVC). J Infect Dis. 1993a;168:1458–65.

Fidel Jr PL, Lynch ME, Sobel JD. Candida-specific Th1-type responsiveness in mice with experimental vaginal candidiasis. Infect Immun. 1993b;61:4202–7.

Fidel Jr PL, Lynch ME, Conaway DH, Tait L, Sobel JD. Mice immunized by primary vaginal C. albicans infection develop acquired vaginal mucosal immunity. Infect Immun. 1995a;63:547–53.

Fidel Jr PL, Lynch ME, Sobel JD. Circulating CD4 and CD8 T cells have little impact on host defense against experimental vaginal candidiasis. Infect Immun. 1995b;63:2403–8.

Fidel PL, Ginsburg KA, Cutright JL, Wall NA, Lennan D, Dunlap K, Sobel JD. Vagina-associated immunity in women with recurrent vulvovaginal candidiasis: evidence for vaginal Th1-type responses following intravaginal challenge with Candida antigen. J Infect Dis. 1997;176:728–39.

Fidel Jr PL, Luo W, Steele C, Chabain J, Baker M, Wormley FL. Analysis of vaginal cell populations during experimental vaginal candidiasis. Infect Immun. 1999;67:3135–40.

Fidel Jr PL, Cutright J, Steele C. Effects of reproductive hormones on experimental vaginal candidiasis. Infect Immun. 2000;68:651–7.

Fidel Jr PL, Barousse M, Espinosa T, Ficarra M, Sturtevant J, Martin DH, Quayle AJ, Dunlap K. An intravaginal live Candida challenge in humans leads to new hypothesis for the immunopathogenesis of vulvovaginal candidiasis. Infect Immun. 2004;72:2939–46.

Filler SG, Pfunder AS, Spellberg BJ, Edwards Jr JE. Candida albicans stimulates cytokine production and leukocyte adhesion molecule expression by endothelial cells. Infect Immun. 1996;64:2609–17.

Han Y, Morrison RP, Cutler JE. A vaccine and monoclonal antibodies that enhance mouse resistance to Candida albicans vaginal infection. Infect Immun. 1998;66:5771–6.

Hurley R. Recurrent Candida infection. Clin Obstet Gynecol. 1981;8:209–13.

Ito K, Ishiguro A, Kanbe T, Tanaka K, Torii S. Characterization of IgE-binding epitopes on Candida albicans enolase. Clin Exp Allergy. 1995;25:529–35.

Ito K, Tanaka T, Tsutsumi N, Obata F, Kashiwagi N. Possible mechanisms of immunotherapy for maintaining pregnancy in recurrent spontaneous aborters: analysis of antiidiotypic antibodies directed against autologous T-cell receptors. Hum Reprod. 1999;14:650–5.

Kalo-Klein A, Witkin SS. Candida albicans: cellular immune system interactions during different stages of the menstrual cycle. Am J Obstet Gynecol. 1989;161:1132–6.

Kelly KA, Gray HL, Walker JC, Rank RG, Wormley FL, Fidel Jr PL. Chlamydia trachomatis infection does not enhance local cellular immunity against concurrent Candida vaginal infection. Infec Immun. 2001;69:3451–4.

Knight L, Fletcher J. Growth of Candida albicans in saliva: stimulation by glucose associated with antibiotics, corticosteriods and diabetes mellitus. J Infect Dis. 1971;123:371–7.

La Valle R, Sandini S, Gomez MJ, Mondello F, Romagnoli G, Nisini R, Cassone A. Generation of a recombinant 65-kilodalton mannoprotein, a major antigen target of cell-mediated immune response to Candida albicans. Infect Immun. 2000;68:6777–84.

Leigh JE, Barousse M, Swoboda RK, Myers T, Hager S, Wolf NA, Cutright JL, Thompson J, Sobel JD, Fidel PL. Candida-specific systemic cell-mediated immune reactivities in human immunodeficiency virus-positive persons with mucosal candidiasis. J Infect Dis. 2001;183:277–85.

Lev-Sagie A, Nyirjesy P, Tarangelo N, et al. Hyaluronan in vaginal secretions: association with recurrent vulvovaginal candidiasis. Am J Obstet Gynecol. 2009a;201:206e.1–5.

Lev-Sagie A, Prus D, Linhares IM, Lavy Y, Ledger WJ, Witkin SS. Polymorphism in a gene coding for the inflammasome component NALP3 and recurrent vulvovaginal candidiasis in women with vulvar vestibulitis syndrome. Am J Obstet Gynecol. 2009b;200:303e.1–6.

Liu F, Liao Q, Liu Z. Mannose-binding lectin and vulvovaginal candidiasis. Int J Gynaecol Obstet. 2006;92:43–7.

Magliani W, Conti S, Cassone A, DeBernardis F, Polonelli L. New immunotherapeutic strategies to control vaginal candidiasis. Trends Mol Med. 2002;8:121–6.

Mendling W, Seebacher C. Guideline vulvovaginal candidosis: Guideline of the German Dermatological Society, the German Speaking Mycological Society and the Working Group for Infections and Infect immunology of the German Society for Gynecology and Obstetrics. Mycoses. 2003;46:365–9.

Mochizuki K, Sato Y, Tsuda N, et al. Immunological evaluation of vaccination with pre-designated peptides frequently selected as vaccine candidates in an individualized peptide vaccination regimen. Int J Oncol. 2004;25:121–31.

Mourad S, Friedman L. Active immunization against Candida albicans. Proc Soc Exp Biol Med. 1961; 106:570–2.

Nohmi T, Abe S, Dobashi K, Tansho S, Yamaguchi H. Suppression of anti-Candida activity of murine neutrophils by progesterone in vitro: a possible mechanism in pregnant women's vulnerability to vaginal candidiasis. Microbiol Immunol. 1995;39:405–9.

Nomanbhoy F, Steele C, Yano J, Fidel Jr PL. Vaginal and oral epithelial cell anti-Candida activity. Infect Immun. 2002;70:7081–8.

Polonelli L, Cassone A. Novel strategies for treating candidiasis. Curr Opin Infect Dis. 1999;12:61–6.

Polonelli L, De Bernardis F, Conti S, Boccanera M, Gerloni M, Morace G, Magliani W, Chezzi C, Cassone A. Idiotypic intravaginal vaccination to protect against candidal vaginitis by secretory, yeast killer toxin-like anti-idiotypic antibodies. J Immunol. 1994;152: 3175–82.

Rigg D, Miller MM, Metzger WJ. Recurrent vulvovaginitis: treatment with Candida albicans allergen immunotherapy. Am J Obstet Gynecol. 1990;162:332–6.

Romani L, Mocci S, Bietta C, Lanfaloni L, Puccetti P, Bistoni F. Th1 and Th2 cytokine secretion patterns in murine candidiasis: association of Th1 responses with acquired resistance. Infect Immun. 1991;59:4647–54.

Rosedale N, Browne K. Hyposensitisation in the management of recurring vaginal candidiasis. Ann Allergy. 1979;43:250–3.

Ruhnke M. Epidemiology of Candida albicans infections and role of non-Candida-albicans yeasts. Curr Drug Targets. 2006;7:495–504.

Sobel JD. Pathogenesis and epidemiology of vulvovaginal candidiasis. Ann N Y Acad Sci. 1988;544:547–57.

Sobel JD. Vaginal infections in adult women. Sex Transm Dis. 1990;74:1573–601.

Sobel JD, Faro S, Force R, Foxman B, Ledger WJ, Nyirjesy PR, Reed PD, Summers PR. Vulvovaginal candidiasis: epidemiologic, diagnostic, and therapeutic considerations. Am J Obstet Gynecol. 1998;178:203–11.

Spencer SE, Valentin-Bon IE, Whaley K, Jerse AE. Inhibition of Neisseria gonorrhoea genital tract infection by leading candidate topical microbicides in a mouse model. J Infect Dis. 2004;189:410–9.

Steele C, Fidel Jr PL. Cytokine and chemokine production by human oral and vaginal ECs in response to Candida albicans. Infect Immun. 2002;70:577–83.

Taylor BN, Saavedra M, Fidel Jr PL. Local Th1/Th2 cytokine production during experimental vaginal candidiasis: potential importance of transforming growth factor-β. Med Mycol. 2000;38:419–31.

Vazquez JA, Sobel JD, Demitriou R, Vaishampayan J, Lynch M, Zervos MJ. Karyotyping of Candida albicans isolates obtained longitudinally in women with recurrent vulvovaginal candidiasis. J Infect Dis. 1994;170:1566–9.

Waldman RH, Cruz JM, Rowe DS. Immunoglobulin levels and antibody to Candida albicans in human cervicovaginal secretions. Clin Exp Immunol. 1971;9: 427–34.

Weissenbacher T. Nachweis von Candida and Bestimmung der Zytokine.Interleukin-4, Interleukin-5 und Interleukin-13 sowie von Prostaglandin E2, Candida-spezifischem IgE und Gesamt-IgE im Vaginalsekret bei Frauen mit Verdacht auf chronisch rezidivierende Vulvovaginalcandidose. München, 2004.

Weissenbacher ER, Weissenbacher T, Spitzbart H. Die Bedeutung der Interleukine und des Candida-IgE bei der chronisch rezidivierenden Vulvovaginalcandidose. Mycoses. 2004;47 Suppl 1:37–40.

Weissenbacher TM, Witkin SS, Gingelmaier A, Scholz C, Friese K, Mylonas I. Relationship between recurrent vulvovaginal candidosis and immune mediators in vaginal fluid. Eur J Obstet Gynecol Reprod Biol. 2009;144:59–63.

White MH. Is vulvovaginal candidiasis an AIDS-related illness? Clin Infect Dis. 1996;22:S124–7.

Witkin SS, Kalo-Klein A, Galland L, Teich M, Ledger WL. Effect of Candida albicans plus histamine on prostaglandin E2 production by peripheral blood mononuclear cells from healthy women and women with recurrent candidal vaginitis. J Infect Dis. 1991;164:396–9.

Wormley Jr FL, Chaiban J, Fidel Jr PL. Cell adhesion molecule and lymphocyte activation marker expression during experimental vaginal candidiasis. Infect Immun. 2001a;69:5072–9.

Wormley Jr FL, Steele C, Wozniak K, Fujihashi K, McGhee JR, Fidel Jr PL. Resistance of TCR δ-chain knockout mice to experimental Candida vaginitis. Infect Immun. 2001b;69:7162–4.

Wormley Jr FL, Cutright JL, Fidel Jr PL. Multiple experimental designs to evaluate the role of T-cell-mediated immunity against experimental vaginal Candida albicans infection. Med Mycol. 2003;41:401–10.

Trichomoniasis

Abraham MC, Desjardins M, Filion LG, Garber GE. Inducible immunity to Trichomonas vaginalis in a mouse model of vaginal infection. Infect Immun. 1996;64:3571–5.

Addis MF, Rappelli P, Pinto De Andrade AM, Rita FM, Colombo MM, Cappuccinelli P, Fiori PL. Identification of Trichomonas vaginalis α-actinin as the most common immunogen recognized by sera of women exposed to the parasite. J Infect Dis. 1999;180:1727–30.

Alderete JF. Does lactobacillus vaccine for trichomoniasis, Solco Trichovac, induce antibody reactive with Trichomonas vaginalis? Genitourin Med. 1988;64: 11–123.

Alderete JF, Kasmala L, Metcalfe E, Garza G. Phenotypic variation and diversity among Trichomonas vaginalis isolates and correlation of phenotype with trichomonal virulence determinants. Infect Immun. 1986;53: 285–93.

Alderete JF, Newton E, Dennis C, Neale KA. Antibody in sera of patients infected with Trichomonas vaginalis is to trichomonal proteinases. Genitourin Med. 1991a; 67:331–4.

Alderete JF, Newton E, Dennis C, Neale KA. The vagina of women infected with Trichomonas vaginalis has numerous proteinases and antibody to trichomonad proteinases. Genitourin Med. 1991b;67:469–74.

Alderete JF, Provenzano D, Lehker W. Iron mediates Trichomonas vaginalis resistance to complement lysis. Microb Pathog. 1995;19:93–103.

Anderson BL, Cosentino LA, Simhan HN, Hillier SL. Systemic immune response to Trichomonas vaginalis infection during pregnancy. Sex Transm Dis. 2007;34: 392–6.

Arroyo R, Engbring J, Alderete JF. Molecular basis of host EC recognition by Trichomonas vaginalis. Mol Microbiol. 1992;6:853–62.

Arroyo R, Gonzalez-Robles A, Martinez-Palomo A, Alderete JF. Trichomonas vaginalis for amoeboid transformation and adhesion synthesis follows cytoadherence. Mol Microbiol. 1993;7:299–309.

Buchvald D, Demes P, Gombosova A, Mraz P, Valent M, Stefanovic J. Vaginal leukocyte characteristics in urogenital trichomoniasis. APMIS. 1992;100:393–400.

Buve A, Weiss H, Laga M, Van Dyck E, Musonda R, Zekeng L, Kahindo M, Anagonou S, Morison L, Robinson NJ, Hayes RJ, The Study Group on Heterogeneity of HIV Epidemics in African Cities. The epidemiology of trichomoniasis in women in four African cities. AIDS. 2001;15 Suppl 4:S89–96.

Caterina P, Lynch D, Ashman RB, Warton A, Papadimitriou JM. Complement-mediated regulation of Trichomonas vaginalis infection in mice. Exp Clin Immunogenet. 1999;16:107–16.

Chang JH, Ryang YS, Morio T, Lee SK, Chang EJ. Trichomonas vaginalis inhibits proinflammatory cytokine production in macrophages by suppressing NF-κB activation. Mol Cells. 2005;18:177–85.

Cogne M, Brasseur P, Ballet JJ. Detection and characterization of serum antitrichomonal antibodies in urogenital trichomoniasis. J Clin Microbiol. 1985;21: 588–92.

Cohen CR, Moscicki AB, Scott ME, et al. Increased levels of immune activation in the genital tract of healthy young women from sub-Saharan Africa. AIDS. 2010;24:2069–74.

Corbeil LB, Anderson ML, Corbeil RR, Eddow JM, Bon Durant RH. Female reproductive tract immunity in bovine trichomoniasis. Am J Reprod Immunol. 1998; 39:189–98.

Cotch MF, Pastorek JG, Nugent RP, Hillier SL, Gibbs RS, Martin DH, Eschenbach DA, Edelmann R, Carey JC, Regan JA, Krohn MA, Klebanoff MA, Rao AV, Rhoads GG. Trichomonas vaginalis associated with low birth weight and preterm delivery. The Vaginal Infections and Prematurity Study Group. Sex Transm Dis. 1997;24:353–60.

Cu-Uvin S, Ko H, Jamieson DJ, Hogan JW, Schuman P, Anderson J, Klein RS. HIV Epidemiology Research Study (HERS) Group. Prevalence, incidence, and persistence or recurrence of trichomoniasis among human immunodeficiency virus (HIV)-positive women and among HIV-negative women at high risk for HIV infection. Clin Infect Dis. 2002;34:1406–11.

Demes P, Gombosova A, Valent M, Fabusova H, Janoska A. Fewer Trichomonas vaginalis organisms in vaginas of infected women during menstruation. Genitourin Med. 1988a;64:22–4.

Demes P, Gombosova A, Valent M, Janoska A, Fabusova H, Petrenko M. Differential susceptibility of fresh Trichomonas vaginalis isolates to complement in menstrual blood and cervical mucus. Genitourin Med. 1988b;64:176–9.

Demirezen S, Korkmaz E, Beksac MS. Association between trichomoniasis and bacterial vaginosis: examination of 600 cervicovaginal smears. Cent Eur J Public Health. 2005;13:96–8.

Fichorova RN. Impact of T. vaginalis infection on innate immune responses and reproductive outcome. J Reprod Immunol. 2009;83:185–9.

Fichorova RN, Trifonova RT, Gilbert RO, et al. Trichomonas vaginalis lipophosphoglycan triggers a selective upregulation of cytokines by human female reproductive tract epithelial cells. Infect Immun. 2006; 74:5773–9.

Gilbert RO, Elia G, Beach DH, Klaessig S, Singh BN. Cytopathogenic effect of Trichomonas vaginalis on human vaginal ECs cultured in vitro. Infect Immun. 2000;68:4200–6.

Gombosova A, Demes P, Valent M. Immunotherapeutic effect of the lactobacillus vaccine, Solco Trichovac, in trichomoniasis is not mediated by antibodies cross reacting with Trichomonas vaginalis. Genitourin Med. 1986;62:107–10.

James JA, Thomason JL, Gelbart SM, Osypowski P, Kaiser P, Hanson L. Is trichomoniasis often associated with bacterial vaginosis in pregnant adolescents? Am J Obstet Gynecol. 1992;166:859–62.

Kigozi GG, Brahmbhatt H, Wabwire-Mangen F, Waver MJ, Serwadda D, Sewankambo N, Gray RH. Treatment of Trichomonas in pregnancy and adverse outcomes of pregnancy: a sub analysis of a randomized trial in Rakai, Uganda. Am J Obstet Gynecol. 2003;189:1398–400.

Klebanoff MA, Carey J, Hauth JC, Hillier SL, Nugent RP, Thom EA, Ernest JM, Heine RP, Wapner RJ, Trout W, Moawad A, Leveno KJ, Miodovnik M, Siai BM, Van Dorsten JP, Dombrowski MP, O'Sullivan MJ, Varner M, Langer O, McNellis D, Roberts JM, National Institute of Child Health and Human Development Network of Maternal-Fetal Medicine Units. Failure of metronidazole to prevent preterm delivery among pregnant women with asymptomatic Trichomonas vaginalis infection. N Engl J Med. 2001;345:487–93.

Kucknoor AS, Mundodi V, Alderete JF. Adherence to human vaginal ECs signals for increased expression of Trichomonas vaginalis genes. Infect Immun. 2005; 73:6472–8.

Malla N, Valadkhani Z, Harjai K, Sharma S, Gupta I. Reactive oxygen intermediates in experimental trichomoniasis induced with isolates from symptomatic and asymptomatic women. Parasitol Res. 2004;94:101–5.

Mendoza-Lopez MR, Becerril-Garcia C, Fattel-Facenda LV, Avila-Gonzalez L, Ruiz-Tachiquin ME, Ortega-Lopez J, Arroyo R. CP30, a cysteine proteinase involved in Trichomonas vaginalis cytoadherence. Infect Immun. 2000;68:4907–12.

Mundodi V, Kucknoor AS, Chang TH, Alderete JF. A novel surface protein of Trichomonas vaginalis is regulated independently by low iron and contact with vaginal ECs. BMC Microbiol. 2006;31:6.

Niccolai L, Kopicko JJ, Kassie A, Petros H, Clark RA, Kissinger P. Incidence and predictors of reinfection with Trichomonas vaginalis in HIV-infected women. Sex Transm Dis. 2000;27:284–8.

Paintlia MK, Kaur S, Gupta I, Ganguly NK, Mahajan RC, Malla N. Specific IgA response, T-cell subtype and cytokine profile in experimental intravaginal trichomoniasis. Parasitol Res. 2002;88:338–43.

Park KJ, Ryu JS, Min DY, Lee KT. Leukocyte chemotaxis to Trichomonas vaginalis. Yonsei J Med Sci. 1984;17:77–88.

Petrin D, Delgaty K, Bhatt R, Garber G. Clinical and microbiological aspects of Trichomonas vaginalis. Clin Microbiol Rev. 1998;11:300–17.

Provenzano D, Alderete JF. Analysis of human immunoglobulin-degrading cysteine proteinases of Trichomonas vaginalis. Infect Immun. 1995;63:3388–95.

Rein MF, Sullivan JA, Mandell GL. Trichomonacidal activity of human polymorphonuclear neutrophils: killing by disruption and fragmentation. J Infect Dis. 1980;142:575–85.

Ryu JS, Kang JH, Jung SH, Shin MH, Kim JM, Park H, Min DY. Production of interleukin-8 by human neutrophils stimulated with Trichomonas vaginalis. Infect Immun. 2004;72:1326–32.

Schwebke JR, Burgess D. Trichomoniasis. Clin Microbiol Rev. 2004;17:794–803.

Shaio MF, Lin PR. Influence of humoral immunity on leukotriene B4 production by neutrophils in response to Trichomonas vaginalis stimulation. Parasite Immunol. 1995a;17:127–33.

Shaio MF, Lin PR. Leukotriene B4 levels in the vaginal discharges from cases of trichomoniasis. Am Trop Med Parasitol. 1995b;89:85–8.

Shaio MF, Chang FY, Hou SC, Lee CS, Lin PR. The role of immunoglobulin and complement in enhancing the respiratory burst of neutrophils against Trichomonas vaginalis. Parasite Immunol. 1991;13:241–50.

Shaio MF, Lin PR, Liu JY, Yang KD. Generation of interleukin-8 from human monocytes in response to Trichomonas vaginalis stimulation. Infect Immun. 1995;63:3864–70.

Sharma P, Malla N, Gupta I, Ganguly NK, Mahajan RC. Antitrichomonal IgA antibodies in trichomoniasis before and after treatment. Folia Microbiol. 1991;36:302–4.

Simhan HN, Anderson BL, Krohn MA, et al. Host immune consequences of asymptomatic Trichomonas vaginalis infection in pregnancy. Am J Obstet Gynecol. 2007;196:591–55.

Sorvillo F, Kerndt P. Trichomonas vaginalis and amplification of HIV-1 transmission. Lancet. 1998;351:213–4.

Street DA, Taylor-Robinson D, Ackers JP, Hanna NF, McMillan A. Evaluation of an enzyme- linked immunosorbent assay for the detection of antibody to Trichomonas vaginalis in sera and vaginal secretions. Br J Vener Dis. 1982;58:330–3.

Thurman AR, Doncel GF. Innate immunity and inflammatory response to Trichomonas vaginalis and bacterial vaginosis: relationship to HIV acquisition. Am J Reprod Immunol. 2011;65:89–98.

Wos SM, Watt RM. Immunoglobulin isotypes of anti-Trichomonas vaginalis antibodies in patients with vaginal trichomoniasis. J Clin Microbiol. 1986;24:790–5.

Yadav M, Dubey ML, Gupta I, Malla N. Nitric oxide radicals in leukocytes and vaginal washes of Trichomonas vaginalis-infected symptomatic and asymptomatic women. Parasitology. 2006;132:339–43.

Zariffard MR, Harwani S, Novak RM, Graham PJ, Ji X, Spear GT. Trichomonas vaginalis infection activates cells through toll-like receptor 4. Clin Immunol. 2004;111:103–7.

Immunology in Reproductive Medicine

5

Contents

5.1   Immunology of Pregnancy

Pregnancy can be described as the symbiosis of two allogeneic individuals that live in intimate contact. Although the fetus provides a panel of MHC antigens derived from both its mother and father, it is not rejected by its mother's immune system. The maternal immune system reacts toward the foreign tissue, but it tolerates, supports, and regulates its development instead of rejecting it. The formation of the placenta is efficiently controlled, ensuring development of the

E.R. Weissenbacher et al., *Immunology of the Female Genital Tract*,
DOI 10.1007/978-3-642-14906-1_5, © Springer-Verlag Berlin Heidelberg 2014

embryo and fetus. In the course of the discovery of the MHC and its role in transplantation, Medawar was the first to compare the immunologically privileged nature of the fetus with an allograft in 1953. He proposed ideas such as the anatomical separation of mother and fetus, antigenic immaturity of the fetus, and maternal immunosuppression, all of which have now been investigated and partly disproved. However, maternal tolerance of a semiallogeneic fetus is a paradox that remains a central theme in the field of reproductive immunology. Although the maternal immune system recognizes the semiallogeneic fetus, it remains in a quiescent state. The potential mechanisms underlying this phenomenon are likely to be complex and may involve several complementary or overlapping pathways to favor reproductive success. Knowledge of the immunoregulatory processes of pregnancy is necessary to understand and treat a variety of disorders that may lead to infertility, premature events, or preeclampsia. Knowledge of the structural basis of the placenta and the immunobiology of the decidua and of trophoblast are important issues to discuss before addressing disturbances in this system, including preeclampsia, preterm labor, or pregnancy loss.

5.1.1   Immunology of Fertilization

An impending pregnancy must prepare the maternal environment to accept a partially foreign body, a semiallograft, which occurs in four distinct phases. The first is the pre-fertilization period in which the egg is surrounded by the follicular fluid with its immunosuppressive activity. This may facilitate the following fertilization process as well as embryo development by minimizing the maternal immune response to the sperm, which has been shown to express foreign antigens.

The second phase comprises fertilization and embryo development until the morula stage in which the sperm penetrates the egg and becomes immunologically invisible to the maternal immune system. No maternal immune reaction occurs during the process of egg and sperm fusion. Once this happens, the fertilized egg is rapidly surrounded by the zona pellucida, which wards off maternal immune cells. Further protection against these cells is provided by maternal cumulus cells for the first days after fertilization.

The third phase consists of the blastocyst and preimplantation trophoblast polarization after the first embryonic cell divisions begin. The surrounding zona pellucida continues to provide a major protection against the maternal immune system so that the development of maternal immune tolerance to the embryo does not take place until the implantation phase, when direct embryo/maternal contact occurs in the uterus. From an immunological point of view, this is the most vulnerable time for the embryo, which is now exposed to maternal endometrial immune cells and cytokines. The uterus is designed to prevent implantation except during a narrow implantation window in which embryonic signals help promote endometrial priming and maternal immune tolerance. The embryo likely plays the more significant role in conditioning the maternal environment toward immune tolerance of pregnancy. The arising questions are how this maternal immune tolerance takes place, what embryo-derived elements are involved and where, if these mechanisms are common to all mammals, and how early embryo tolerance can be detected in the maternal organism.

The developing fetus is not directly exposed to maternal blood except in the placenta as the newly formed organ at the fetomaternal interface. The placenta plays the key role in maintenance of local tolerance and allows the mother to accept the embryo during pregnancy. At the fetal side of the placenta, the villous trophoblast forms a continuous barrier that physically separates the mother from the fetus but is exposed to maternal immunocompetent cells present in the circulating blood of the intervillous space. Syncytiotrophoblast and villous cytotrophoblast can also be found in the maternal circulation and lung providing additional antigenic stimuli for the mother. Trophoblast cells are also present in the decidua where they contribute to further stimulating the mother with fetal antigens. This physiological condition of close physical contact between maternal immune system and fetal cells with paternal antigens is unique and normally does not trigger a maternal immune reaction that would lead to fetal death.

Earlier studies suggest that shortly after fertilization, certain changes that favor immune tolerance take place in the maternal environment, possibly due to early pregnancy factor (EPF) and platelet-activating factor (PAF). EPF is an immunosuppressive factor with growth-regulatory properties that interacts with T lymphocytes and suppresses cellular immune responses and the early expression of cell surface membrane IgG. It was first described more than 20 years ago as a very early serum marker of fertilization and is now known to be essential for the initiation and maintenance of pregnancy. It displays the regulated production and pleiotropic function typical of many cytokines and growth factors. On the one hand, it may maintain a successful pregnancy, but on the other hand, its immunosuppressive activity might cause some adverse impact. Studies have proved that EPF activity is detectable in serum, amniotic fluid, and cervical mucus of pregnant women. Therefore, EPF may provide wide clinical applications, such as detecting the occurrence of fertilization in vivo, predicting the prognosis of pregnancy, and evaluating embryo quality in in vitro fertilization–embryo transfer treatment.

These factors have since been found not to be specific to pregnancy: they are found in a nonpregnant state as well, and they do not appear to be critical in initiating maternal recognition of the embryo. Therefore, the unique embryo-derived compounds are involved in creating the unique maternal immunological response to the embryo. Shortly after fertilization, the viable embryo starts to emit signals that promote maternal recognition of pregnancy and immune tolerance. Recent studies have found that the cumulus cells surrounding the embryo might be able to serve as a relay system because they contain active immune cells that secrete cytokines. This proximity between the putative embryo-derived compounds and the maternal immune system would permit rapid diffusion of embryonic signals leading initially to a local immune response, followed by a systemic maternal immune recognition. This conclusion is based on the observation that preimplantation factor (PIF) peptide expression modulates but does

not suppress the maternal immune system, allowing the mother to maintain her ability to fight diseases. With respect to PIF, the presence of its activity in maternal serum within 4 days after embryo transfer indicated a >70 % chance of successful pregnancy outcome, whereas the absence of PIF activity indicated that pregnancy would not develop in 97 % of cases (unpublished data).

5.1.2   Immunobiology of the Trophoblast

As already described, the fetal–placental unit initially is a semiallograft due to paternal genetic contributions. Subsequently, there is a maternal immune reaction to the allogeneic pregnancy. The constituents of the maternal immune reaction to the allogeneic stimulus are not different from any other immune reaction, and the allogeneic conceptus, the trophoblast, is like all other allogeneic tissue grafts.

However, trophoblast is an unusual cell type. It is extraembryonic and has several distinctive properties such as the expression of endogenous retrovirus products, oncofetal proteins, and imprinted genes. In addition, the DNA in trophoblast is relatively unmethylated. All these properties could have some relevance in interaction with the maternal immune system. The special characteristic, however, that distinguishes the trophoblast from other tissues is its ability to eliminate abortogenic maternal B-cell and T-cell responses. The trophoblast induces an immunomodulation and thus actively defends itself from the maternal immune attack. The presence of progesterone, and its interaction with progesterone receptors at the decidual level, appears to play a major role in this defense strategy. Indeed, trophoblasts can influence the immune system during pregnancy through their expression of soluble and cell surface-associated immunomodulatory molecules. For example, trophoblasts secrete indoleamine 2,3-dioxygenase (IDO), which limits the availability of the essential amino acid tryptophan, consequently limiting lymphocyte proliferation and protecting the conceptus from rejection. IDO is an enzyme from the tryptophan catabolic pathway that depletes tryptophan in local tissue environments, thereby suppressing proliferation of cells in the vicinity. IDO may not only inhibit T-cell proliferation but also may be bactericidal via this mechanism. LPS and the inflammatory cytokines IL-1 and TNF-α act synergistically with IFN-γ to further increase IDO expression in human DCs, while anti-inflammatory cytokines IL-4, IL-10, and TGF-β inhibit IDO expression.

It has been shown experimentally that cells at the maternal–fetal interface expressing IDO may establish local microenvironments in which reduced tryptophan concentration precludes T-cell proliferation, thus protecting the conceptus from rejection.

Regulation of the expression of CD200 might play an immunoregulatory role at the maternal–fetal interface. CD200 is another DC-associated molecule that has been shown to contribute to the successful outcome of organ and tissue allografts in mice. CD200 is upregulated in rodent transplantation models where successful inhibition of rejection is accomplished and is believed to signal immunosuppression following engagement of a receptor, CD200R. The investigation of CD200 expression in implantation sites of different strains of mice revealed an elevated abortion rate in mice due to anti-CD200, and infusion of a CD200 immunoadhesin reduced the abortion rate. CD200 mRNA expression was demonstrated in fetal trophoblast and certain areas of decidua. Reduction in CD200 has proven essential for fgl2 prothrombinase triggering of abortions in the mouse model, but the mechanism behind it remains unclear.

There is growing evidence that trophoblast cells are able to recognize and respond to pathogens through the expression of TLRs. Normal term placental tissue has been shown to express TLR1–10 at the RNA level. Term syncytiotrophoblast and intermediate trophoblast cells express TLR2 and TLR4 at the protein level. In contrast, TLR4-positive placental cells express extravillous and intermediate trophoblasts. The first-trimester trophoblast cell populations expressing these receptors are the villous cytotrophoblast and extravillous trophoblast cells, while the first-trimester syncytiotrophoblast cells do not express these TLRs. This suggests that the placenta serves as a highly specialized barrier, protecting the developing fetus against infection.

These findings suggest that trophoblast cells may interact with microorganisms present at the implantation site and may be able to initiate an immune response. The trophoblast may thus function as an active member of the innate immune system.

Trophoblast cells from term placental explants have been demonstrated to produce IL-6 and IL-8 following ligation of TLR2 or TLR4 by LPS. Activation of TLR4 by LPS triggers first-trimester cytotrophoblast and villous trophoblast cells to generate a classical TLR response, characterized by the increased production of both pro- and anti-inflammatory cytokines.

It has been found that TLR4 ligation promotes cytokine production, while ligation of TLR2 induces apoptosis in first-trimester trophoblast cells. Therefore, a pathogen may directly promote elevated trophoblast cell death via TLR2 that is observed in a number of pregnancy complications. TLR2-mediated trophoblast apoptosis may provide a novel mechanism of pathogenesis by which certain intrauterine infections may contribute to conditions such as preterm labor or preeclampsia.

Remarkably, in contrast to most other somatic tissues, invasive trophoblast cells lack not only the classical MHC class I but also MHC class II, which might be important in avoiding the attack of maternal T-cell-mediated rejection. Among the polymorphic classical class I molecules, they only express HLA-C and, additionally, the nonclassical HLA-E, HLA-F, and HLA-G class I molecules. Membrane-bound HLA-G1 and soluble HLA-G1 and HLA-G2 have also been detected in extravillous trophoblast. Additionally, trophoblasts have been shown to express the nonclassical MHC class I molecule, CD1d, on the surface of first-trimester human trophoblasts.

Increasing evidence suggests that placental expressed MHC molecules may play an important role in modulating the innate branch of the maternal immune system. These molecules have several characteristics, which suggest that antigen presentation is not their primary function, including limited tissue expression, relatively short half-life at the cell surface, and limited genetic polymorphism. It is assumed that the nonclassical HLA-G class I may contribute to the immunological mechanisms that protect the fetus against maternal alloimmune response. HLA-G expression may promote allograft survival. HLA-G was found to inhibit cytotoxicity by NK cells via HLA-E and is thought to be important when considering the presence of atypical CD16+ NK cells in successful pregnancy and increased presence of classical CD16+ NK cells in pregnancy failure. Recent evidence suggests that soluble HLA-G1 is immunosuppressive and induces apoptosis of activated CD8+ T cells and downmodulates CD4+ T-cell proliferation. Thus, soluble HLA-G1 could also play a role during implantation.

In addition, the trophoblast also protects itself by expression of FasL. In mice, FasL is also expressed on uterine glandular ECs and decidual cells in placental trophoblasts. Predominant expression of FasL in mice is found in the uterus, which shifts to the placenta at later gestation days during pregnancy. FasL expression has also been reported in first-trimester and term human placental villi. Thus, expression sites of FasL may be positioned to induce apoptosis in maternal Fas-positive immune cells, such as NK and T cells, at the fetomaternal interface.

The relationship between FasL expression and NK cell infiltration in human placenta during early pregnancy has been also evaluated. The findings suggested that a reduction in FasL expression seems to be closely associated with activation and infiltration of maternal NK cells and destruction of uterine glands, resulting in rejection of the fetus. Thus, expression of FasL in the uterine glands and cytotrophoblasts may play a role in the downregulation of the maternal immune response, thereby maintaining pregnancy at early stage.

5.1.3 Immunology at the Fetomaternal Interface

5.1.3.1 Antigen-Presenting Cells

APCs are often regarded as the responsible inducers of maternal tolerance against fetal antigens. Studies in mice or rats and humans showed that the population of APCs in the decidua of pregnancy comprises classical macrophages, classical mature DCs (CD83+), immature or intermediate macrophage/DC-like cells (CD83−), and myeloid DCs (121, 157, 158, 439, 579, 657, 659, 660, 808, 900, 952, 1047, 1385). However, the exact functions of decidual APCs are unclear. In their function of presenting antigens to lymphocytes, it could be assumed that they would be ideally located at the fetomaternal interface to present fetal antigens in a tolerance-inducing manner. Decidual APCs are able to either acquire functions of classical mDCs that can activate T cells or rest in an immature state that likely induces tolerance.

5.1.3.1.1 Dendritic Cells

The specific presence of DCs in the maternal decidua has pointed to a biological role of APCs in maternal–fetal interactions. DCs in the pregnant human uterine mucosa are likely to regulate immune responses to both uterine infections and placental trophoblast cells. In studies on pregnant rat and mouse uteri, the first hints for a possible role of APCs in creating a local environment prohibitive of maternal lymphocyte stimulation against the embryo were observed. Macrophages from the rat uterus were shown to be depleted shortly after implantation, being actually immunosuppressive. A high population of early pregnancy human decidual cells to be HLA-DR+ has been found, concluding that these HLA-DR+ cells mainly were macrophages. These macrophages increase premenstrually and make up to 35 % of the decidual leukocytes around implantation. Interestingly, 21–32 % of maternal decidual cells were positive for HLA class I and II molecules. The class II+ cells were identified as macrophages by antibody staining. Isolated decidual macrophages were able to present soluble antigens in an MHC-restricted manner but also possessed suppressive activity for maternal immune responses. However, another study showed that cultured human decidual stromal cells expressed HLA-DR and the activation markers CD80 and CD86 but not the classical macrophage marker CD14 and were able to stimulate allogeneic T cells. In recent years, classical mature CD40+ CD45+ CD83+ DCs similar to those of other mucosal surfaces were demonstrated in human endometrium and early pregnancy decidua. CD83 has been shown to be a suitable and selective cell surface marker for mDCs.

In addition, the immature precursors of decidual DCs, DC-SIGN-positive HLA-DR+ decidual cells that also stained for CD14 and CD68 as classical macrophage markers, were detected. The maturation of CD14+ DC-SIGN+ decidual cells into CD25+ CD83+ mDCs upon inflammatory cytokine treatment resulted in downregulation of antigen uptake capacity and effective stimulation of resting T cells. A small population of decidual DC expressing DC11c, a marker for myeloid DC, but not expressing other classical leukocyte lineage markers was detected. These decidual DCs comprised about 1.7 % of CD45+ cells in the isolates. A bidirectional cross talk between decidual CD56 NK cells and decidual CD83+ cells was shown, resulting in activation and proliferative response of autologous NK cells. In experiments with mice, the majority of uterine DCs were of myeloid lineage and that the relative number of CD11c+ uterine cells is not constant during pregnancy. There was an increase occurring simultaneously with implantation.

Decidual mDCs secrete less of the proinflammatory cytokine, IL-12, than blood monocyte-derived DCs and induce Th2 cells when cocultured with naïve CD4+ T cells, which suggests an immunosuppressive phenotype of decidual DCs. A significantly higher number of mDCs in human decidual tissue from abortions than in normal pregnancies could be observed, which leads to speculation that mDCs may play a role in recurrent abortions.

The systemic response of DCs and their cytolytic products was studied and reported that the frequency of myeloid DCs in the early and middle stages of human pregnancy was comparable with that of lymphoid DCs, while in the late stage of pregnancy, the frequency of myeloid DCs significantly increased. They also showed that in the presence of human chorionic gonadotropin (hCG), both peripheral blood DC subsets can be activated to respond to invading pathogens that affect DC subtypes. Myeloid DCs can produce

IL-12 and IFN-γ in response to hCG. Thus, IL-12 produced from myeloid DCs can stimulate the production of IFN-γ as a positive feedback loop, while lymphoid DCs might be directly activated by hCG to produce IFN-γ.

5.1.3.1.2 Macrophages

Macrophages constitute 20–30 % of the decidual cells at the site of implantation and, unlike NK cells, remain high throughout pregnancy. Indeed, macrophages are one of the major cell types in both the maternal and fetal compartments of the uteroplacental unit. In humans, during the first weeks of implantation, macrophages are found in high numbers in the maternal decidua and in tissues close in proximity to the placenta, especially in the stroma surrounding the transformed spiral arteries and extravillous trophoblast.

This suggests that the innate immune system is not indifferent to the fetus and may have a role not only in host protection to infections but also as important players in the fetomaternal immune adjustment. Macrophages are also a main source of cytokines and growth factors and contribute to the maintenance of the balance between Th1 and Th2 cytokines at the placental bed.

There are also several indications that macrophages are often more closely associated with trophoblast than uterine NK cells, with close associations between macrophages and extravillous trophoblast in decidua basalis, and a recent study of rhesus monkey decidua also highlights the close association of macrophages, rather than uterine NK cells, with trophoblast. Although decidual macrophages are activated in vivo, as indicated by their expression of HLA class II, CD11c, and CD86, they have recently been reported to express markers such as DC-SIGN that may aid in immune evasion or are associated with macrophage alternative activation, a phenotypic state of immunosuppressive activity. Early in vitro studies of the suppressive functions of decidual cell mixtures pointed to maternal macrophage production of prostaglandin E2. Decidual macrophages have also been shown to elicit reduced allogeneic and autologous T-cell responses when compared to their blood counterparts. The question then arises as to how decidual

APCs are driven into immune inhibitory profiles. Several studies have indicated that placental HLA-G as a product of infiltrating fetal cytotrophoblast cells may suppress APC functions, but reports published to date fail to show that HLA-G is acting specifically at the level of the APC. Macrophages and DCs both express the HLA-G receptors, ILT2 and ILT4, which can suppress activation signals in order to induce immunosuppressive activities by APCs.

The dense macrophage infiltration at the maternal–fetal interface suggests that these cells are also involved in specific pregnancy-associated functions and not only to perform their usual immunological tasks. Interestingly, maternal macrophages probably assist in the tissue remodeling necessary to accommodate expansion of extraembryonic tissue. Macrophages actively orchestrate apoptosis of unwanted cells during tissue remodeling through cytokines and the influence of hormonal factors. During implantation, apoptosis is important for the appropriate tissue remodeling of the maternal decidua and invasion of the developing embryo. Apoptosis has been described in the trophoblast layer of placentas from uncomplicated pregnancies throughout gestation, suggesting that there is a constant cell turnover at the site of implantation necessary for the appropriate growth and function of the placenta. In addition, the incidence of trophoblast apoptosis is higher in third-trimester villi compared to first-trimester placenta, suggesting that increasing placental apoptosis may be involved in the process of parturition.

However, the clearance of apoptotic bodies represents the critical step in tissue homeostasis, preventing the release of intracellular contents, which may cause tissue damage and the possibility to initiate an inflammatory reaction that may have lethal consequences in pregnancy. During the period of implantation and trophoblast invasion with its induction of apoptosis in maternal tissue, numerous macrophages are present at the implantation site that was originally thought to represent an immune response against the invading trophoblast. Alternatively, it is suggested that macrophage engulfment of apoptotic cells prevents the release of potentially proinflammatory and proimmunogenic intracellular contents that occurs during secondary necrosis. Trophoblast cells are carriers of proteins, which are antigenically foreign to the maternal immune system and if released, as a result of cell death, may initiate or accelerate immunological responses with lethal consequences for the fetus. Therefore, the appropriate removal of dying trophoblast cells by macrophages prior to the release of these intracellular components is critical for the prevention of fetal rejection. During normal pregnancy, the uptake of apoptotic cells suppresses activated macrophages from secreting proinflammatory cytokines such as TNF-α and IFN-γ and promotes the release of Th2-type, anti-inflammatory, and immunosuppressive cytokines with protective effects on trophoblast survival and immunological tolerance (Fig. 5.1).

Changes in the cytokine milieu, owing to elevated levels of apoptotic bodies and inefficient clearance, will result in a proinflammatory microenvironment that in turn may result in changes in trophoblast resistance to Fas-mediated apoptosis and the maternal immune system (Fig. 5.2). Further explanations are to be discussed in the chapter on disturbances in maternal–fetal interactions later.

5.1.3.2 Leukocytes

Already in the final part of the menstrual cycle, a large number of maternal leukocytes can be found in the endometrium. As the mucosal lining of the uterus is transformed from endometrium in the nonpregnant state to the decidua of pregnancy by the influence of sex hormones, these leukocytes further increase in number and are found in close contact with trophoblast. CD56+ leukocytes make up 70 % of the immunocompetent decidual cells. The predominant type of these cells is uterine NK cells (46 %), followed by macrophages (19 %) and T cells (8 %), mainly CD8+ T cells, whereas B cells are virtually absent. In general, cells of the innate immune system seem to dominate this tissue, since the levels of T and B lymphocytes are relatively low (1–3 %). Extravillous trophoblast cells interact with maternal immune cells at the implantation site in the decidua basalis, including the abundant NK cells, APCs, and T cells.

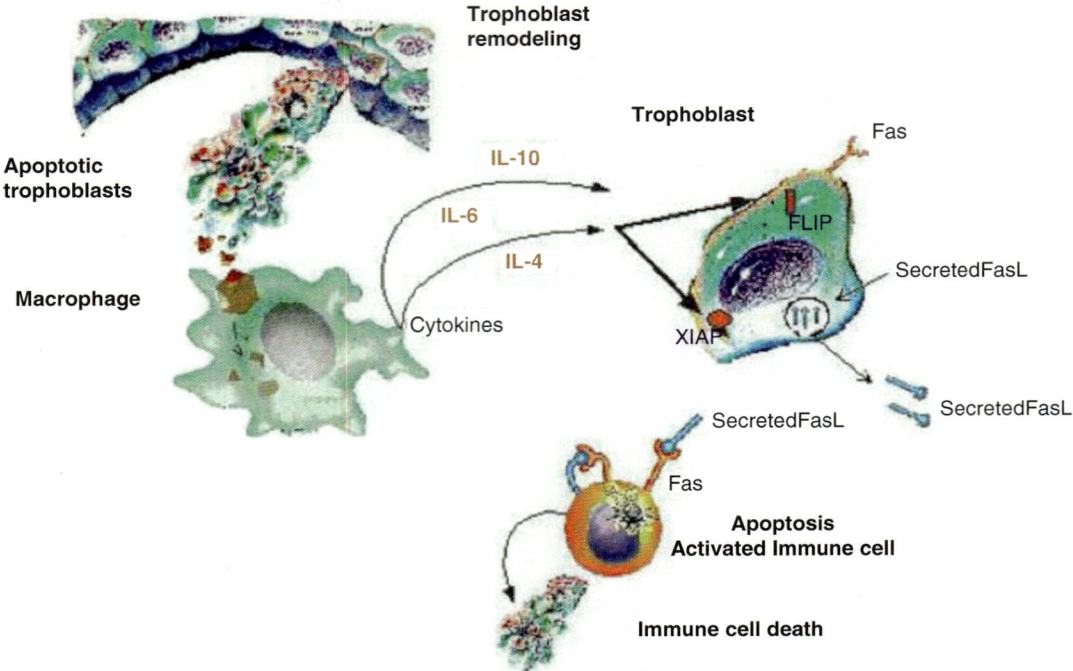

Fig. 5.1 Clearance of apoptotic cells by macrophages in normal pregnancy (Mor G, Abrahams VM. Potential role of macrophages as immunoregulators of pregnancy. Reprod Biol Endocrinol. 2003;1:119–27)

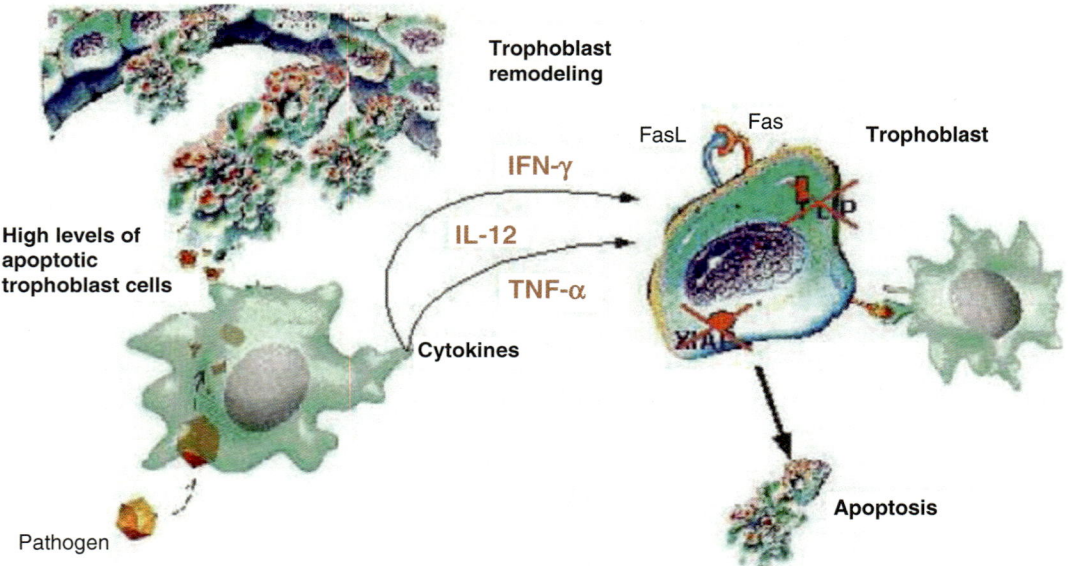

Fig. 5.2 Proinflammatory environment by inefficient clearance of apoptotic bodies in complicated pregnancy (Mor G, Abrahams VM. Potential role of macrophages as immunoregulators of pregnancy. Reprod Biol Endocrinol. 2003;1:119–27)

5.1.3.2.1 NK Cells

Analysis of the leukocytes in the uterus has shown that NK cells are the predominant population, but their total number in the uterine mucosa varies throughout the menstrual cycle with an increase throughout the secretory phase and in the decidua during the early stages of gestation.

There is a massive recruitment of NK cells at the embryonic site of implantation that makes them the dominant cell type of maternal immune cells in the decidua basalis in early pregnancy. As gestation proceeds, NK cell numbers decline and at term these leukocytes are absent. This reduction of uterine NK cells in later pregnancy remains unexplained. Death by both apoptosis and necrosis has been proposed for the loss of uterine NK cells in the late stages of mouse pregnancy, but no information is available regarding the fate of the cells in human pregnancy.

Results of studies that have compared the distribution of uterine NK cells between decidua basalis, which underlies the placenta and is infiltrated by trophoblast, and decidua parietalis, which lines the remainder of the uterine cavity, have been inconsistent. Some have reported increased numbers of uterine NK cells in decidua basalis and considered this to support a role in the control of trophoblast invasion, but others have failed to detect any difference in the different decidual areas (unpublished data). However, the possibility of a functional difference between the two sites has not been considered in detail. Since uterine NK cells express receptors for the nonclassical HLA antigens expressed by extravillous trophoblast, contact with trophoblast in decidua basalis could lead to altered function such as a differing cytokine profiles. Increased IFN-γ levels have been reported in decidua basalis.

Phenotypically, decidual NK cells (CD56bright CD16– CD160–) differ from NK cells in peripheral blood (CD56dim CD16+ CD160+), which suggests that either decidual NK cells represent a distinct subpopulation of circulating NK cells or they have undergone some tissue-specific differentiation.

There are also morphological differences between CD56bright NK cells in decidua and those present in low numbers in peripheral blood.

All the peripheral CD56bright NK cells are small and agranular, whereas those in decidua are mostly large granular lymphocytes. However, decidual NK cells can change into classical CD16-expressing cells after IL-2 stimulation which can result in cytotoxicity and an alloimmune reaction. Women with recurrent abortions have high numbers of NK cells of the conventional CD16+ CD56+ type in the uterus. This underlines the possibility that decidual NK cells exert different functions with the priority of contributing to placental development and pregnancy outcome.

After blastocyst implantation and decidualization, decidual NK cells are activated and secrete IFN-γ, perforin, and angiogenic factors in order to control trophoblast invasion through their cytotoxic activity and also initiate vessel instability and remodeling of decidual arteries to increase the blood supply to the fetoplacental unit. Moreover, they take part in regulation of the maternal immune response producing Th2- and Th3-type cytokines, which results in placental augmentation and local immunosuppression.

Decidual NK cells express receptors for classical and nonclassical HLA class I which are expressed on the cell surface of, or secreted by, extravillous trophoblast. The extravillous cytotrophoblast attracts decidual NK cells by producing MIP-1α chemokines so that the HLA class I molecules on the trophoblast interact with MHC class I-dependent receptors present on the surface of decidual NK cells. These receptors on decidual NK cells comprise four different families with both activating and inhibitory members. The specific ligands for most NK cell receptors are the only HLA molecules expressed on extravillous trophoblast, HLA-C, HLA-E, and HLA-G. These are the KIRs for which HLA-C and HLA-G molecules are the ligands: the Ig-like receptor ILT2, which is expressed by 20–25 % of decidual NK cells and interacts with HLA-G; the CD160 receptor with its major ligand HLA-C, which is expressed on a minor set of decidual NK cells; and the CD94/NKG2 receptor, which binds HLA-E. Among the different interactions of NK receptors with their specific counterparts on trophoblast, the inhibitory KIR–HLA-C interactions appear to be those mainly involved in the functions of an NK cell-mediated allorecognition system in pregnancy.

The functions for decidual NK cells in pregnancy are still not exactly clear, but there are some hints for a possible control of placental development and pregnancy maintenance. Due to the high abundance of uterine NK cells in the decidua in the first and second trimesters of pregnancy, and their association with extravillous trophoblast cells, it has been proposed that they play an active role in the regulation of trophoblast invasion. Several mechanisms have been suggested for this regulation including cytotoxicity, local cytokine production, and induction of trophoblast apoptosis. There is strong evidence that decidual NK cells are unlikely to play a role in cytotoxicity. Results from in vitro studies have proposed the involvement of NK cell receptor–HLA class I interactions in protection of the trophoblast. HLA-G antigen was thought to be the main factor for protection of the fetus from decidual NK cell lysis. NK cells in decidua express a noncytotoxic phenotype lacking CD16 and CD160 as markers of cytotoxicity.

Although expression of granzyme A, granzyme B, and perforin was detected in decidual NK cells, these cells had a very low cytotoxic effect on K562 target cells. Moreover, the extravillous trophoblast may not express enough triggering ligands of activating NK cell receptors such as NKG2D and natural cytotoxicity receptors. Trophoblast cells are resistant to cell lysis unless decidual NK cells have been stimulated with IL-2 which is not present in the decidua. However, no in situ evidence of trophoblast lysis by uterine NK cells in early decidua has as yet been detected. Another argument is the exposure of decidual NK cells to progesterone. A mediator of progesterone, progesterone-induced blocking factor (PIBF), was shown to block decidual NK cytolytic activity. Therefore, the general consensus is that the cytotoxic activity of uNK cells is reduced compared to peripheral blood NK cells.

As there is considerable interest in the role of cytokines in pregnancy, attention has also focused on uterine NK cell cytokine production. Studies detected transcripts for various cytokines and growth factors including GM-CSF, TNF-α, IFN-γ, IL-10, IL-1β, TGF-β, VEGF, and LIF in decidual NK cells. At present the functional importance of these cytokines and growth factors in normal pregnancy is not known. The cytokine profile of uterine NK cells does, however, appear to differ dependent on the phenotype of the surrounding cells, such as HLA-G-expressing cells. Altered production of IFN-γ has been reported in decidua basalis compared with decidua parietalis, and an increased production of IFN-γ and VEGF by uterine NK cells in response to HLA-G was also demonstrated.

Current interest is directed toward the role of uterine NK cell-derived cytokines, particularly IFN-γ, in the control of trophoblast invasion by a noncytotoxic mechanism and remodeling of uterine spiral arteries in the first half of normal pregnancy. These cytokines may influence trophoblast growth since their receptors have been found in human trophoblast cells. In the placental bed of uncomplicated pregnancies during early gestation, up to 30 % of the extravillous trophoblast cells are undergoing apoptosis, and many of these apoptosing trophoblast cells are surrounded by uterine NK cells. A possible explanation for this may be that the trophoblast cells which undergo apoptosis recruit uterine NK cells after apoptosis has been initiated. If uterine NK cells regulate trophoblast invasion, then the most likely mechanism by which this occurs is mediated by uterine NK cell cytokine secretion. Also cytokine production by decidual NK cells might play a role in defense against virus spreading to the fetus in case of uterine infection, for example, secreted IFN-γ might control cytomegalovirus spreading.

Uterine NK cells have also been proposed to play a role in spiral artery transformation. Murine studies on NK cell-deficient mice also showed abnormal decidual vasculature including abnormal thick spiral arteries, suggesting an additional role in uterine vascular remodeling. These abnormalities could be reversed after injection of allogeneic NK cells. It has also been demonstrated that the major uterine NK cell product responsible for spiral artery remodeling defect is IFN-γ.

These results may be also true in humans as decidual NK cells are closely aggregated around maternal spiral arteries. However, much less is known about the mechanisms involved in spiral artery remodeling in humans, but it is likely that they are, at least in part, different from those controlling trophoblast invasion. Early structural changes in decidual spiral arteries, including dilation and medial disorganization, occur before cellular interaction with trophoblast, but at a time when uterine NK cells are present. Uterine NK cells reduce in number after 20 weeks' gestation when vascular changes are generally complete.

5.1.3.2.2 Granulocytes and Monocytes

It appears that other components of the immune system, especially the innate immune system, are activated during pregnancy. Monocytes are activated in pregnancy, and data showed elevated surface expression of CD11b, CD14, and CD64 antigens on monocytes from third-trimester pregnant women. In addition, an increased expression of CD11a, CD49d, and CD54 on monocytes was also observed in pregnant women.

Granulocytes from pregnant women show increased surface expression of both activation markers and adhesion molecules, for example, of CD11b and CD64. These cells also show increased production of intracellular ROS and enhanced phagocytosis, as compared to nonpregnant women. Baseline intracellular ROS and oxidative burst were higher in both granulocytes and monocytes from pregnant women than in the control group.

Together, these data are consistent with the idea that pregnancy is a proinflammatory state. However, granulocytes from pregnant women in other studies had reduced microbial killing activity and chemotaxis as well as a decreased respiratory burst activity and intracellular H_2O_2 production when challenged. In contrast, there was no increase in CD11b expression and no upregulation of CD18 or downregulation of CD62L expression, both of which are needed for appropriate priming and activation of granulocytes. During pregnancy the percentage distribution of granulocytes was significantly increased, with a consequent reduction in the percentage of lymphocytes and monocytes as compared to nonpregnant women. Data on pregnant women followed longitudinally throughout gestation showed that an increase in the proportion of granulocytes and a decrease in the proportion of lymphocytes appeared from the second trimester onward. Neutrophils were located near the placenta where they are available to phagocytose cellular debris from decidual cells killed by invading trophoblast.

5.1.3.2.3 T Lymphocytes

In early pregnancy, T cells comprise about 10–20 % of the leukocytes in the uterine mucosa. Their proportion, however, increases with gestational age, followed by a decline in at term. A significant increase in the frequency of CD8+ T lymphocytes and a decrease in the frequency of CD4+ T lymphocytes were evident in pregnant women. Furthermore, an increase in the frequency of CD8+ T cells was observed in pregnant women during labor together with a concomitant reduction in the CD4/CD8 ratio. Th1- and Th2-type cytokines produced by maternal T lymphocytes present at the fetomaternal interface seem to play a role in the development of pregnancy. In humans, the success of pregnancy seems to be associated with the production of IL-4, IL-10, and M-CSF by T cells. Both IL-4 and IL-10 can inhibit the development and function of Th1 cells and macrophages, thus preventing allograft rejection.

There is direct evidence that the pregnancy-associated hormones progesterone and estradiol modify the cytokine production pattern of human antigen-specific T cells. Progesterone is a potent inducer of the production of Th2-type cytokines and of LIF and M-CSF production by T cells, mediated by IL-4. Estradiol and hCG both have no effect on T-cell differentiation to Th1 or Th2 cells. In summary, results suggest a hormone–cytokine–T-cell network at the fetomaternal interface, with progesterone partly responsible for the T2 switch. Defects in this network can result in fetal loss.

T cells have also been detected in surrounding cell masses of the oocyte during ovulation, the so-called cumulus oophorus. In women with blocked fallopian tubes, CD4+ T cells and macrophages were found in cumuli, but only few NK cells. Cumulus T cells produce higher levels of IL-4 and LIF than peripheral blood or ovarian T cells. Hormones can also modulate the cytokine profile of these cumulus oophorus T cells. Progesterone produced by cumulus granulosa cells may favor IL-4 production by T cells, which in turn can produce LIF.

5.1.3.2.4 T Regulatory Cells

Treg cells, representing 2–5 % of CD4+ cells, are believed to be important by maintaining natural self-tolerance and negative control of pathological, as well as physiological, immune responses. Recently, in mice the absence of CD4+CD25+ Treg led to a failure of gestation due to immunological rejection of the fetus, suggesting that CD4+CD25+ Treg cells mediate maternal tolerance to the fetus. With only the CD4+ T-cell population that expresses high levels of CD25 demonstrating regulatory function in humans, it was first reported in 2003 that decidual and peripheral blood CD4+CD25 T cells increased during early pregnancy. Recently, an increase in circulating CD4+CD25+ T cells during early pregnancy was observed, peaking in the second trimester and then declining in postpartum. The population of CD4+CD25 T cells rose from 6 % in the peripheral blood of nonpregnant subjects to 8 % in normal early pregnancy subjects, but this elevated CD4+CD25 T-cell ratio decreased to a nonpregnancy level in miscarriage cases. They reported also that the population of CD4+CD25 T cells to CD4+ T cells increased to over 20 % in early pregnancy decidua, and this population rate decreased to 6 % in spontaneous abortion cases.

However, the factors regulating CD4+CD25+ Treg cells are largely unknown. Data suggest that estrogen promotes maternal tolerance to the fetus by increasing the number of CD4+CD25+ Treg cells. Decidual CD4+CD25high T cells express a high frequency of intracellular CTLA-4, and 5–7 % of these cells express surface CTLA-4, suggesting that decidual CD4+CD25high T cells are stimulated by some antigens such as fetal antigens. Because antigen stimulation by dendritic cells induced the surface expression of CTLA-4, these activated CD4+CD25high Treg cells should mediate maternal tolerance to the fetus. Recently, it was reported that labor is associated with a decrease in CD4+CD25+ cells in decidua, suggesting that the disappearance of the CD4+CD25+ T-cell population may contribute to the induction of labor, although the study did not explicitly investigate CD4+CD25high cells.

Interestingly, CD4+CD25+ Treg cells express TLR4, TLR5, TLR7, and TLR8. Recent data showed that microbial induction of the Toll pathway, partly mediated by inflammatory IL-6, blocks the suppressive effect of CD4+CD25+ Treg, allowing activation of pathogen-specific adaptive immune responses. Interestingly, DC-based tumor vaccines ablate tumor-specific T-cell tolerance only after removal of CD4+CD25+ Treg cells. However, to ablate tumor-specific T-cell tolerance in the presence of CD4+CD25+ Treg cells by DC-based tumor vaccines, persistent TLR signals are required to reverse CD4+CD25+ Treg-mediated CD8+ T-cell tolerance.

These data suggest that chronic inflammation in recurrent spontaneous abortion, preterm labor, and preeclampsia might disturb the suppressive effects of CD4+CD25+ Treg cells, resulting in induction of fetal rejection responses.

Several scientific groups have focused on a subset of Treg cells, the CD8+ regulatory T cell, which were described originally in the intestine where they are activated by a combination of the nonclassical class I molecule CD1d and a costimulatory molecule of the carcinoembryonic antigen family. CD1d and a form of this costimulatory molecule were also expressed by trophoblasts during the early stages of pregnancy. Furthermore, isolated trophoblasts preferentially activated clonal populations of CD8+ T cells. The authors suggest the possibility that, in vivo, CD8+ T-cell subsets may have a role in regulating B cells, potentially protecting the fetus from deleterious antibody effects.

Altogether, the decidua is a highly complex tissue containing unique, highly specialized leukocyte subpopulations for each stage of gestation that may play a role in determining the nature of local immune responses at the fetomaternal interface. The specific leukocyte composition is controlled at the level of cell trafficking with different expression of cellular adhesion molecules involved in leukocyte recruitment which has been demonstrated in the mouse. Switches in vascular specificity or partial loss of microenvironmental specialization during the second half of mouse development results in dramatic changes in leukocyte populations recruited to the fetomaternal interface.

Studies showed a generalized activation of peripheral blood leukocytes in the third trimester of normal pregnancy, which is not reflected in the leukocyte populations within the decidua. Although a Th2 phenotype predominates within the decidua during pregnancy, this is not the case in the peripheral circulation. As the vast majority of maternal–fetal interactions during gestation occur within the uterus, it is not surprising to find a discrepancy in the phenotype of leukocytes between the two compartments.

Future studies are needed to get a more integrated understanding of how these different cell types in the decidua interact with each other and with trophoblast to create the correct environment for implantation to be a success from both the maternal and the fetal perspectives (Fig. 5.3).

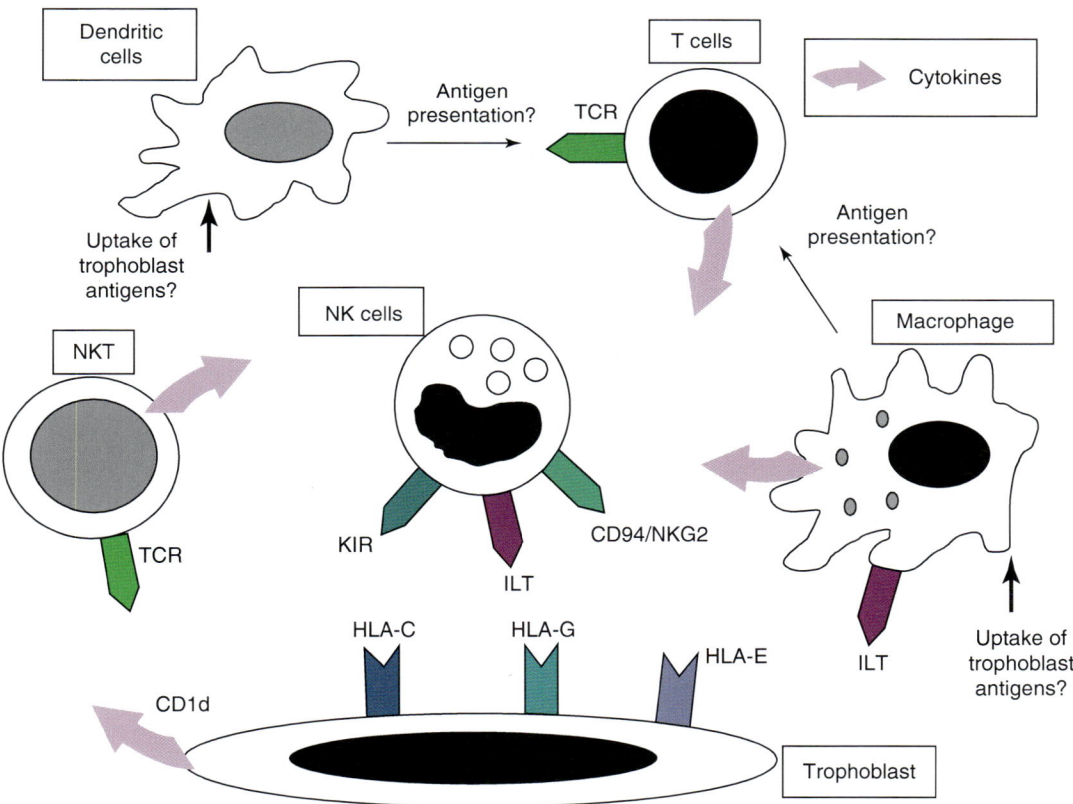

Fig. 5.3 A schematic representation of some of the interactions at the human implantation site. Trophoblast cells expressing HLA-C, HLA-G, HLA-E, and possibly CD1d invade into the decidua. Different leukocytes in the decidua can detect the presence of trophoblast through their various HLA receptors. APCs may take up trophoblast antigens and present them to T cells whose recognition would then result in the production of cytokines from the maternal immune cells. These cytokines contribute to controlling the immune response against trophoblast and may also control trophoblast invasion. *ILT* immunoglobulin-like transcript, *KIR* killer immunoglobulin-like receptor, *TCR* T-cell receptor (Trundley A, Moffett A. Human uterine leukocytes and pregnancy. Tissue Antigens. 2004;63:1–12)

5.1.3.3 Complement System

The observation that NK cells and macrophages, and not T and B cells, comprise the major population of leukocytes in the uterus lends support to the idea that implantation is likely to involve an innate immune response that is distinct from that seen in clinical organ transplantation, where rejection is mediated by cells of the acquired immune system, T and B lymphocytes.

Pregnancy is characterized by enhancement of the innate immune system and suppression of the acquired immune response. There is accumulating evidence in support of this view, for example, an increased number of granulocytes in maternal blood as well as phenotypic and metabolic changes in granulocytes and monocytes including increased expression of adhesion molecules, intracellular reactive oxygen, and oxidative burst. Moreover, an increased concentration of acute-phase proteins such as fibrinogen, clotting factors, or globulin and a shift of the Th1- to the Th2-type cytokine profile is observed. Complement activation could potentially harm the developing fetus. Recent evidence in murine models has implicated a deficiency of a C3 convertase inhibitor and C3 products in the mechanisms of pregnancy loss. Additionally, fetal injury and pregnancy loss in experimental antiphospholipid antibody syndrome have been attributed to the effects of complement, mainly C5a. Therefore, it has been proposed that inhibition of the complement system is an absolute requirement for normal pregnancy. The placental tissue contains a fully organized complement system that is mostly contributed by the complement factors in the maternal blood circulating in placental vessels, although some components may also be produced locally. As the placenta as a newly formed organ undergoes the process of tissue remodeling, the role of the complement system in the clearing of potentially destructive debris products may be essential.

In the placenta, deposits of complement components can be detected in physiological pregnancy, whereas at other tissue levels, these are usually seen in association with diseases. Many years ago, the complement components C1q, C4, C5, C6, and C9 were detected in normal human placenta. These were found to be associated with stromal cells as well as in the wall of fetal stem vessels and co-localized with fibrin on trophoblast plasma membranes and perivillous fibrin. C3d and C9, but not C4, were seen associated with trophoblast basement membranes, which suggested that activation pathways leading to complement disposition on trophoblast basement membrane and on perivillous fibrin may be different. Deposits of complement components were also detected on spiral arteries in normal pregnancy, with the highest staining for C3d and C9, suggesting that the complement system is likely to be activated through the classical pathway. A humoral immune response leading to complement activation may thus be involved in the physiological changes of spiral arteries in early pregnancy. The terminal C complex as the final end product of all three pathways was also found to localize in the fibrinoid material of the basal decidua, in chorionic villi stroma, and in vessel walls.

As the placenta as a newly formed organ undergoes the process of tissue remodeling, the role of the complement system in the clearing of potentially destructive debris products may be essential. However, the exact mechanism of complement activation in the placenta has not been clarified. Potential local activators including cellular and tissue debris could be responsible. Another study demonstrated that normal pregnancy is associated with activation of the complement system as determined by maternal plasma C3a, C4a, and C5a concentrations remaining elevated from 20 weeks' gestation to term.

Fetal protection against maternal complement activation products is achieved by surface expression of complement regulators that act at different steps in the activation cascade. These regulators, including DAF, MCP, and CD59, are present in the placenta about 6 weeks from gestation until term, and syncytiotrophoblast is protected from complement attack by expressing these three regulatory molecules. CD59 is distributed on all types of trophoblast, while DAF and MCP are preferentially expressed on giant decidual cells. The effect of complement on trophoblast is not necessarily cytotoxic and may

Table 5.1 Changes in innate immunity during pregnancy

Monocytes	Increase in number
	Increase in phagocytosis activity
	Increase in IL-12 production
Neutrophils	Increase in number
	Increase in phagocytosis activity
NK cells	Decrease in number
	Decrease in cytotoxicity
	Decrease in IFNγ production
Complement system	Increase of C1q, C3, C4. C4d
Acute phase proteins	Decrease of albumin
	Increase of ceruloplasmin/fibrinogen/globulins/alpha-1 antitrypsin/clotting factors

Adapted from Herz U, Renz H. Fetomaternale Immunität. Neue Konzepte zur Plastizität des Immunsystems während der Schwangerschaft Gynäkologe. 2001;34:494–502

result either in impairment or in stimulation of the cell function caused by the membrane attack complex (MAC).

Table 5.1 shows a summary of the changes in the innate immune system during pregnancy.

5.1.3.4 Cytokines and Growth Factors

The local environment of the maternal–fetal interface is characterized not only by the cell types present but also by the soluble factors produced therein. A wide range of cytokines and growth factors is present in the decidua physiologically, including LIF, TNF-α, IFN-α, IL-1, IL-2, IL-4, IL-5, IL-6, IL-8, IL-10, IL-11, IL-12, IL-13, IL-15, IL-16, and IL-18. These mediators are able to act on lymphocytes and NK cells expressing a variety of receptors. The production and effects of these cytokines at the implantation site are important for the regulation of trophoblast cell growth, differentiation, and invasion. APCs and T lymphocytes in the maternal decidua are potentially able to promote rejection of the fetal allograft, which is first mediated by the recognition of paternal MHC antigens by APCs and then by the activity of effector T cells via the release of cytokines. Therefore, changes in cytokine production by activated T cells may play an important role in the immunological tolerance of the conceptus.

5.1.3.4.1 Th1/Th2 Cytokine Dichotomy

Placental and decidual tissues from normal pregnancies have been shown to express both pro- and anti-inflammatory cytokines. In normal pregnancies, particularly at the maternal–fetal interface, anti-inflammatory Th2-type cytokines predominate over proinflammatory Th1-type cytokines, and, therefore, an appropriate balance between proinflammatory and anti-inflammatory cytokines is thought to be crucial for determining the success or failure of a pregnancy. Interestingly, clinical disease activity of several T-cell-mediated autoimmune disorders, such as rheumatoid arthritis, Crohn's disease, or multiple sclerosis, is reduced during pregnancy but flares again in the postpartum period. As disease activity in these disorders is often associated with increased Th1-type cytokine responses in the blood, it was suggested that a cytokine shift during pregnancy may be a protective process.

Evidence for a dichotomous Th response in reproduction originated from murine models, which showed that pregnancy rejection is mediated by Th1 cytokines, whereas a Th2 cytokine response confers protection. There have been only few ex vivo studies on cytokine production in human pregnancy, which yielded conflicting results and were unable to detect the expected early Th1/Th2 shift during pregnancy initially. A study in vivo demonstrated that women with recurrent miscarriage exhibit primarily Th1 cytokines, whereas healthy women exhibit decreased Th1 cytokines and increased Th2 cytokines which suggests a potential role for a dichotomous Th response in the mediation of subsequent reproductive events. Interestingly, significantly reduced IL-2, IL-18, and IFN-γ mRNA expression levels are already observed during the first trimester of normal pregnancy. The mRNA levels for IL-4 and IL-10 also declined during pregnancy could be observed, although this reduction was only marginal. Calculating the cytokine ratios revealed a shift from a Th1-type to a pronounced Th2-type response, which was at the highest level during the second trimester.

Other studies showed that proinflammatory Th1 cytokines appear to be potentially harmful to pregnancy since excess production of TNF-α or

IFN-γ has been associated with preterm delivery. Low concentrations of LIF, IL-4, IL-6, and IL-10 in endometrial tissue and deciduas were described in women with multiple failures of implantation and habitual abortions. Similarly, low levels of decidual IL-4 and IL-10 have been observed in women suffering from unexplained recurrent abortions and where spontaneous abortion has occurred during the first trimester of pregnancy. Moreover, a defect of IL-4 production by decidual CD4+ and CD8+ T cells and a defect of IL-10, LIF, and M-CSF by decidual CD4+ T cells were observed in women with recurrent abortions. IL-4, IL-5, and IL-10 were detected at the fetomaternal interface throughout gestation in mice, whereas IFN-γ was only present in the first period.

It is currently believed that for the continuous normal development of pregnancy, production of inflammatory cytokines such as IL-2, TNF-α, and IFN-γ is suppressed, whereas production of anti-inflammatory cytokines such as IL-4, IL-6, or IL-10 is enhanced. Therefore, the conception of Th2 overbalance during pregnancy has been a paradigm for immunology of reproduction for many years, while Th1 activity has been presented as unwanted component. However, the broadening knowledge of immunological mechanisms working for successful pregnancy and birth of the viable fetus brings nowadays the necessity to verify the "Th2 phenomenon" in favor of conception of "Th1/Th2 cooperation" in which Th1-type activity is no longer only a destructive component of physiological pregnancy.

This fine-tuned cytokine balance between Th1 and Th2 seems to be modulated at the intracellular signaling level which is regulated again by a complex of cytokines and other factors, for example, the JAK/STAT system. Intracellular signals from cytokine receptors are mostly transduced via the Janus kinases (JAK) and signal transducers and activators of a transcription (STAT) system. Only little is known, however, about the specific intracellular signals in decidual lymphocytes during pregnancy that may support fetomaternal tolerance. Important regulators of cytokine signals in lymphocytes are suppressors of cytokine signaling (SOCS) which are constitutively expressed in

naïve T cells. They have also been detected in gestational tissues, and their differential regulation is associated with the onset of labor, but there is so far no information about their role in decidual lymphocytes in pregnancy.

5.1.3.4.2 Th2 Cytokine Activity in Pregnancy

CD4+ T lymphocytes of Th2 activity are the source of IL-4, IL-5, IL-6, IL-10, IL-13, and GM-CSF, whereas CD4+ T lymphocytes of Th1 activity produce mainly IL-1, IL-2, IL-12, IL-15, IL-18, IFN-γ, and TNF-α. Already during the luteal phase of the menstrual cycle, endometrial cells have increased mRNA expression for Th2 cytokines including IL-4 and IL-6 compared to Th1 cytokines such as IL-2, IL-12, and IFN-γ.

IL-4, known to be the essential anti-inflammatory cytokine for Th2 differentiation, IL-6, and IL-10 are constantly present in high numbers at the fetomaternal interface where they are involved in pregnancy-supporting mechanisms. IL-4, which is secreted by endometrium-infiltrating lymphocytes, stimulates production of LIF in endometrial tissue, another cytokine of great significance for peri-implantation period as it together with TGF-β facilitates the processes of trophoblast invasion, endometrial decidualization, regulation of interactions between decidual lymphocytes and trophoblast, and, together with IL-6, controlling angiogenesis inside trophoblastic villi. During labor at term as well as premature labor even when the onset of contractions was not connected with intrauterine infection, increased concentration of IL-6 was found in serum, placental villi, decidua, and fetal membranes. IL-10 is crucial for survival of the fetal allograft and counteracts the effects of inflammatory cytokines. High levels of IL-12 during pregnancy are associated with preterm labor, preterm birth, or recurrent abortions.

It was also found that peripheral blood lymphocytes of pregnant women in the first trimester secrete "in vitro" more Th2, i.e., IL-4 and IL-10, and less Th1, i.e., IL-2 and IFN-γ cytokines, compared to nonpregnant patients. Also the number of IL-4-secreting cells rises progressively in the course of pregnancy. Probably alloantigens localized on trophoblast are the signal for peripheral lymphocytes to initiate Th2 activity which is supported by the observation that in subsequent trimesters peripheral lymphocytes of pregnant women differentiated to Th2 cells and secreted IL-4 after recognition of paternal alloantigens in mixed lymphocyte culture.

Progesterone seems to be another possible inducer of Th2 overactivity during pregnancy. Progesterone influences the cytokine network by decreasing Th1 activity of TNF-α in luteal phase endometrial tissue and by inducing synthesis of TGF-β in endometrial cells. It stimulates lymphocytes to produce progesterone-induced blocking factor (PIBF) which has the potential to intensify production of Th2 cytokines (IL-3, IL-4, IL-10) and to block IL-12 secretion by peripheral blood lymphocytes from pregnant women; hCG also seems to play a role in regulation of endometrial Th1/Th2 balance.

5.1.3.4.3 Th1 Cytokine Activity in Pregnancy

CD4+ T lymphocytes of Th1 activity produce mainly IL-1, IL-2, IL-12, IL-15, IL-18, IFN-γ, and TNF-α. The significance of these Th1 cytokines on the implantation period was defined by studies in mice. Components of seminal plasma influenced the expression of chemokines by endometrial cells which activated elements of innate immunity, including neutrophil and macrophages homing to the endometrial stroma and uterine cavity. In a local inflammatory reaction, activated neutrophils secreted ROS and phagocyte cellular debris, while activated macrophages became the most important source of Th1 cytokines, IL-1β and TNF-α. The uterine cavity is cleared of sperm elements and accompanying microorganisms.

A Th1-biased reaction produces an adequate environment for presentation of paternal alloantigens to maternal immunocompetent cells, and it also induces changes in the number and composition of endometrial leucocytes, activates angiogenic and growth factors, rebuilds extracellular matrix, and activates endothelial and stromal cells, thus preparing maternal tissues for embryo implantation. Th1 activity triggers endometrial leucocytes

and the embryo itself to produce Th2 cytokines, LIF, and TGF-β and activates angiogenic factors and endothelial cells, thus preparing maternal tissues for embryo implantation. Th1 cytokines stimulate cytolytic activity of decidual NK cells and lymphokine-activated "killer" T lymphocytes which are able to restrict excessive trophoblast proliferation and invasion. Similar mechanisms have been studied during the peri-implantation period in humans. Th1 cytokines present inside the uterine milieu as a result of an inflammatory response to paternal seminal components can stimulate trophoblastic MMP-9. It can thus enhance its invasive properties and can mediate neoangiogenesis by inducing VEGF gene transcription. IL-1β together with TNF-α stimulates secretion of LIF which has a positive impact on trophoblastic growth and differentiation. Embryonic cells are also capable of secreting IL-2 which seems to play a stimulating role for decidual NK cells and with macrophages. It can restrict the depth of trophoblastic infiltration, as Th1 cytokines are potent inductors of trophoblast apoptosis.

IFNs, especially upon GM-CSF stimulation, can be secreted by cyto- and syncytiotrophoblast. All isoforms of IFNs are present in human placenta, mostly in extravillous trophoblast, but also in villous syncytiotrophoblast. They play a role as immunomodulators since they can decrease proliferative activity of maternal T and B lymphocytes as well as induce soluble HLA shedding from the surface of trophoblast cells. Soluble HLA functions as an immunosuppressive factor for maternal macrophages and cytotoxic lymphocytes. IFNs can also increase expression of HLA-G molecules on cytotrophoblast; augment Th2 cytokine production, i.e., IL-6 and GM-CSF in endometrial stroma; and, together with IL-12, IL-15, IL-18, and VEGF, influence local angiogenesis in the uterus. These facts lead to the hypothesis that Th1 activity plays an important role in promotion of the Th2 response, regulation of the placentation process, defense against infections, and initiation of delivery. Together with Th2 activity, it is a necessary component of immunological reactions during pregnancy.

IL-15 is one of the critical cytokines controlling uterine NK cell cytokine production and cytolytic potential. Moreover, IL-15 has been implicated in differentiation and proliferation of uterine NK cells and plays a possible role in induction of IFN-γ production as a mediator in vascular remodeling during early pregnancy. It was detected in the nonpregnant endometrium, decidua, and placenta but also in uterine macrophages, stromal cells, chorion, and amnion. IL-15 was found in glandular ECs and endometrial stroma during the late stages of the menstrual cycle with the highest levels in perivascular cells surrounding the decidual spiral arteries. Expression of IL-15 during early pregnancy is most prominent in endothelial cells of spiral arteries. Decidualization elevates IL-15 levels which promote survival of pre-NK cells present in and mobilizing into the uterus. Recent studies demonstrated that IL-15 is essential for the support of NK cell differentiation in the decidualizing uterus. IL-15-deficient mice revealed a complete absence of uterine NK cells, poor development of decidua, and unmodified spiral artery structure.

Progesterone induces IL-15 expression, and, therefore, when progesterone levels fall as a result of failing pregnancy, the manifestation of apoptotic NK cells could be the result of a decreasing level of IL-15. IL-15 seems to stimulate GM-CSF production by resting CD56+ NK cells and, together with IL-12, induces IFN-γ and TNF-α as macrophage-activating factors. NK cells also produce MIP-1α and MIP-1β after stimulation with IL-15 which may be a mechanism for trafficking of additional NK cells to the site of implantation. IL-15 is essential for Th2 cytokine production by NK cells, and it stimulates uterine NK cell production of IFN-γ and IL-10. Concerning cytotoxicity, IL-15 was found to activate cytotoxicity by decidual NK cells. IL-15 appears to directly induce upregulation of perforin and FasL expression on human decidual NK cells at the fetomaternal interface suggesting that IL-15-activated decidual CD56+ cells use perforin and FasL mediated against transformed or infected cells.

IL-18 at the fetomaternal interface is produced by the entire decidua on gestation day 4. In murine studies, production starts in the basal proliferative stroma followed by glandular cells in peri-implantation uterus and appears early in murine spongiotrophoblast. IL-18 does not appear early in human villous trophoblast cells but later persists in giant extravillous trophoblast cells and in rare activated macrophages. IL-18 enhances innate immunity and both Th1- and Th2-driven immune responses. IL-18 is essential for induction of IFN-γ production from Th1 cells, NK cells, B cells, and DCs, often in combination with IL-12. IL-18 alone has the potential to induce IL-4 and IL-13 production by T cells and NK cells and promotes a Th2-mediated response. It also plays a role in regulating GM-CSF production and induction of IL-8 and TNF-α. Therefore, IL-18 at the peri-implantation site is able to stimulate murine uterine NK cells to produce IFN-γ that plays a key role in vascular remodeling during early pregnancy. Therefore, IL-18 might be essential for proper vascularization of the implantation site.

Only a few studies have investigated the role of IL-18 on the cytolytic potential of decidual NK cells. IL-18 directly upregulates cytotoxic activity of NK cells and CD8+ T cells and induces perforin and FasL receptor expression on NK cells. Stimulation of decidual lymphocytes with IL-18 increased perforin expression and perforin-mediated cytotoxicity of NK cells. IL-18 serum levels in pregnant women also show a significant increase from the first trimester to labor and remain at high levels until at least day 3 afterward. IL-18 may have an important role during implantation. However, there are also high serum IL-18 levels in women with implantation failure, fetal growth restriction, or recurrent abortions. An increased level of IL-18 promotes strong NK cell activation and probably excessive IFN-γ production. It seems that a tight regulation of IL-18 is important for normal implantation and decidual remodeling in early pregnancy.

Th1 cytokines also play a positive role for initiation of labor at term. In sera of delivering women, elevated concentrations of IFN-γ and IL-1β were observed. Th1 cytokines stimulate decidual prostaglandins which are responsible for the onset of uterine contractions. Proinflammatory cytokines together with mechanical stimuli induce

Il-8 production, whose concentration in cervical mucus is positively correlated with the progress of cervical ripening and opening.

5.1.3.4.4 Leukemia Inhibitory Factor

Leukemia inhibitory factor (LIF) is required for implantation and embryo development. This is shown in studies on mice lacking the LIF gene; they are fertile but their blastocysts fail to implant and do not develop unless the animals are treated locally with LIF. LIF is produced by endometrial ECs, NK cells, and T cells. However, LIF expression by glandular epithelium is dramatically downregulated after implantation, whereas expression by leukocytes is upregulated in the decidua. Most of the LIF expression was assigned to NK cells, but decidual NK cells in culture did not produce LIF. Therefore, production of decidual LIF seems to be assigned to T cells. LIF secretion is inhibited by Th1 cytokines such as IL-12 and IFN-γ in vitro.

5.1.3.5 Humoral Immunity in Pregnancy: Asymmetric Antibodies

It has been established that the synthesis of asymmetric antibodies is increased under different physiopathological situations involving Th2 responses, including pregnancy. These are asymmetrically glycosylated IgG molecules which are affected in their antigen interaction, turning them into functionally univalent and blocking antibodies. As a consequence, they are not capable of triggering immune effector mechanisms.

An asymmetric proportion of 10–20 % of IgG molecules has been demonstrated in nonimmune sera. Their existence could be either beneficial or harmful to the host, depending on the self or non-self nature of the antigen. They act as protective antibodies if binding self-antigens, but when they are specific for a foreign aggressor, for example, in chronic infections, they block antigens of the pathogen, leading to its survival and chronicity.

In murine pregnancy, antibodies with antipaternal specificity, predominantly of the IgG1 subclass, were detected both in serum and on the placenta. In an analysis of the humoral immune response in pregnant females, the predominance of antipaternal blocking IgG antibodies was demonstrated. Multiparous women had a marked increase in asymmetric IgG in serum during the first trimester followed by a decrease after delivery. Antibody activity was located in both symmetric and asymmetric IgG in a 1:5 ratio, which indicates the prevalence of asymmetric antibodies in this immune response.

Experiments showed that IL-6 is the main responsible factor for the glycosylation of asymmetric IgG molecules and therefore regulates the quality of the humoral immune response during pregnancy. It has been hypothesized that during pregnancy, in the context of a predominant Th2 immune response, the quality of IgG antibodies synthesized is modified by IL-6 of placental origin. If the IL-6 levels secreted by placental cells are normal, there is a preferential synthesis of asymmetric glycosylated antibodies which have a blocking activity and participate in the protection of the fetal antigens, whereas if IL-6 levels are abnormal, there is a predominance of aggressive antibodies.

5.1.3.6 The Role of Progesterone as an Immunomodulator in Pregnancy

The best-studied immunomodulator at the maternal–fetal interface is progesterone, which clearly has a role in survival of the fetal allograft. Numerous studies have demonstrated that progesterone blocks mitogen-stimulated lymphocyte proliferation, improves allograft survival time, and modulates antibody production, besides affecting other phases of the immune response.

While the mechanism by which progesterone exerts its immunomodulatory actions in reproductive tissues is unclear, it may involve both direct and indirect actions on immune cells. Progesterone can induce the production of LIF and M-CSF by T cells, which is mediated by IL-4. Moreover, it can decrease the Th1 activity of TNF-α in luteal phase endometrial tissue, which is at least partly regulated by increased levels of PIBF. PIBF is secreted by lymphocytes of pregnant women in the presence of progesterone and mediates the latter's biological effects. PIBF concentrations in pregnancy urine are

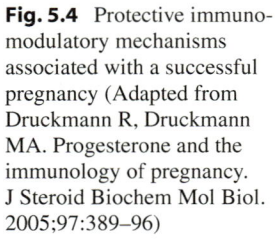

Fig. 5.4 Protective immunomodulatory mechanisms
associated with a successful
pregnancy (Adapted from
Druckmann R, Druckmann
MA. Progesterone and the
immunology of pregnancy.
J Steroid Biochem Mol Biol.
2005;97:389–96)

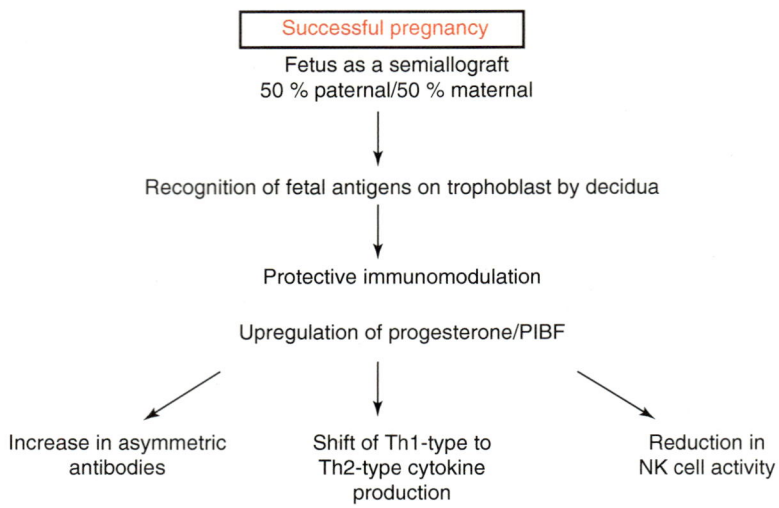

related to pregnancy outcome as PIBF levels
have been found to increase up to term in normal
pregnancies but fail to increase in pathological
pregnancies. Therefore, a PIBF concentration
correlates with positive or negative pregnancy
outcome, and premature pregnancy termination
is predictable by below normal PIBF values.

PIBF affects B cells and induces increased production of asymmetric antibodies which has a regulatory effect on antifetal immune responses during
pregnancy. In animal experiments, blockade of the
progesterone receptor resulted in reduced PIBF
production together with a reduced amount of
asymmetric antibodies and elevated fetal resorption rates. PIBF inhibits arachidonic acid release
which results in a reduced cytotoxic NK activity
and therefore favors a normal pregnancy outcome.
NK activity in pregnant women is inversely related
to the rate of PIBF-positive lymphocytes. PIBF
keeps NK activity at a low level both by controlling
IL-12 production and also by inhibiting perforin
liberation. Decidual NK cells express a high level
of perforin; however, they have low cytotoxic activity. In vitro studies in decidual cells obtained from
elective pregnancy termination suggest that it is
PIBF that inhibits the cytotoxicity of NK cells via
blockade of degranulation and thus contributes to
the low decidual NK activity.

PIBF also alters the profile of cytokine secretion by activated lymphocytes and increases the

production of IL-3, IL-4, and IL-10. PIBF seems
to induce a Th2-type cytokine production and
inhibits IL-12 production by lymphocytes, which
was shown to be pregnancy protective as an
increased lymphocyte IL-12 production correlated with pathological pregnancies and high NK
activity.

In summary, results suggest a hormone–cytokine–T-cell network at the fetomaternal interface,
with progesterone partly responsible for the T2
switch there. Defects in this network can result in
fetal loss. Numerous studies have also demonstrated that progesterone via PIBF blocks
mitogen-stimulated lymphocyte proliferation,
improves allograft survival time, reduces NK cell
cytotoxicity, and modulates antibody production
as well as besides affecting other phases of the
immune response.

Figure 5.4 serves to summarize the results of
this last section by elucidating the immunological requirements for the maintenance of a successful pregnancy.

5.1.4   Immunology of Labor
and the Postpartum Period

Some of the physiological processes involved in
labor seem to be mediated by proinflammatory
cytokines, suggesting the immune privileges that

the fetal–placental unit has enjoyed during pregnancy are revoked at the time of labor. An inflammatory response during labor may also help to remove placental fragments and prepare the uterus for the pathogens that it will undoubtedly encounter during the immediate postpartum period. In the following, the immunological changes during the three important processes in parturition will be briefly described.

The process of cervical ripening appears to be an inflammatory reaction associated with catabolism of the cervical extracellular matrix by enzymes released from infiltrating leukocytes. During cervical ripening and remodeling, IL-8, IL-1β, IL-6, and TNF-α production was increased in the human cervix. IL-1β is produced predominantly by leukocytes; IL-6 by leukocytes, glandular ECs, and surface ECs; and IL-8 is produced primarily by leukocytes, glandular ECs, surface ECs, and stromal cells. During labor there is an influx in the number of leukocytes in the cervix, due primarily by increased numbers of neutrophils and macrophages (CD68+ cells) but not T (CD3+ cells) or B cells (CD20+ cells).

The ripening of the cervix is induced by proinflammatory cytokines in different ways. IL-1β and TNF-α increase production of MMP-1, MMP-3, MMP-9, and cathepsin S. IL-1β acts on a number of cell types to increase the production of cyclooxygenase (COX)-2 and prostaglandin E2, the most effective compound for inducing cervical dilation in women. Prostaglandin E2 may then further stimulate labor by increasing production of proteinases or indirectly by increasing the permeability of blood vessels for leukocyte trafficking. NO, another proinflammatory mediator that is increased at term, may also contribute to vasodilatation to facilitate leukocyte trafficking.

Besides prostaglandin E2, IL-8 also attracts neutrophils from the periphery to migrate toward the cervix and activates them to release MMP-8 (neutrophil collagenase) and neutrophil elastase that can digest the extracellular matrix produced by cervical fibroblasts. Increased concentrations of G-CSF in the cervix during labor may also stimulate proliferation of the neutrophil subset. Possible roles for IL-6 in the cervix could be to

stimulate neutrophils, macrophages, or other cells present in the local tissues to produce additional proinflammatory cytokines that aid the process of cervical ripening, such as prostaglandin E2 or NO. IL-6 has been used as an effective biomarker for predicting labor. The process of weakening and rupture of the membranes in the region that overlies the cervix also involves a similar proinflammatory process as in the cervix. During labor, the production of IL-8, TNF-α, IL-6, IL-1β, and MMP-9 increases in the membranes and levels of TIMPs decrease; with regard to the latter, IL-1β has in particular been found to downregulate the expression of TIMP-2, an endogenous inhibitor of MMP-2, which can digest the collagen and elastin fibers in the extracellular matrix of the cervix to further increase cervical compliance. TNF-α and IL-1β increase the production of MMP-9 by amnion, but not chorion, explants in vitro.

Increased collagenase activity can weaken the strength of the membranes and lower their threshold for rupture. Stimulation of amnion and chorion cells with IL-1β and TNF-α also increases the production of prostaglandin E2 via COX-2. Prostaglandin E2 may then either cause increased production of MMP-9 or it can cross the membranes to stimulate cervical ripening in the cervix or stimulate contractions by the myometrium. Hormones and cytokines associated with labor, such as cortisol, TNF-α, and IL-1β, have been shown to inhibit production of the enzyme 15-hydroxyprostaglandin dehydrogenase by chorion and trophoblast, which may contribute to increased prostaglandin production during labor.

The initiation of rhythmic contractions of increasing amplitude and frequency as another component of labor in the myometrium is also associated with these cytokine-induced changes. Increased protein concentrations of IL-1β, TNF-α, and IL-6 have been detected in myometrium at labor and immunolocalized to the leukocytes. The increased concentrations of leukocytes in the myometrium during labor could be due to increased expression of chemokines such as MCP-1 and IL-8 that are also increased during labor and may recruit macrophages and neutrophils to the myometrium. IL-1β and TNF-α stimulate arachidonic acid release, activate phospholipid metabolism, and increase the production of prostaglandins by myometrial cells. These effects of IL-1β on myometrial cells are similar to the effects of oxytocin which also upregulates COX-2 and prostaglandin E2 production by myometrial cells. IL-1β and TNF-α can also increase the production of MMP-9 by myometrial cells, which may be important for detachment of the placenta.

IL-6 has no effect on prostaglandin production by myometrial cells and is unable to stimulate myometrial contractions. However, this cytokine may play a role in labor by increasing the expression of oxytocin receptors on myometrial cells like IL-1β; it can also increase oxytocin secretion by myometrial cells.

The postpartum period of about 1 year has been considered as a time for immunological recovery from the profound immunological changes of pregnancy. The immunology of the postpartum period is often viewed as a restoration of Th1/Th2 balance; this concept has been useful, but it is not the only explanatory model for autoimmune diseases such as rheumatoid arthritis that, as Th1-driven diseases, remit during pregnancy but exacerbate during the postpartum period.

Delivery is associated with increased serum levels of inflammatory cytokines such as IL-6 and IL-1. The early postpartum period is also characterized by upregulated inflammatory responses. Both Th1 and Th2 ex vivo cytokine production rise during the postpartum period compared to pregnancy, with increased Th1/Th2 ratios observed through the postpartum months 1–12. Increased levels of T-helper cells, cytotoxic T cells, and NK cell subsets with weak cytotoxicity (CD16+ CD57+) were identified in the first months postpartum. An increase in suppressor T cells and CD5+ B cells follows during months 7–10 postpartum, which may also be related to the postpartum aggravation of autoimmune diseases. The three immune activation markers neopterin, soluble IL-2 receptor (both elevated during allograft rejection or autoimmune disorders), and soluble CD8 antigen were found to be elevated at delivery and postpartum. Moreover, every serum cytokine measured and all proinflammatory macrophage and acute-phase proteins (TNF-α, IL-6, CRP, and neopterin) were higher in postpartum mothers along with a higher lymphocyte proliferative response and the secretion of higher levels of S-IgA.

All these data suggest a broad state of immune activation and an upregulated general and mucosal immunity whose functions are unclear at this time. One can speculate that innate inflammatory activation is both protective and related to the stage of uterine involution. There is increased risk for maternal uterine contamination during birth, and the endometrium is protected from infection by activated macrophages. Uterine involution is associated with myometrial shrinkage, elimination of microorganisms, and repair and restoration of the endometrium that is also associated with both apoptosis and proliferation. This process probably involves inflammatory and immune mediators.

5.1.5 Disturbances in Maternal–Fetal Interaction of the Immune System

The following section deals with pathological conditions during pregnancy including preeclampsia, intrauterine growth restriction (IUGR), preterm labor (PTL), and recurrent spontaneous abortion (RSA), which are some of the leading causes of maternal and fetal morbidity and mortality worldwide. There are several histological similarities between IUGR and other pregnancy disorders such as preeclampsia and RSA, which has led to the suggestion of a common etiology for these pregnancy disturbances. An increased decidual cellular immunity limiting trophoblastic invasion and leading to failure of placentation has been reported to be involved in the pathogenesis of several pathological conditions in pregnancy such as spontaneous abortion, preeclampsia, and IUGR. Probably, pregnancy complications such as IUGR, abruptio placentae, and fetal death are all clinical signs of placental ischemia and inflammation due to an inadequate trophoblast invasion and defect remodeling of spiral arteries (Fig. 5.5).

Fig. 5.5 Mechanism of placental development in pathological pregnancies (Adapted from Matthiesen L, Berg G, Ernerudh J, Ekerfelt C, Jonsson Y, Sharma S. Immunology of preeclampsia. Chem Immunol Allergy. 2005;89:49–61)

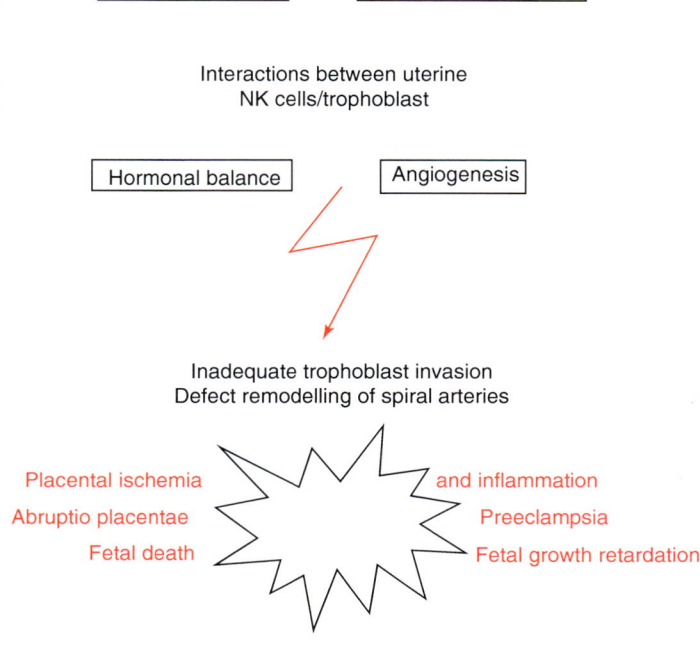

5.1.5.1 Immunological Aspects of Preeclampsia

Preeclampsia is a placenta-dependent disorder with both local intrauterine and systemic anomalies resulting in maternal and fetal morbidity and mortality. Worldwide it affects about 3–7 % of all pregnancies; it is often detected in the second half of pregnancy but most probably has its onset during early pregnancy. To date, there is no reliable, cost-effective screening test for this disease, and there are no widely accepted or proven measures for primary prevention.

As histological features such as restrained trophoblast invasion, placental ischemia, and vasculitis are similar to those observed in other pregnancy complications, including IUGR, RSA, and abruptio placentae, a common immune etiology with local subclinical inflammation at the placental bed and systemic immune responses in the maternal circulation has been suggested. However, an endothelial cell dysfunction as a pathophysiological denominator has been also suggested. Thus, a two-stage process is proposed, with an excessive maternal inflammatory response, probably against foreign fetal antigens, resulting in an impaired trophoblast invasion, defective spiral artery remodeling, and reduced placental perfusion. Consequently, placental hypoxia and infarction lead to the release of inflammatory cytokines and placental fragments into the maternal circulation. This ends in systemic vascular endothelial disruption and eventual clinical manifestations of preeclampsia.

Preeclampsia is likely, at least in part, the consequence of an abnormal maternal immune response to antigenic challenge by the fetoplacental allograft. In the 1970s, studies indicated that histological changes in the placental beds of preeclamptic women resembled those of acute allograft rejection. Epidemiological evidence also pointed convincingly toward an immunogenetic basis for preeclampsia. Although exposure to paternal antigens through a prior pregnancy had a protective effect against development of preeclampsia, exposure to new or different paternal antigens because of change in paternity was associated with an increased risk of preeclampsia. Consistent with these findings, the hypothesis of immune maladaptation contends that certain reproductive practices, such as barrier contraception and oocyte embryo donation, that minimize maternal exposure to seminal fluid may be associated with an increased risk of preeclampsia. A recent paper by Feinberg presents the thesis of a minimal excess of placental immune complex production versus removal as the cause of a proinflammatory autoamplification cascade of trophoblast apoptosis and oxidative stress, culminating in clinical preeclampsia.

For years, there have been discussions on the question of primiparity versus primipaternity in the etiology of preeclampsia. For some researchers, preeclampsia is associated with the first pregnancy, with oxidative stress as the main cause of vascular defects. For others, it may be associated with the first pregnancy with a particular father.

The first occurrence of preeclampsia, or its recurrence in primiparous women, seems to be associated with a change of partner. Furthermore, its incidence is inversely correlated with the duration of sexual cohabitation. In other studies oral sex seemed to be protective; a possible immunological explanation is that both local and, more importantly, systemic tolerance can be obtained by oral administration of an antigen. Although exposure to paternal antigens through a prior pregnancy has a protective effect against the development of preeclampsia, exposure to new or different paternal antigens because of change in paternity is associated with an altered risk of preeclampsia. Certain reproductive practices that minimize maternal exposure to seminal fluid are associated with increased risk of preeclampsia; these include barrier contraception, brief sexual cohabitation, nonpartner donor insemination, oocyte embryo donation, absence of preconceptual oral sex, or intracytoplasmic sperm injection with surgically obtained sperm. Thus, an accumulating body of epidemiological evidence points convincingly toward an immunogenetic basis for preeclampsia.

Perhaps the greatest barrier to clarification of the etiology of preeclampsia is the still incomplete understanding of the immunological basis for normal pregnancy. The success of human reproduction depends on the ability of the mother and fetus to control allogeneic immune responses through multiple, overlapping mechanisms, while maintaining the capacity to mount a defense against infectious organisms. Evidence suggests that site-specific suppression, whereby maternal immune responses are controlled locally at the maternal–fetal interface, plays a fundamental role. As mentioned above, in normal pregnancy the ratio of proinflammatory Th1 to suppressor Th2 lymphocytes is shifted toward the suppressor phenotype, which is believed to facilitate maternal immune tolerance of the fetus by suppressing activity of the cytotoxic Th1 cytokines, which are capable of attacking the fetal allograft and impairing trophoblastic invasion.

In the following subsections, studies addressing the role of macrophages, lymphocytes, and cytokines in the pathogenesis of preeclampsia are summarized.

5.1.5.1.1 Macrophages

In pregnancy, pathologies like preeclampsia, an increase in trophoblast apoptosis, possibly because of infection, may initiate an inflammatory event that further promotes trophoblast cell death. This prevents normal trophoblast invasion and spiral arteries transformations and negatively affects fetal survival. In pregnancies complicated by preeclampsia or IUGR, activated macrophages secrete proinflammatory cytokines such as TNF-α and IFN-γ and induce apoptosis in extravillous trophoblast. This hypothesis is supported by finding a higher incidence of cell clusters secreting TNF-α, probably macrophages, in the placental bed of patients with severe forms of preeclampsia. Studies of placental bed specimens demonstrated changes in the distribution of macrophages during pathological conditions such as preeclampsia. While in normal pregnancies macrophages are located in the stroma surrounding the transformed spiral arteries and extravillous trophoblast, in preeclampsia macrophages are located within and around the spiral arteries separating them from the trophoblast cells.

In addition, it was reported that macrophages residing in excess in the placental bed of preeclamptic women are able to limit extravillous trophoblast invasion of spiral arteries segments

Normal

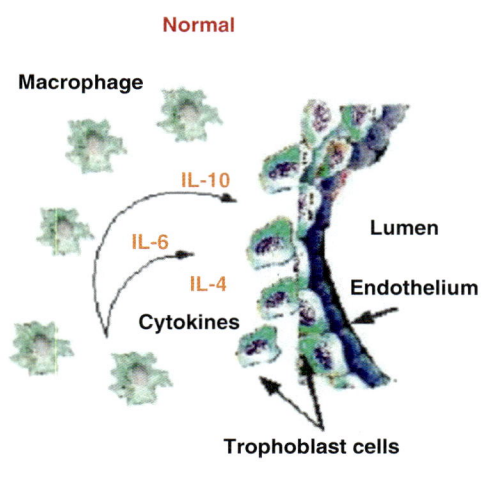

IUG/pree Clampsia

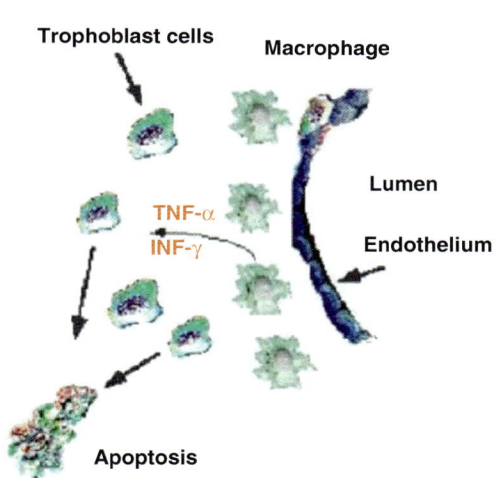

Fig. 5.6 Difference in macrophage distribution in normal and complicated pregnancies with preeclampsia and IUGR (Mor G, Abrahams VM. Potential role of macrophages as immunoregulators of pregnancy. Reprod Biol Endocrinol. 2003;1:119–27)

through apoptosis mediated by the secretion of TNF-α. Whereas in normal pregnancies macrophages function as support cells by facilitating trophoblast invasion through the placental bed, they seem to function as a barrier for trophoblast invasion and differentiation by inducing trophoblast apoptosis and therefore preventing spiral arteries transformation in pathological conditions (Fig. 5.6).

Increased trophoblast apoptosis would increase the amount of trophoblast debris and syncytial knots that leak into the maternal circulation and generate a systemic endothelial activation as seen in preeclampsia. Trophoblast debris can activate TNF-α and IL-12 production from monocytes in vitro, which further pushes the systemic immune response toward excessive inflammation instead of normal immune activity.

5.1.5.1.2 T Lymphocytes and T Regulatory Cells

An increased number of classical cytotoxic NK cells were described in third-trimester decidua of preeclamptic patients. Preeclamptic pregnancies are also characterized by an increase in the percentage of CD8+ decidual T lymphocytes. This would be consistent with a dominance of Th1

cytokine activation, which stimulates NK cells and CTLs.

In preeclamptic patients, the T-cell activation marker HLA-DR is extremely highly expressed on CD8+ T cells. Lymphocyte subsets have been characterized in the decidua of patients with preeclampsia and reported an increased percentage of CD3-/CD56+CD16+ NK cells and cytotoxic CD8+/CD28+ T cells and a decreased percentage of T CD3+, B CD19+, and suppressor/inducer T CD4+/CD45RA+lymphocyte subsets. Increased levels of activated/memory cells (CD4+CD45RO+ and CD4+CD29+) are interpreted as T cells activated by antigens. CD4+CD25+ Treg cells have been investigated, and it has been found that the ratio of CD4+CD25+/CD4+ cells is markedly decreased in preeclampsia cases compared to normal pregnancy subjects and even nonpregnant controls. Also there is a general consensus that there are increased levels of activated/memory cells (CD4+CD25RO+ and CD4+CD29+) and decreased levels of naïve/suppressor cells (CD4+CD45RA+), whereas there is a switch to naïve/suppressor T cells in normal pregnancy. A possible explanation is that antigens have activated these T cells in preeclampsia, indicating inflammatory activity. Systemic immunological deviation toward suppression seen during normal pregnancy is absent not only in peripheral blood but also locally in decidua of preeclamptic women. Moreover, this is consistent with the dominance of Th1 cytokine activation in preeclampsia, which stimulates NK cells and CTLs.

5.1.5.1.3 Cytokines

As preeclampsia is often regarded as a syndrome of an excessive inflammatory response similar to that seen during septic shock, the question of the role of superantigen involvement with a predominant Th1-type cytokine production has arisen. Endothelial dysfunction in preeclampsia is found to be associated with excessive release of Th1 cytokines like TNF-α, IL-1, and IL-8 and the Th2 cytokine, IL-6, which has proinflammatory properties. The imbalance of Th1- and Th2-type cytokines has been found in peripheral lymphocyte and placenta in preeclampsia, with an increased TNF-α, IL-2, and IFN-γ in PBMCs from preeclamptic patients compared to controls. A shift to Th1 activity with elevated IFN-γ levels and low IL-6 and IL-10 secretion has been also observed in third-trimester decidua of preeclamptic patients.

IFN-γ secreted by activated T cells activates specialized uterine NK cells with regulatory properties for physiological trophoblast invasion in decidua. IFN-γ affects the Th1/Th2 cytokine balance and increases proinflammatory potential. High levels of IFN-γ, together with TNF-α, can lead to apoptosis of trophoblasts.

IFN-γ upregulation could also involve superantigen-like stimulation of decidual lymphocytes by an infectious factor. IL-12 stimulates the production of IFN-γ that activates lymphocytes and neutrophils. In an inflammatory environment, macrophages secrete high levels of IL-12 that stimulate IFN-γ secretion by NK cells, thereby inhibiting angiogenesis. Increased serum concentrations of IL-12 in peripheral blood of preeclamptic women have been observed which points to a local dysregulation in IL-12 production.

Interestingly, an upregulated leptin expression in placental tissue in preeclampsia was observed. Leptin is an obesity-regulating protein that also induces the production of large amounts of IFN and IL-2 and decreases IL-4 production. However, the dichotomous role of IL-4 has been demonstrated also during pregnancy. Normotensive pregnancy was associated with a high increase in IL-4 in the first half of the pregnancy, but in the second half of pregnancy and puerperium, high levels of IL-4 were associated with preeclampsia. This may be a compensatory attempt to control or balance the effect of proinflammatory cytokines like TNF-α. In conjunction with an overexpression of TNF-α in placenta and in plasma, as is observed in preeclampsia, an enhanced plasma and placental expression of IL-1 has been reported. Both cytokines promote functional and structural changes in endothelial cells including oxidative stress, complement activation, and microthrombosis.

The role of TGF-β in trophoblast invasion might be also dysregulated in preeclampsia. An increase of placental oxygen during the second physiological invasion normally results in a decrease of TGF-β, which prevents excessive trophoblast invasion. In case of hypoxia, TGF-β does not decrease which results in insufficient trophoblast invasion. However, no changes in expression of TGF-β in placenta or placental bed in preeclampsia compared with normal pregnancy could be observed, which has put the impact of an overexpression of TGF-β on trophoblast invasion into question.

Elevated levels of IL-18 in preeclampsia, especially in women with HELLP syndrome, have been reported as well. IL-18 induces IFN-γ production and diverts immunity toward Th1 when IL-12 is present.

IL-10 as an anti-inflammatory cytokine promotes the termination of Th1 rejection reactions against the fetal–placental unit. A deficiency in IL-10 expression in placenta and decidua was observed during preeclamptic pregnancy which was interpreted as a modified immune balance consistent with inflammatory responses in preeclampsia. However, in some preeclampsia cases, high peripheral and placental levels of IL-10 were observed, which might be a compensatory response to elevated levels of IFN-γ, TNF-α, and IL-12.

Additionally, serum levels of granulysin, a cytotoxic granule protein of NK cells and CTLs, were significantly elevated in preeclamptic patients compared to normal pregnancies. Levels were also associated with mean blood pressure, percentage of peripheral blood Th1 cells, and the Th1/Th2 ratio. Serum granulysin would thus be a useful marker to evaluate the Th1/Th2 balance in preeclampsia. In the search for an early marker of preeclampsia, an increased expression of soluble IL-2 receptor in plasma of first-trimester pregnancies that later developed preeclampsia was observed.

Despite the fact that there is a shift to a Th1 response in preeclampsia, accompanied by a systemic inflammatory response, there is also a marked systemic inflammatory response in normal pregnancy, and the question has been raised as to whether the Th1/Th2 paradigm is too simplistic. The state of preeclampsia could be seen as an exacerbation of the inflammation during normal pregnancy. They demonstrated that the first signs of a systemic inflammatory cytokine response characteristic of pregnancy begin before implantation and deduced that its origins may not necessarily involve immune recognition of the fetal allograft. Their data show that the predominant changes are in NK and NK T-cell populations, whereas T lymphocytes show minimal or no changes. These changes are observed especially for IL-18, which is interesting since there is a Th1 storm in fulminant preeclampsia characterized by excess IL-18 which, with IL-12, stimulates IFN-γ secretion and creates a vicious loop. They then presented data suggesting the systemic stimulus triggering the innate immune system is due to the circulating fetal cells in maternal blood, plus the release of placental debris from syncytiotrophoblast. This shedding of syncytiotrophoblast microparticles is increased in preeclampsia, and these syncytiotrophoblast microvillous membrane particles increasingly bind to maternal DCs. They likely interact with TLRs and thus trigger Th1 cytokine production.

Some investigators have proposed that preeclampsia represents a defect in immunological masking that normally allows trophoblast cells to evade maternal immune recognition.

A dysregulation of the expression of HLA-G and MMP-9 on human trophoblast in preeclampsia has been described. Interestingly, lower expression of HLA-G on trophoblast could result in local IFN-γ and NK cell upregulation, which may be the main factors underlying pregnancy failure in preeclampsia. Defects in the immunosuppressive functions of HLA-G contributing to the control of CD4+ and CD8+ T-cell activity in preeclampsia may alter the local cytokine profile which is normally controlled by T cells. The expression pattern of TLR4 and TLR2 at the fetomaternal interface, the placental bed, has been evaluated in both normal and complicated pregnancies. TLR4 protein expression was found to be increased in interstitial trophoblasts of patients with preeclampsia, which suggests that dangerous host or microbial signals at the fetomaternal interface, which are recognized by trophoblasts through TLR4, may play a key role in creating a local abnormal cytokine milieu leading to the development of preeclampsia.

5.1.5.1.4 Other Immunological Mediators of Endothelial Cell Injury

Also important for the pathogenesis of preeclampsia are other mediators of inflammation such as ROS which are generally found to be increased. In the case of preeclampsia, the balance between antioxidants and free radicals is disturbed. Free radicals and levels of lipid peroxidation are increased in preeclampsia and probably evoke systemic endothelial activation and increased TNF-α production. Autoantibodies may also contribute functionally to vascular and placental dysfunction associated with preeclampsia. Studies have confirmed the presence of higher levels of antiphospholipid as well as anti-endothelial cell antibodies in serum of preeclamptic women compared to controls. Some authors found that autoantibodies against angiotensin II type 1 receptor are present in sera of preeclamptic patients.

5.1.5.1.5 Summary

Preeclampsia is based on a cascade of complex immunological events originating from the placenta. During normal pregnancy, trophoblast cells interact with uterine NK cells, modifying their cytokine repertoire, which results in cellular homeostasis and angiogenesis. Preeclampsia is characterized by the inability of the trophoblast to accomplish this. Trophoblast apoptosis prevents adequate trophoblast invasion into the decidua and results in defect remodeling of spiral arteries, hypoxia, placental ischemia, and an excessive inflammatory reaction. Leakage of increasing amounts of placental fragments and cytokines into the maternal circulation and a systemic endothelial activation lead to the clinical signs of preeclampsia. Important for future studies are the further identification of these complex immune factors, perhaps with the help of animal studies, and discovery of possible early markers for preeclampsia. Treatment options for preeclampsia, which are still focused on signs like hypertension, could be widened with respect to modification of immune responses.

5.1.5.2 Immunology of Preterm Labor and Preterm Birth

Preterm labor (PTL) or preterm birth (PTB), defined as labor or birth before 37 weeks' gestation, is preceded in 30 % of cases by preterm, premature rupture of membranes (PPROM), which is defined as membrane rupture prior to the initiation of labor at less than 37 weeks of gestation. Previously, all babies that were born less than 2,500 g were considered to be premature, but it was revealed that many of these infants were actually delivered at term but were small because of intrauterine growth restriction (IUGR). PTL is probably the final common pathway of a number of pregnancy complications due to causes such as infection, smoking, or coagulation disorders. Inflammation at the maternal–fetal interface, mediated by proinflammatory cytokines including TNF-α and IL-1β (345, 346, 1105, 1187), is considered the main common component and can be caused by intrauterine infections, lower genital infections, or distant infections such as periodontitis in pregnancy. The consequence is fetal loss of immunological privilege.

According to the literature, about 50 % of spontaneous preterm births are associated with

Table 5.2 Kinds of infection with examples predisposing to preterm birth

Intrauterine infection, clinical or subclinical	Mostly polymicrobial
Lower genital infection	BV, trichomoniasis
Distant infection	Periodontitis

M. Wirth 2006, Personal communication

ascending genital tract infection. The earlier in pregnancy at which spontaneous preterm labor occurs, the more likely it is due to an infection and the earlier in pregnancy at which abnormal genital flora is detected, the greater the risk for a subsequent infective adverse outcome. Different infections significantly predispose to spontaneous preterm birth (Table 5.2).

Multiple studies have led to the hypothesis that ascending lower genital tract infection can result in preterm labor. Bacterial entry into the decidua is followed by recruitment of leukocytes and cytokine production which in turn leads to prostaglandin synthesis in the amnion, chorion, decidua, and myometrium and MMP synthesis by chorion and amnion. MMPs are involved in cervical ripening and degradation of fetal membranes, while triggering prostaglandin synthesis results in cervical dilation, uterine contractions, and even greater entry of microbes. In the following, aspects of different lower genital infections and intrauterine infection are discussed.

Long considered a "minor" STD with few associated complications, infection with *T. vaginalis* has recently been implicated as a cause of preterm delivery in several studies. In a large multicenter study, trichomoniasis was significantly associated with low birth weight, premature rupture of membranes, and preterm delivery. A significant correlation between trichomoniasis and premature rupture of membranes with an incidence of 27.5 % in women with *trichomoniasis* versus 12.8 % in those without this microorganism has been observed. A more recent randomized treatment trial has, however, lent controversy to this area. Pregnant women with asymptomatic trichomonal infection were randomized to placebo versus treatment with metronidazole. Unexpectedly, women in the treatment group were found to have higher rates of preterm birth than those who received placebo; a possible explanation is that dying trichomonads could release inflammatory mediators that trigger PTL. This study, however, is flawed and results may be difficult to extrapolate to the clinical care of pregnant woman with trichomoniasis as only women with asymptomatic infections were included in the study and much higher doses of metronidazole were used than is the standard of care. It is also possible that women with symptomatic trichomoniasis have a different response to treatment than women with asymptomatic infection as a result of organism burden or host factors. Similar results with increased low birth weight and a trend toward increased preterm birth were reported from a recent randomized trial from Uganda. Further studies may be warranted to resolve the conflicting findings. Only symptomatic trichomoniasis should therefore be treated during pregnancy.

Bacterial vaginosis (BV) increases the risk of preterm delivery and low-birth-weight children, first-trimester miscarriage among women undergoing IVF, chorioamnionitis, and other infections. BV is associated with a twofold increased risk of preterm birth, presenting the greatest risk when detected before 16 weeks' gestation; this implies a critical period during early gestation where pathogens can ascend the genital tract. Screening for BV and treatment has been considered a strategy to reduce the rate of preterm birth, but recent meta-analyses revealed no reduction in overall preterm birth with routine screening and treatment for BV. In both studies, however, oral BV treatment did lead to a decrease in PPROM and low birth weight in a subgroup of patients with a history of preterm birth. Treatment of low-risk women with BV with an intravaginal clindamycin cream resulted in a decrease in preterm birth. Another trial with oral clindamycin showed similar results. A difference between these two trials and others was that all patients were enrolled and treated before 22 weeks of gestation, which suggests that early treatment of BV may be the key to prevention of preterm birth. These results have to be proved in high-risk populations such as women with prior preterm delivery.

Other genital tract infections found to be associated with an increased preterm birth rate are *C. trachomatis* and *N. gonorrhoeae*. The Preterm Prediction Study found that chlamydial infection detected at 24 weeks' gestation doubled the risk for preterm birth. However, trials to treat *C. trachomatis* during pregnancy have failed to demonstrate a consistent reduction in the preterm birth rate. *N. gonorrhoeae* was found to be associated with a 2.9-fold increased risk of preterm birth. Other vaginal colonizations including *Candida, Ureaplasma urealyticum,* and group B streptococci have not been found to be associated with increased risks for preterm birth. Intrauterine infection was found to be another frequent cause of PPROM and PTL, based on pathological studies of placentas. Signs of chorioamnionitis were found in 94 % of placentas of infants delivered at 21–24 weeks compared to 5 % of all placentas. The main mechanism for this infection is ascending microbial invasion by lower genital tract organisms which could produce local inflammation, i.e., subclinical chorioamnionitis leading to PPROM, PTL, and possibly preterm birth.

There is a strong association between elevated vaginal pH and the presence of vaginal neutrophils and early third-trimester PPROM. Depending on which laboratory technique is performed, the prevalence of intra-amniotic infection in the setting of preterm labor ranges from 0–24 % to 30–55 %. Many infections are polymicrobial. *Ureaplasma urealyticum, Mycoplasma hominis*, group B streptococci, *G. vaginalis*, and gram-negative bacteria such as *Escherichia coli* have been identified as pathogens commonly associated with PTL.

The main mechanism of such infections is, as already mentioned, ascending microbial invasion by lower genital tract organisms, which may produce local inflammation caused by proinflammatory cytokines and prostaglandins, i.e., subclinical chorioamnionitis leading to PPROM, PTL, and possibly preterm birth. It is also important to mention the higher probability of respiratory distress, sepsis, and cerebral palsy in preterm infants due to fetal inflammatory responses in cases of clinical chorioamnionitis. Once intra-amniotic infection has been diagnosed, the standard care is administration of intravenous antibiotics and delivery regardless of gestational age. However, a recent meta-analysis assessing 11 trials among 7,428 patients in PTL with intact membranes showed that overall use of antibiotics did not decrease preterm birth or perinatal morbidity. Routine administration of antibiotics to women with preterm labor and intact membranes is therefore not recommended as there are no clear improvements in neonatal outcomes.

5.1.5.2.1 Cytokines

The administration of bacteria or bacterial products to rodents or primates during late pregnancy induces PTL that is preceded by increased production of proinflammatory cytokines including TNF-α and IL-1β. Treatment with IL-1β was able to mimic the effects of bacteria by causing PTL, suggesting a causal role for this cytokine in infection-induced PTL. Studies both in primates and mice have demonstrated that intra-amniotic or systemic maternal infusion of IL-1β readily induced preterm labor and delivery which suggests the possibility that fetal or maternal conditions leading to elevated levels of IL-1β or other proinflammatory cytokines might precede and predict the later occurrence of preterm labor.

Many bacteria involved in ascending infection produce phospholipases A2 and C, proteinases and endotoxins which activate placental, decidual, amnion, and fetal membrane cells. This in turn may stimulate these cells to produce proinflammatory cytokines and prostaglandins which play an important role in the initiation of parturition, especially in cases related to chorioamnionitis. Cytokines such as TNF-α and IL-1β may originate from trophoblast cells as well as fetal or maternal macrophages, as cultures of amnion, chorion, and decidual cells produce proinflammatory cytokines such as MIP-1, IL-6, and IL-8 in response to bacteria or bacterial products. However, it is also possible that macrophage-derived cytokines can interact with receptors on placental cells, which augment the production of proinflammatory cytokines at the maternal–fetal interface.

Recent human studies have demonstrated that fetal carriage of a polymorphism in the IL-1 receptor antagonist gene is associated with elevated second trimester intra-amniotic IL-1β levels and an increased rate of spontaneous preterm birth, as well as with a history of spontaneous abortions. Fetal carriage of polymorphism in genes coding for IL-1 receptor antagonist, IL-4, and TNF-α, as well as a maternal IL-4 polymorphism, is associated with PPROM and preterm birth in multifetal gestations. In a further study by the same group, differences between singleton and twin gestations in immune mediators in midtrimester amniotic fluid were investigated. Concentrations of IL-1β, TNF-α, and IL-4 were increased in amniotic fluid from twins, which may contribute to the increased rate of PPROM and spontaneous preterm birth in twin populations.

Recent findings indicate that midgestation maternal immune hyporesponsiveness, as represented by low cervicovaginal concentrations of various proinflammatory cytokines, also constitutes an increased risk for subsequent preterm delivery among women with lower genital tract pathological microflora. The highest risk of preterm delivery was observed among women with low cervicovaginal concentrations of IL-1α and IL-1β; lower but still elevated risk was found for women with genital tract infection and low cervicovaginal levels of IL-6 and IL-8. The increased risk for preterm delivery was found only in the group of women with lower genital tract infections who had low cervicovaginal concentrations of proinflammatory cytokines. The latter condition may also imply a lower reactivity of the maternal immune system that should normally result in diminishing the growth of pathological bacteria in the genitourinary tract. Probably, pregnant women with an inadequate, i.e., hypo- or hyperimmune, response are at risk for subsequent infection-related preterm birth. Increased concentrations of free radicals such as proinflammatory NO and prostaglandin E2 in amniotic fluid are also associated with intrauterine infection. Furthermore, a COX-2 inhibitor blocked LPS-induced PTL in mice.

5.1.5.2.2 Anti-inflammatory Effects of IL-10 and Progesterone

IL-10 may be helpful in reducing the incidence of PTL and resulting neonatal morbidity. Administration of LPS to pregnant rats between gestation days 14 and 17 causes extensive IUGR, fetal death, and low birth weight and is associated with increased production of TNF-α and NO in the placenta and increased numbers of apoptotic cells. However, coadministration of IL-10 to LPS-treated dams improved fetal outcome by restoring birth weight and decreasing placental TNF-α, NO, and apoptosis. Intravenous administration of IL-10 also prevented preterm birth caused by intrauterine infusion of LPS in rats. IL-10 may function by decreasing LPS-stimulated IL-1ß production that could prevent the induction of COX-2 and ultimately lead to decreased prostaglandin E2 in gestational tissues. Furthermore, IL-10 blocked IL-1β-induced PTL in rhesus monkeys, probably mediated by a decrease in prostaglandin E2 production.

Progestins have also been shown to be effective in preventing PTL and delivery. Administration of pharmacological, but not physiological, levels of progesterone to mice delayed PTL in response to intrauterine injection of *E. coli*. In women with a history of preterm birth, the weekly injection of synthetic progestin, 17α-OH progesterone caproate, significantly reduced the rate of delivery at 30, 32, or 37 weeks' gestation.

Figure 5.7 shows a model for the immunological mechanisms involved in PTL and PPROM.

5.1.5.3 Immunology of Intrauterine Growth Restriction

IUGR is a main cause of perinatal morbidity and mortality. It is a heterogeneous condition that includes abnormal situations, most of them related to placental insufficiency or other physiological events leading to small-for-gestational-age babies. There are many reports studying the role of immunological mechanisms in the genesis of spontaneous abortion and preeclampsia, but only a few concerning IUGR.

An increased production of antibodies and a chronic activation of the lymphoid system similar to those found in other placental disorders seem likely in women with IUGR. Patients with IUGR presented numbers of circulating lymphoid cells positive for cytoplasmic IgM, IgG, and IgA at least tenfold higher than in normal pregnancies. Higher levels of B lymphocytes in women with IUGR compared to women with normal pregnancies have been observed, while a higher absolute number and percentage of B cells in women with IUGR has been also suggested. There have been only a few studies on the subpopulations of peripheral lymphocytes in IUGR. The percentage of circulating CD4+ cells and the CD4/CD8 ratio were found to be decreased, while the percentage of CD8+ cells is increased in women with IUGR with respect to normal pregnancies.

Serum TNF-α is increased in women with IUGR and placental insufficiency but normal in those with IUGR and normal placental perfusion. It was suggested that elevations in TNF-α could be a specific phenomenon of certain subsets of IUGR, identifying cases with placental dysfunction. This was supported by studies showing an increased TNF-α secretion in placentas of intrauterine growth-restricted fetuses was related to enhanced vasoconstriction of the fetal placental vascular bed. In addition, when they perfused normal placentas with the vasoconstrictor angiotensin II, TNF-α production was increased, which supports the finding of elevated TNF-α levels in cases of IUGR with increased umbilical artery resistance.

Serum autoantibody against the angiotensin type 1 receptor in a high percentage of pregnant women with preeclampsia and IUGR was detected. This autoantibody may be causative for pathological uteroplacental perfusion and thus be associated with distinct types of pregnancy disorder resulting from impaired placental development. Further studies have to be undertaken to investigate whether it could serve as an early marker for these disorders.

Cytokine mRNA expression in term human placentas of patients with IUGR was determined and found higher IL-1α as well as higher PDGF-A and PDGF-B levels compared to normal placentas but no clear correlation of these differences with clinical observations.

5.1.6 Immunological Aspects of Early Pregnancy Loss

The physiology of human reproduction, including the immune mechanisms that permit pregnancy,

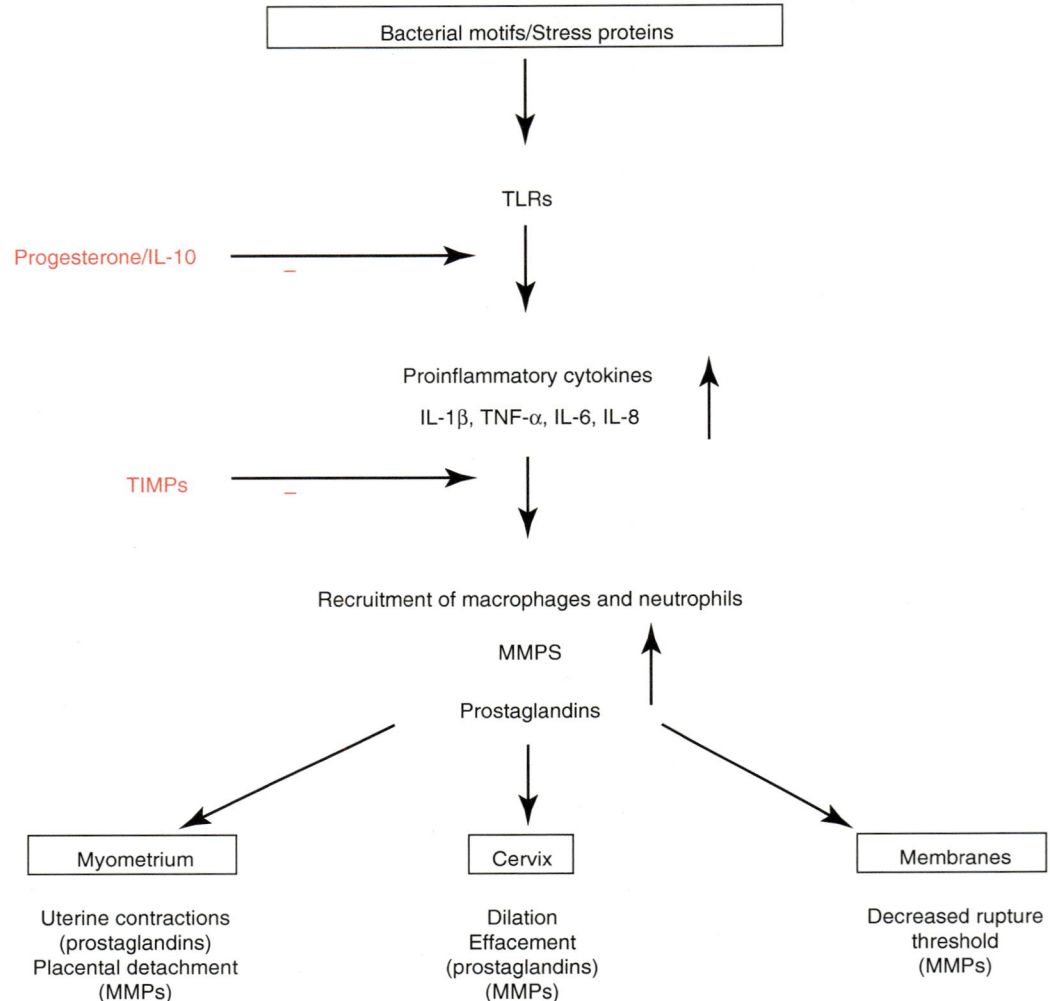

Fig. 5.7 Cascade of immunological events in the pathomechanism of PTL and PPROM (Adapted from Peltier MR. Immunology of term and preterm labor. Reprod Biol Endocrnol. 2003;1:122–33)

is extremely complex and inefficient. Spontaneous miscarriage (abortion) occurs in 15 % of all clinically recognized pregnancies, primarily in the first trimester, and is the most common complication of pregnancy. A highly sensitive C-terminal peptide of hCG assay for pregnancy indicates that an additional 20 % of conceptions terminate as "occult losses" before pregnancy is detected clinically. While most spontaneous miscarriages are sporadic and nonrecurrent, RSA, defined as two consecutive or more than three spontaneous abortions prior to the 20th week of gestation, occurs in approximately 1–3 % of women with

diagnosed pregnancies. Approximately 50–60 % of spontaneous pregnancy losses can be explained by chromosomal anomalies of the fetus, infectious etiologies or maternal endocrinology, or anatomical comorbidity; 40–50 % remain unexplained. A substantial portion of these unexplained cases could be attributable to an abnormal, abortogenic immune response of the mother toward antigens on the fetus.

There is considerable evidence that pregnancy activates the maternal immune system. Already over 20 years ago, antibodies with paternal specificity were found in sera from multiparous women, and immunosuppressive activity has been described in supernatants of oocytes after in vitro fertilization. As early as 1977, it was suggested that HLA matching between parents was associated with spontaneous abortion, a hypothesis confirmed in a more recent 10-year prospective study.

To study the role of immune cells and molecules in the etiology of RSA, we would need first-trimester placental tissues of human pregnancy, which is clearly not possible. Various alternative approaches have been adopted instead, including the analysis of immune cell populations and cytokines in the peripheral blood of women with RSA and normal fertile women either before pregnancy or at the time of miscarriage. Moreover, studies have compared endometrial tissue obtained from women with RSA and normal fertile women in the peri-implantation period in the nonpregnant state and placental tissue obtained at the time of miscarriage from women with a history of RSA, from women with spontaneous abortions, and from women requesting terminations of normal pregnancy.

While the study of placental tissue might appear to be the best approach, there are difficulties, particularly with respect to components of the immune system, in determining whether observed differences are due to proinflammatory events as a consequence of the miscarriage. One must also emphasize the importance of the compartment, i.e., peripheral blood, endometrium, or decidua, in which the cells and molecules are measured. The measurement of factors such as cytokines in peripheral blood may have little significance as this compartment is far removed from where the important interactions are taking place. In addition, the peripheral blood cell population is considerably different to that in the endometrium and decidua. Other important factors are the timing of the sampling with respect to the menstrual cycle and pregnancy and whether sampling is at the time of or just after miscarriage: both of these factors will affect the expression of these cells and molecules and have critical relevance for the interpretation of results.

Recurrent miscarriage is normally defined as three or more miscarriages, but some studies also include women with only two miscarriages. In addition, the timing of the fetal loss may differ between studies and may result in the study of different populations. It must also not be neglected that the immune mechanisms responsible for infertility, which are discussed further in a separate section, and early pregnancy loss might overlap. Moreover, there is a tendency to extrapolate directly from animal models, particularly those of rodents, to humans, and this has led to assumptions regarding mechanisms for which the evidence is incomplete. Lastly, it has recently been suggested that the importance of chromosomal abnormalities in RSA has been vastly underestimated. Karyotyping of the fetus is also important and should be carried out in future studies so that miscarriages which result from chromosomally abnormal pregnancies can be considered separately from those resulting from chromosomally normal pregnancies.

In the following, the most important approaches concerning immunological aspects in RSA are discussed.

5.1.6.1 Complement System

Evidence collected over the last few years suggests that dysfunction of the innate immune system, including uncontrolled complement activation, may induce fetal loss. Complement inhibition is an absolute requirement for normal pregnancy, as has been demonstrated by the finding that a deficiency of Crry, an intrinsic complement regulatory protein, in utero leads to progressive embryonic lethality in mice. Although the presence of complement components in the villi and in decidua is a common finding in physiological pregnancy, the quantity of proteins deposited increases substantially in pathological pregnancies. Preeclampsia is an example of a pathological condition associated with marked deposition of both early and late complement components. However, complement is also thought to play a pathogenetic role in RSA following the observation that Crry deficiency in mice is associated with fetal loss and C3 deposition. There is some indication that an abnormal expression of complement regulators may account for the occurrence of abortions in patients with a history of RSA.

The involvement of complement at placental levels is also suggested by the finding of increased deposition of C3 and TCC on the wall of decidual vessels in patients with RSA. An interesting observation was that the complement activity progressively declined prior to fetal loss in about 25 % of patients with RSA. The trophoblast tissue collected from hypocomplementemic patients was responsible for complement consumption through the alternative pathway and had a reduced level of DAF as compared to the tissue obtained from patients with normal complement activity.

Besides the reduced expression of complement regulatory molecules, antibodies directed against surface antigens on trophoblast may also be implicated in complement activation in patients with RSA. Antiphospholipid antibodies (APAs) are the antibodies that are more frequently encountered in these patients and are dealt with in detail in the next section. However, APAs are not the sole antibodies found in these patients. During the screening of a large number of sera obtained from primary and secondary aborters that did not contain APA, complement-fixing antibodies in 10–20 % of the sera that were cytotoxic for syncytiotrophoblasts could be detected.

5.1.6.2 Cell-Mediated Immune Mechanisms

5.1.6.2.1 NK Cells

NK cells, as the predominant leukocyte population in decidua during early pregnancy, may play an important role in RSA when too high in concentration. High concentrations of classical CD56+ CD16+ NK cells have been found in the uterus of women with abortions. Studies have shown increased numbers of CD56+ cells among a general increase of various lymphocyte populations (CD4+, CD8+, CD14+, CD16+/CD56+) in the nonpregnant endometrium of women with RSA, and lower numbers were seen in women with RSA who subsequently had a live birth compared with those who miscarried. This is in contrast to a flow cytometric study which showed similar numbers of CD56+ cells in the endometrium of women with RSA and control subjects,

although the women with RSA did have increased numbers of endometrial CD56dim CD16+ cells compared with control subjects. However, a decreased number of decidual CD56+ NK cells are reported in the placental tissue from spontaneous miscarriages in RSA women compared with tissue from spontaneous miscarriages in women without RSA and women requesting termination. A decreased cytotoxic capability of decidual CD56+ NK cells in placental tissue from spontaneous aborters was demonstrated, though women with RSA were not included in this study. The fact that there appears to be decreased numbers of CD56+ cells in the decidua and increased numbers in the endometrium could be due to the presence of two different populations of CD56+ cells, either CD16+ or CD16-. The increased number in the endometrium could be due to CD56+, CD16+ cells as suggested previously, while the decreased number reported in decidua could be the CD56+, CD16− population, which is supported by the study showing increased numbers of CD16+ cells in early pregnancy decidua of women with RSA.

Studies have shown increased numbers of CD56+ cells among a general increase in various lymphocyte populations (CD4+, CD8+, CD14+, CD16+/CD56+) in the nonpregnant endometrium of women with RSA, and lower numbers were seen in women with RSA who subsequently had a live birth compared with those who miscarried. This is in contrast to a flow cytometric study which showed similar numbers of CD56+ cells in the endometrium of women with RSA and control subjects, although the women with RSA did have increased numbers of endometrial CD56dim CD16+ cells compared with control subjects. However, the latter report suggested that CD3+ cells were the major leukocytes within the endometrial leukocyte population, both in women with RSA and in fertile controls. This is in disagreement with numerous in vivo immunocytochemical studies and suggests that flow cytometry may not be the best means of studying these endometrial leukocyte populations.

The above results suggest that there are alterations in the CD56+ population of leukocytes in women with RSA, but whether these are increased or decreased depends on whether peripheral blood, first-trimester decidua, or peri-implantation endometrium is analyzed. The fact that there appears to be decreased numbers of CD56+ cells in the decidua and increased numbers in the endometrium could be due to the presence of two different populations of CD56+ cells, either CD16+ or CD16–. The increased number in the endometrium could be due to CD56+, CD16+ cells as suggested previously, while the decreased number reported in decidua could be the CD56+, CD16– population, which is supported by a study showing increased numbers of CD16+ cells in early pregnancy decidua of women with RSA.

Moreover, normal human pregnancy is characterized by low peripheral NK cell activity, whereas spontaneous pregnancy termination is linked to increased NK cell activity. Some women with RSA show an abnormal cellular immune response with a marked increase in peripheral CD56+ CD16+ NK cells. Increased peripheral blood NK cells are described both in absolute and in percentage values, in RSA pregnant and nonpregnant women. A significantly increased number of circulating CD56+ NK cells was found in RSA women who miscarried compared with RSA women who delivered, and other studies have also shown that levels of peripheral blood CD56+ cells both prior to and during pregnancy can predict pregnancy outcome in women with RSA. Moreover, high preconceptional peripheral NK cell activity in women with RSA is found to associate with subsequent abortion. However, no differences in the levels of peripheral blood CD56+ CD16+ NK cells in normal pregnancies and missed abortions with normal and abnormal chromosomes could be established.

Despite the above findings, it is not the presence of NK cells that is detrimental to the trophoblast as it is able to resist NK-mediated lysis in vitro. In fact, NK cells are able to induce trophoblast lysis and cause fetal loss only if they are converted to lymphokine-activated killer cells by IFN-γ, TNF-α, and IL-2. As NK cells are not only the target of cytokines but also producers of proinflammatory cytokines such as IFN-γ, this can result in the initiation of a vicious circle. Interactions between trophoblast HLA-C,

HLA-E, and HLA-G with inhibitory receptors like KIR and CD94/NKG2 in NK cells normally block NK cell cytotoxicity against trophoblast cells.

Recent studies further suggest that a divergence of the specific NK cell repertoire in peripheral blood might be related to the etiology of RSA. NK cells in peripheral blood of women with RSA expressed higher levels of the activation marker CD69 but significantly less of the inhibitory receptor CD94 compared with fertile controls. The same authors investigated the expression of inhibitory and activating receptors in peripheral NK cells of women with RSA, found an imbalance, with increased expression of CD161-activating receptor, and decreased expression of CD158-inhibiting receptors. HLA-G polymorphisms in couples with RSA were analyzed and compared their results with normal fertile couples. Although no significant difference was found in the distribution of HLA-G alleles between controls and RSA couples, 15 % of the women who aborted carried the HLA-G*0106 allele compared to 2 % of those that did not. Additionally, the role of HLA-G polymorphisms in 113 women with RSA was evaluated, showing a significant association with increased risk for RSA. It is proposed that women with alloimmune abortions have a limited inhibitory NK cell receptor repertoire, resulting in the recognition of trophoblast HLA class I molecules by decidual NK cells. The relationship between uterine NK cell populations and RSA is still unclear.

5.1.6.2.2 Macrophages

No significant differences have been found in the number of macrophages in first-trimester decidua from women with RSA either with chromosomally normal and abnormal fetuses or in first-trimester decidua from spontaneous abortions and controls. However, an increase in the number of macrophages in the nonpregnant endometrium of women with RSA, together with an increased number of endometrial macrophages in RSA women who subsequently miscarried compared with those who had a live birth, has been reported.

5.1.6.2.3 Lymphocytes

Results concerning the numbers of CD3+ T cells as the second most abundant population in endometrium and decidua in RSA patients are also partly inconsistent. Some studies showed no differences in numbers of CD3+ T cells in peripheral blood of women with RSA and normal fertile women prior to pregnancy, but others found a significantly decreased number of CD3+ T cells in the peripheral blood of pregnant women with RSA who subsequently miscarried compared with those who had a live birth and normal pregnant controls. Two recent studies have investigated a subpopulation of CD3+ T cells that also express the CD56+ uterine NK cell marker and have shown a decrease in the number of CD56+CD3+ cells in the peripheral blood prior to pregnancy. No differences in the numbers of CD3+ T cells in the endometrium from RSA and control women have been reported; neither were there any differences in numbers of CD3+ cells in early pregnancy decidua from normal fertile women and women with RSA and in decidua from normal pregnancies and after spontaneous abortion. However, a decreased number of CD56+CD3+ cells in the decidua of women with RSA compared with control women have been reported. Thus, although there appear to be no differences in the total T-cell numbers in women with RSA, there may be differences in subpopulations of T cells, which may be important.

T cells can also be classified according to protein components of their TCR. The majority of peripheral blood T cells express $\alpha\beta$, but $\gamma\delta$ T cells are found in EC layers where they are thought to play a role in preventing the invasion of infectious agents. Extensive studies have suggested that these different populations of T cells play important roles in successful pregnancy outcome in mice, with $\alpha\beta$ cells being important immediately after implantation and decidual $\gamma\delta$ T cells being important in preventing RSA. In abortion-prone mice the production of IL-10 and TGF-β2 by Vγ1.1δ6.3 T cells, which infiltrate into the decidua on day 8.5, has been shown to be important in preventing miscarriage. In humans, the ratio of specific subpopulations of peripheral blood $\gamma\delta$ T cells, Vγl4Vδl and Vγ9Vδ2,

is reported to be different in pregnant women with a history of RSA compared with controls. Although several reports have suggested the presence and importance of $\gamma\delta$ T cells in the human decidua, other investigations have shown that most human decidual T cells are $\alpha\beta$ positive, with only 5–10 % of T cells expressing $\gamma\delta$.

Thus, although there appear to be no differences in the total T-cell numbers in women with RSA, there may be differences in subpopulations of T cells that may be important.

Lymphocyte subsets in peripheral blood in women with a history of unexplained RSA during the first trimester of pregnancy were analyzed, demonstrating significant changes in T-cell subpopulations in pregnant RSA women. Interestingly, the proportions of T-helper/memory cells (CD4+ CD45RO+), T-killer/effector cells (CD8+ S6F1+), and HLA-DR-positive T cells (CD3+ HLA-DR+), all markers of T-cell activation, were increased compared with normal pregnant controls. In contrast, the T-suppressor/inducer population (CD4+CD45RA+) was decreased compared with normal pregnant controls. Thus, RSA women reveal the opposite phenotype compared to the state of suppression/nonactivation during normal pregnancy, indicating that women with RSA have an activated immune system during pregnancy. However, it is not known whether this aberration in T-cell subsets is pathogenetically involved in RSA or whether it represents an epiphenomenon. In addition, the proportion and number of B cells (CD19+) were found to be significantly increased in the first trimester of pregnancy in RSA women compared with normal pregnant controls.

In older studies, no significant changes in the CD4/CD8 ratio in RSA women were observed. In a recent study 15 % of RSA women had an increased CD4/CD8 ratio. These patients had normal levels of CD4+ T cells but low or absent suppressor/cytotoxic CD57+ CD8+ T cells suggesting lack of suppression, i.e., activation. The activation status of both T cells and CD56+ has been investigated by measurement of expression of CD25 as T-cell activation marker and CD69 as NK cell activation marker. Interestingly, levels of CD25 in peripheral blood obtained from women with RSA in the first trimester of pregnancy were higher than those of healthy pregnant and healthy nonpregnant women. An increased number of CD25+ cells have been shown in the first-trimester decidua of women with RSA with chromosomally normal fetuses compared with decidua from elective terminations and women with RSA with chromosomally abnormal fetuses.

During normal pregnancy, the absolute leukocyte number rises due to increased numbers of granulocytes with unchanged numbers of lymphocytes and monocytes. The proportion and number of B cells (CD19+) were found to be significantly increased in the first trimester of pregnancy in RSA women compared with normal pregnant controls.

5.1.6.2.4 Fas–FasL Interaction

The critical role of Fas–FasL interaction between activated mother's immune cells and trophoblast during pregnancy leads to apoptosis of activated immune cells that may block alloreactive responses and prevent pregnancy failure. This mechanism is generally regulated by two specific proteins, bcl-2 and bax, that can promote or inhibit the apoptosis process. However, the decreased expression of bcl-2 and increased expression of bax in the decidua are among the characteristic features of pregnancy failure in women with RSA. Hence, reduction of Fas or FasL during pregnancy may be associated with fetal loss in women with RSA.

5.1.6.3 Cytokine and Growth Factors
5.1.6.3.1 The Th1/Th2 Bias

Studies in rodents during the early 1990s provided strong evidence that successful pregnancy is associated with a predominant Th2 cytokine profile and that Th1 cytokines are detrimental to pregnancy. Subsequently, even in mice the Th1/Th2 hypothesis represents an oversimplification of the situation. Experience in humans, however, confirms the role of Th1 cytokines. Concentrations of Th1-type cytokines, both at the maternal–fetal interface and in PBMC, are higher in women with unexplained recurrent abortion. A Th1-type reaction at the maternofetal interface mainly triggers the inflammatory response with increases in IFN-γ, TNF-β, IL-2, and TNF-α, which contribute to trophoblast toxicity and failure of pregnancy

in women with RSA. These Th1-type cytokines may damage the placenta directly or indirectly via the activation of certain immune cells. In addition, Th1-type cytokines induce NK cells and lymphokine-activated killer cell activity, whereas Th2-type reaction triggers the secretion of anti-inflammatory cytokines (IL-3, IL-4, IL-5, IL-10, and IL-13) during normal pregnancy that promotes the success of pregnancy by alloantibody induction, counter inflammation, and suppression of the NK cell activity. Th1 and Th2 cytokines are mutually inhibitory and a shift toward a Th1 bias tends to further downregulate Th2 reactivity.

Further studies have provided seemingly convincing evidence for an abnormal Th1 cellular immune response with higher levels of IFN-γ and lower levels of IL-6 and IL-10 to reproductive antigens in women with RSA. It has been shown that stimulation of PBMC with autologous placental cells results in production of Th2 cytokines by women in term labor and Th1 cytokines by patients with spontaneous miscarriage. PBMCs from women with RSA produce TNF-α and IFN-γ in response to stimulation from trophoblast cell extracts, while cells from healthy nonpregnant women and men produce IL-10. Similar studies have also shown decreased production of IL-4, IL-5, IL-6, and IL-10 and increased production of IFN-γ, IL-2, TNF-α, and TNF-β in supernatants of phorbol-12-myristate-13-acetate-stimulated PBMCs obtained from women with RSA at the time of miscarriage compared with stimulated PBMCs obtained during the first trimester of ongoing pregnancies in women with a normal reproductive history. However, a recent study of cytokine production by peripheral blood cells of women with RSA taken during early pregnancy before miscarriage has shown opposite effects, with increased IL-4 and IL-10 and decreased IFN-γ in women with RSA. In contrast to other studies, the results of this study are not complicated by comparing results from blood samples taken with and without miscarriage and during the first trimester of pregnancy and at birth, both of which are likely to affect cytokine production.

Compared to controls, the secretion of Th1 cytokines from immune cells was increased in

RSA patients and was associated with tropho-blast apoptosis. There was a positive correlation between apoptosis and increased IFN-γ production by PBMCs. These results suggest that women with evidence of Th1 immunity to trophoblast stimulation undergo apoptosis of trophoblast cells, offering a potential pathological mechanism of Th1-mediated reproductive failure. Higher serum levels of IL-6 and IL-10 were detected in women at normal delivery than in patients with RSA at the time of abortion, and increased concentrations of TNF-α were detected in this group of women with RSA compared to those with successful pregnancy. Some studies have evaluated women at the time of abortion, during pregnancy, or at labor, and these reports have also shown lower levels of IL-6 in RSA patients compared to healthy women.

Some evidence for differences in endometrial and decidual Th1 and Th2 cytokine production in RSA patients and in particular decreased production of cytokines such as IL-4, IL-6, and IL-10 have been recently provided. However, although the cells in this study originated from the decidua, they underwent considerable in vitro manipulations before cytokine measurement. In addition, the T-cell population from which these clones were derived comprises only a small percentage of cytokine-producing cells in the decidua.

Significantly higher levels of IFN-γ could be detected, and a trend toward increased TNF-α in whole blood cultures from nonpregnant RSA women as compared to nonpregnant controls but no significant difference in IL-6 and TGF-β1 was detected between the two groups. Under experimental conditions, the outcome of pregnancy can also be influenced by modulating the cytokine balance. Administration of TNF-α, IFN-γ, or IL-2 to normal pregnant mice caused abortion, whereas anti-TNF-α antibody reduced the resorption rate in a murine model of spontaneous immunologically mediated abortion.

5.1.6.3.2 Interleukin-12 and Other Interleukins

As already mentioned, there has been an increased interest in newly identified cytokines such as IL-12, IL-15, IL-16, IL-17, and IL-18 in relation to RSA. Elevated serum levels of IL-12 and IL-18 were found in RSA patients who miscarried compared with healthy or delivering RSA women. IL-12 is known to be a Th1-inducer cytokine and IL-18 can synergize with IL-12 in the induction of Th1 immune response resulting in pregnancy loss. The endometrium of women with RSA also expresses elevated levels of IL-13 and IL-15 that might induce a proliferative response in decidual NK cells and augment their cytolytic activity. These findings await further investigation.

5.1.6.3.3 Granulocyte–Macrophage Colony-Stimulating Factor

IFN-γ has been shown to inhibit the secretion of GM-CSF, an immune mediator that promotes the growth and differentiation of trophoblast, during normal pregnancy as compared to women with RSA. Studies in mice have also suggested that GM-CSF and CSF-1 are important in successful pregnancy outcome. Implantation is compromised in CSF-1 mutant mice that have both a lower rate of implantation and fetal viability, both of which can be restored to normal by administration of exogenous CSF-1. Decreased expression of uteroplacental CSF-1 mRNA has also been shown in mice with spontaneous and induced pregnancy loss compared with control mice.

5.1.6.3.4 Tumor Growth Factor-β

TGF-β is produced by Th3 cells and has been suggested to play an essential role both in promoting and in limiting placental development. TGF-β2 also induces decidual antiproliferative activity and is reduced in decidua from women with RSA at the time of miscarriage compared to women at first trimester with induced pregnancy termination. Significantly higher levels of TGF-β1 both in nonpregnant and pregnant women with RSA compared to nonpregnant and pregnant controls, respectively, were recently demonstrated. They suggested that TGF-β1 is necessary for pregnancy development but may also represent a risk factor for recurrent abortions.

5.1.6.3.5 The Role of TNF-α in Early Embryonic Death

TNF-α is synthesized throughout the female reproductive tract as well as in the placenta and embryo practically at all stages of development. Data suggest that this multifunctional cytokine is involved in triggering immunological pregnancy loss, i.e., death of embryos, owing to failure of defense mechanisms preventing rejection of the semiallogeneic fetoplacental unit.

The injection of TNF-α into pregnant mice resulted in embryonic death, and, moreover, in a mouse model with high incidence of embryonic death, there was an elevated level of TNF-α in supernatants of decidual cell cultures. TNF-α also influences preimplantation development of embryos. Embryo transfer studies addressing the in vivo development of blastocysts that were exposed to TNF-α revealed that TNF-α treatment caused a 17 % decrease in the proportion of implanted embryos and that the proportion of embryos that died after implantation was 40 % higher in the TNF-α pretreated group compared to controls. Results suggested that TNF-α acting on blastocysts mainly decreased their ability to differentiate into fetuses after implantation rather than their ability to implant in the uterus. Uterine cells may also serve as targets for the toxic effect of TNF-α. Experiments in the mouse uterine EC line WEG-1 revealed that TNF-α had a dose- and time-dependent cytotoxic effect on these cells while stimulating apoptosis.

TNF-α might also be involved in pathological processes leading to pregnancy loss by disturbing normal trophoblast endocrine functions. TNF-α may also be involved in the pathogenesis of stress-induced early embryonic death. An elevated TNF-α expression was observed in the uterine epithelium, stroma, and in giant and spongiotrophoblast cells of mouse placenta exposed to DNA-damaging cyclophosphamide. In mice exposed to ultrasonic sound stress, TNF-α-producing cells at the fetomaternal interface appeared to be activated and increased their TNF-α production. In a study with diabetic mice, there was a much higher decrease in the pregnancy rate in severely diabetic TNF-α +/+ mice than in TNF-α-deficient mice.

Recently, it has been proposed that LIF is another proinflammatory cytokine that may be involved in mediating TNF-α-induced stress-induced early embryonic death. LIF knockout mice were shown to produce normal blastocysts, but implantation of the embryos did not occur. When transferred to wild-type pseudopregnant recipients, the blastocysts could implant and develop. These results suggest that implantation failure in LIF-deficient mice was not due to some defects specific to the embryos but to those arising in the uterus that resulted in the total loss of its receptivity.

There is the possibility that LIF signaling may be affected due to alterations in TNF-α expression. Observations showed that LIF must be expressed in the uterus at the right time and at the right level, with activated receptors and signaling pathways, to guarantee a successful implantation. Data reported that a sustained increased TNF-α expression in the reproductive tract of females exposed to stress can alter the temporal pattern of LIF expression.

5.1.6.3.6   Activation of Thrombotic Events

Recent studies have suggested that the way in which Th1 cytokines bring about pregnancy loss is via upregulation of a newly described procoagulant, fg12. Fg12 converts prothrombin to thrombin, which in turn leads to deposition of fibrin and activation of polymorphonuclear leukocytes that can destroy the vascular supply to the placenta. In mice, anti-fg12 antibodies completely prevent spontaneous abortion and dramatically reduce the effects of TNF-α and IFN-γ on abortion rates, while TNF-α and IFN-γ upregulate the production of fg12 by both fetal trophoblast and maternal decidua. In humans, increased expression of fg12 in trophoblast cells from failing pregnancies with chromosomally normal embryos, but not in trophoblast tissue from chromosomally abnormal embryos, has also been reported.

5.1.6.4   Humoral Immunity: Alloimmune and Autoimmune Antibodies

The majority of unexplained RSA cases are found to be associated with certain autoimmune and alloimmune antibodies that may play a major role in the immunological failure of pregnancy and may lead to abortion. Indeed, infertility and recurrent miscarriages can be a manifestation of subclinical autoimmune disease, and a variety of autoantibodies have been found at increased frequencies in women with pregnancy failures. Autoimmune abortions are characterized by maternal autoimmune reactions where antibodies or autoreactive cells target decidual or trophoblast molecules and affect placental and fetal growth. Alloimmune abortions are characterized by impaired maternal immune reactions against paternally derived molecules on trophoblast resulting in rejection of the fetus.

5.1.6.4.1 Autoimmune Factors

Autoimmune factors represent the immunological response of the mother to a pregnancy that can cause fetal rejection in 30 % of women with RSA. Different types of APAs, including lupus anticoagulant, anticardiolipin β2-glycoprotein IgG/IgM/IgA, anticardiolipin IgG/IgM/IgA, antiphosphatidylserine prothrombin IgG/IgM, and anti-phosphatidylethanolamine IgG/IgM, have been reported in women with RSA.

As phospholipid molecules are normal components of cell membranes holding the dividing cells together, the production of antibodies to phospholipid molecules may inhibit the development of placenta at the maternofetal interface. These antibodies can specifically damage the inner wall of the blood vessel, which allows blood cells to adhere to the site of the injury and cause blood clot formation. The combination of blood clots and constricted blood vessels may impair blood supply to the fetus and placenta resulting in complete fetal demise or growth retardation in women with RSA.

In a study over 20 years by Makino, antiphosphatidylethanolamine antibodies and anti-annexin antibodies were more common factors in RSA patients than were anticardiolipin antibodies in terms of induction of recurrent pregnancy losses. The association of IgG antiprothrombin antibodies with pregnancy loss and in particular early pregnancy loss in a cohort of patients with antiphospholipid syndrome was recently demonstrated. Women with RSA of unknown etiology were shown to have a higher incidence of antinuclear antibodies (ANA) which indicates that there may be an underlying autoimmune process

that affects the development of the placenta and can lead to early pregnancy loss.

The incidence of thyroid antibodies (ATA) in women with RSA was significantly increased compared to controls. Women with ATA doubled their risk of miscarriage as compared to women without these antibodies. Increased levels of thyroglobulin and thyroid microsomal (thyroid peroxidase) autoantibodies were associated with an increased miscarriage rate, and as many as 31 % of women experiencing RSA were positive for one or both antibodies. The risk of fetal loss increased to 20 % in the first trimester of pregnancy, and there was also an increased risk of postpartum thyroid dysfunction. A high percentage of women with RSA were also shown to have anti-endothelial cell antibodies, which suggests that the migration of endovascular trophoblast may be inhibited by anti-endothelial cell antibodies in women with RSA.

5.1.6.4.2 Alloimmune Factors

The observation that trophoblast expresses MHC antigens on its surface which when recognized by the maternal immune system triggers an alloimmune mechanism essential for the development of maternal immunotolerance has led to suggestions that RSA of unknown etiology could be attributed to alloimmune characteristics that determine whether the fetus will survive or be rejected.

In normal pregnancy, the maternal immune system recognizes paternal HLA as being different from its own and induces the expression of several alloantibodies including antipaternal cytotoxic antibodies (APCA), anti-idiotypic antibodies (Ab2), and mixed lymphocyte reaction blocking antibodies (MLR-Bf) that may coat and protect the fetus from the cytotoxic maternal immune responses. Several investigators reported that the absence or decreased expression of APCA, Ab2, and MLR-Bf might lead to abortion in women with RSA. Less than 8.7 % APCA positivity in women with poor pregnancy outcome was also shown. APCA were present only in 8.5 % of women with RSA as compared to 33–46 % in women with normal pregnancy. Anti-anti-HLA antibodies (Ab2) and seemingly clonotypic antibodies recognize alloantigen receptors on T lymphocytes and induce suppression in allo-immune responses during normal pregnancy. The prevalence of Ab2 in women with RSA as well as in women with normal pregnancy was recently evaluated. A 30 % Ab2 positivity in women with normal pregnancy was found as compared to none in women with RSA, which indicated a role for Ab2 in maintenance of pregnancies. The same group also observed a similar fetoprotective effect of MLR-Bf.

A MLR-Bf positivity in 82.4 % women with normal pregnancy opposites 10 % of women with RSA. They also demonstrated that a blocking effect of MLR-Bf was enhanced as the pregnancy progressed and once it is developed may also be helpful with subsequent pregnancies. A study on time kinetics of MLR-Bf during the course of a successful pregnancy showed maximum levels during the first trimester and a progressive decline through the subsequent trimesters and postdelivery. However, there are also several studies that reported that MLR-Bf does not play a protective role in the maintenance of pregnancy, as blocking antibodies have no predictive value for the pregnancy outcome in RSA patients.

5.1.6.4.3 Symmetric Antibodies

Approximately 80 % of the IgG specifically reactive with endometrial antigens are symmetric antibodies, which can be cytotoxic in women with habitual abortion; in healthy pregnant women, the percentage is much lower at approximately 25 %. According to a recent study, women with a history of recurrent abortions have significantly lower proportions of asymmetric IgG antibodies (3 % of total IgG) compared with healthy pregnant women (29 % of total IgG) and nulliparous and multiparous women. In addition, among antibodies reactive with endometrial antigens, recurrent aborters had significantly lower proportions of asymmetric antibodies than healthy pregnant women. Some investigators consider that the lower levels of the non-precipitating asymmetric type of antibodies in RSA patients that would allow immunological tolerance are the major determining factor for unsuccessful pregnancy.

5.1.6.5 The Role of Progesterone in Recurrent Abortion

The immunomodulatory effects of progesterone in the maintenance of pregnancy were already described in Sect. 5.1.3.6. Chronic exposure of immunocompetent maternal cells to allogeneic embryonic antigens progressively increases the number of PR on maternal lymphocytes, whereas cases of spontaneous abortion and preterm labor are associated with decreased numbers of maternal PR-positive immune cells. A specific T-cell subpopulation, the γ/δ TCR+ cell, is likely to play a role in recognizing embryonic antigens, as they are able to recognize unprocessed antigens without MHC. In the decidua, the proportion of γ/δ TCR+ cells significantly increases and is under hormonal control; 90 % of these cells express PRs and overlap to a high degree with the CD56+ population.

Trophoblast recognition is TCR dependent and is mediated by the hsp60 reactive Vγl subset of γ/δ T lymphocytes. Within this subset, specific differences in the ratio of Vγl4Vδl and Vγ9Vδ2 cells in peripheral blood have been detected between healthy pregnant women and recurrent aborters. Signaling via the Vγl4Vδl receptor induced a Th2 response, whereas activation of the lymphocytes via the Vγ9Vδ2 receptor resulted in increased IL-12 production and NK cell activity. The immunomodulatory effect of progesterone by PIBF stimulation, as mentioned above, leads to the inhibition of NK cell activity and induction of the Th2 response, especially IL-10 production. Both progesterone and its stereoisomer dydrogesterone are thought to inhibit the activity of NK cells at the fetomaternal interface in humans via PIBF. PIBF production by lymphocytes is induced by both progesterone and dydrogesterone in a dose-dependent manner and can be inhibited by equimolar concentrations of RU-486 (mifepristone). The absence or decreased expression of PIBF during pregnancy in RSA patients may cause abortion.

Inhibiting the effects of progesterone by receptor blockade, or neutralizing PIBF effects with a specific antibody, significantly reduced the production of asymmetric antibodies in mice as well. Progesterone-associated endometrial proteins or

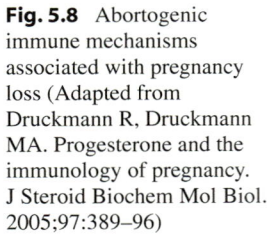

Fig. 5.8 Abortogenic immune mechanisms associated with pregnancy loss (Adapted from Druckmann R, Druckmann MA. Progesterone and the immunology of pregnancy. J Steroid Biochem Mol Biol. 2005;97:389–96)

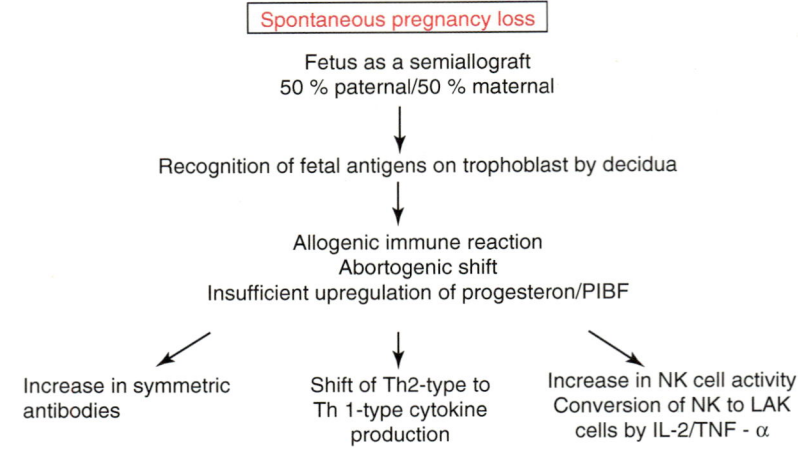

placental-derived glycodelins found in epithelial glands of endometrium, endometriotic tissues, ECs of umbilical cord, human fallopian tube, decidua amniotic fluid, and normal and ovarian tumors also act as immunosuppressive agents during pregnancy. Low levels of these proteins might lead to RSA and termination of pregnancy.

To conclude, the following diagram summarizes the immunological mechanisms leading to early pregnancy loss in women with RSA (Fig. 5.8).

5.1.6.6 Influence of Stress on Pregnancy-Related Immune Mediators

A well-balanced interaction of the nervous, endocrine, and immune systems is crucial for the maintenance of successful pregnancy. The exposure of pregnant mice to a defined stressor during the peri-implantation period has been shown to induce neurotransmitter substance P-mediated activation of T cells, mast cells, and macrophages in the uterus, resulting in decreased levels of TGF-β2 and increased secretion of TNF-α. One recent study revealed a positive correlation between increasing stress scores and the number of decidua basalis mast cells, CD8+ T cells, and TNF-α expression in women with RSA. However, no significant differences between individuals with lower or higher stress scores could be observed with respect to decidual CD56+ NK cells and CD3+ T cells. It is proposed that the

increase in CD8+ decidual cells observed in miscarriage patients with higher stress scores may reflect an attempt to abrogate the imminent or present failure of pregnancy.

Interestingly, the increase in maternal stress perception has recently been shown to cause a decrease of the pregnancy-supporting hormone progesterone and subsequently PIBF. PIBF is produced by peripheral CD8+ T lymphocytes of pregnant women, and recent findings on immune parameters in stress-scored miscarriage patients further suggest an involvement of CD8+ cells.

Psychotherapy has also been reported to result in successful pregnancy outcome in patients with a history of RSA. Furthermore, relaxation therapy, another strategy to improve stress management, has been shown to decrease peripheral levels of TNF-α. Therefore, women with recurrent pregnancy loss who received psychological counseling may have a better power to manage stress, resulting in decreased levels of abortogenic Th1 cytokines, such as TNF-α.

5.2   Immunological Infertility

Infertility is defined as a failure to conceive after 12 months of unprotected intercourse. The causes of infertility, which affects about 18–20 % of couples in reproductive age, include endocrine, tubal, uterine, cervical, and male factors. Unexplained infertility occurs when no cause of infertility can be identified after full clinical investigation of both partners: a thorough evaluation of the infertile couple will demonstrate no explanation for infertility in approximately 10 % of cases, whereas the evaluation of RSA will demonstrate no cause in as many as 60 % of cases. Recent studies in humans suggest that an unexplained reproductive failure can be influenced by some immunological abnormalities, similar to the causes described for RSA; therefore, the term "immunological infertility" has been created.

Immunological infertility is considered an incapability to conceive due to immunological disturbances in the reproductive tract. Reproductive failure and infertility in association with autoimmune diseases has been recognized for decades but only recently has it been demonstrated that specific autoantibodies are involved. Autoantibodies, such as APA, ATA, and ANA, are considered responsible not only for recurrent miscarriages and some pregnancy complications but for infertility. Antisperm antibodies (ASA) which can affect the transport of sperm cells, the process of capacitation, and the acrosome reaction as well as fertilization, postfertilization, and preimplantation processes are also associated with reproductive failure.

Recent attention has focused on a range of immunological tests for the infertile couple based on the hypothesis that a portion of unexplained infertility results from immune-mediated reproductive failure. Several immunological tests purport to identify autoimmune abnormalities, e.g., APA, ATA, and ASA, or more generalized immune defects, e.g., an NK cell dysregulation, postulated to cause reproductive failure (Table 5.3). However, this has to be evaluated critically for several reasons. The precise mechanisms by which these alloimmune or autoimmune disorders contribute to infertility remain to be established. Furthermore, there is considerable variability in the methodologies utilized, their validity, and the standardization for many of the above-mentioned tests. Similarly, the interpretation of test results is inconsistent. The rationale for valid testing in clinical practice should include the ability to secure a diagnosis and to

Table 5.3 Immunological tests in fertility practice

| Antiphospholipid antibodies (anticardiolipin, antiphosphatidyl antibodies) (APA) |
| Lupus anticoagulant |
| Antisperm antibodies (ASA) |
| Antithyroid antibodies (ATA) |
| Antinuclear antibodies (ANA) |
| Anti-smooth muscle antibodies (SMA) |
| Embryotoxicity assay |
| NK cells |

M. Wirth 2006, Personal communication

Table 5.4 Immune cells in the normal human testis

Macrophages	++	NK cells	?
Mast cells	+	DCs	?
Lymphocytes	(+)	Granulocytes	?

M. Wirth 2006, Personal communication

guide clinical decision making and a treatment plan.

The following gives an overview of the most important disorders in immunological infertility, the presence of ASA, anti-ovarian antibodies (AOA), and the group of non-organ-specific antibodies including APA. Further, the latest approaches in treatment options in immunological infertility and abortion are outlined.

5.2.1 Immunological Infertility in Males

5.2.1.1 Immunology of the Male Reproductive System

The testis is one of the few organs in the human body that is capable of sustaining foreign grafts over a period without evidence of rejection. This "immunological privilege" is derived from the need to prevent immune responses against meiotic germ cells expressing nonself antigens that first appear long after the establishment of self-tolerance during puberty. However, innate and adaptive immune responses are not generally impaired in the testis as demonstrated by the capability of inflammatory responses to infections. In addition, immune cells are found in considerable numbers within the interstitial compartment of the normal human testis (Table 5.4).

Macrophages are the second most abundant cell type next to Leydig cells; mast cells can be found as well. There are a small number of lymphocytes, whereas there is no clear evidence for the presence of NK cells, DCs, and granulocytes.

Macrophages in the testis have considered being potential effector cells activating innate immune responses and inflammation. Testicular macrophages also express MHC class II antigens indicating a capacity for antigen presentation to CD4+ Th cells. However, their ability to produce proinflammatory cytokines such as IL-1, IL-6, and TNF-α was reduced in rats compared to macrophages at other sites. Probably, resident macrophages in the testis mainly exert anti-inflammatory activities. Similar to mast cells, macrophages also seem to be involved in the local regulation of testicular functions. Only a few lymphocytes were detected in testicular tissue. The lining epithelium showed more CD8+ than CD4+ T cells and the intertubular tissue more CD4+ than CD8+ T cells. Immunotolerance in the testis has long been explained because Sertoli cells can mechanically segregate all germ cell autoantigens by means of the so-called blood–testis barrier. However, tissue barriers and mechanical sequestration are important but not sufficient to protect male germ cells from autoimmune attack as circulating antibodies, T cells, can enter and soluble sperm antigens can exit at the level of the rete testis. The presence of an immunosuppressive activity in testicular fluid was confirmed by a study that showed that Sertoli cells secrete molecules capable of inhibiting the proliferation of B and T lymphocytes. These lymphocytes produced drastically lower levels of IL-12, which shows that Sertoli cells contribute to the maintenance of immunological privilege in the testis. Expression of FasL by Sertoli cells has also been implicated in maintaining testicular immune privilege. CD8+ T cells migrating into the testis are capable of mounting an immune response against foreign tissue grafts but undergo apoptosis at an increased level via upregulation of Fas on their surface. However, the role of FasL in the immune privilege in the testis remains controversial. Local anergy of T lymphocytes may also play a key role. Constitutive expression of MHC molecules is found in the testis, whereas costimulatory molecules such as ICAM-1, CD80, and CD86 are absent which would leave naïve T cells refractory to antigen-specific activation.

Resident macrophages as well as nonimmune testicular cells have been shown to produce both pro- and anti-inflammatory cytokines such as IL-1, IL-6, TNF-α, and TGF-β even in the absence of inflammation. The overlap between testicular functions including steroidogenesis and spermatogenesis and immune regulatory functions of these cytokines helps to understand testicular immune privilege and the processes leading to inflammation-mediated damage in the testis. Consequently, local upregulation of cytokine expression during infection or injury may contribute to the disruption of testicular function and fertility.

5.2.1.2 Influence of Male Genital Tract Infection on Fertility

In men, infection and inflammation of the reproductive tract including the testes are widely accepted as important etiological factors of infertility. Invasion of microorganisms into the male genital tract has been frequently shown to be associated with impaired sperm function and, thus, persistent infertility. Bacteria present in semen may act directly on sperm cells causing agglutination of motile sperm, reducing the ability of inducing the acrosome reaction, and causing alterations in cell morphology.

Recently a statistically significant deteriorated semen volume, sperm concentration, motility, morphology, and vitality in ejaculated samples of men with *Escherichia coli, Ureaplasma urealyticum,* and *Staphylococcus aureus* in their genital tract in comparison to healthy controls have been demonstrated. Moreover, the inflammatory process in the genital tract may lead to deterioration of spermatogenesis and obstruction of the seminal tract, worsening characteristics of semen and sperm density. Microorganisms trigger a local inflammatory reaction, activating leukocytes and inflammatory mediators such as cytokines and ROS, which are known to be important in the etiology of male infertility.

The influence of bacteriospermia on the antioxidant status and proinflammatory cytokine levels in seminal plasma of infertile males with genital tract infection to those of fertile controls with genital tract infection has also been the purpose of several studies. Results suggested that urogenital infection in the latter phase in normozoospermic patients may lead to the predominance of antioxidant levels in seminal plasma, creating a positive environment for the recovery of complete function of sperm cells, whereas genital tract infection in infertile patients may cause a pro-oxidant overbalance in semen that may additionally impair the fertilization ability of spermatozoa and worsen the prognosis for future fertility. In addition, the significantly enhanced IL-6 concentration in the seminal plasma of normozoospermic patients may indicate that normozoospermic semen recovers better from infection, whereas in semen of infertile patients, leukocytes may be an additional factor worsening the fertility prognosis.

The impact of *Chlamydia trachomatis* as one of the most common STDs on semen quality and its role in male infertility is still controversial, probably due to different study designs. It is thought that up to 50 % of men infected with *Chlamydia* might be asymptomatic, and in those with symptoms, the most common presentation is urethritis. Many upper genital tract infections in young men, including epididymitis as a cause for infertility, are also attributable to *Chlamydia*. Data suggest that a *C. trachomatis* infection of the male reproductive system may contribute to the formation of ASA. Antichlamydial antibodies in women's sera correlated with detection of IgA antibodies in the male ejaculate and not with antichlamydial antibodies in the corresponding men's sera. The presence of antichlamydial antibodies in semen has been correlated with the development of autoimmunity to spermatozoa.

Overall, in vivo studies of *C. trachomatis* in men have provided conflicting evidence as to whether it is associated with reduced fertility. By contrast, in vitro studies show that coincubation of spermatozoa with *Chlamydia* causes a significant decline in numbers of motile sperm and results in premature sperm death possibly due to the action of chlamydial LPS. Prospective long-term investigations regarding the fertility of men after acute infections with *C. trachomatis* are lacking. The

effect of *C. trachomatis* infections on male fertility may be related to the quality of the immune response of the host. Thus, cell-mediated immunity must be studied more accurately. No doubt exists that female partners carry a major risk of infertility from chlamydial infection.

Chronic inflammatory reactions following acute orchitis are characterized by multifocal lymphocytic infiltrates and tubular changes that finally result in complete disruption of spermatogenesis as reflected by testicular atrophy and persistent infertility. A symptomatic orchitis due to bacterial or viral pathogens is considered rare, but a high prevalence of asymptomatic testicular inflammatory reactions could be demonstrated among infertile men.

Only a few studies have investigated testicular inflammatory reactions among infertile males. Tissue specimen from asymptomatic patients with impaired fertility showed a testicular infiltration of lymphocytes in about 56 % of the cases, predominantly CD4+ and CD8+ T cells, mast cells, and nonresident CD68+ macrophages. The degree of infiltration correlated with characteristic signs of tubular damage. These testicular inflammatory reactions in infertile men were associated with significantly reduced testicular volume and impaired spermatogenesis. This indicates a significant disturbance of local immunoregulation and testicular immune privilege. The disbalance of locally produced cytokines toward a proinflammatory profile, impairment of Sertoli cell function, and subsequent breakdown of the blood–testis barrier appear to be important features of testicular inflammatory reactions, which finally result in deterioration of spermatogenesis and infertility. The pattern of lymphocyte infiltration and concomitant damage of seminiferous tubules also supports the concept that activation of autoreactive T cells is involved.

5.2.2 Autoimmune Processes in Infertility

5.2.2.1 Antisperm Antibodies

ASA are one of the main causes of immunological infertility by binding to the sperm membrane and impairing sperm functions and can be present in males and females. They occur in seminal plasma, bound to the sperm surface, in sera of men and women and in cervical mucus and follicular fluid of women. The incidence of ASA in infertile couples ranges between 9 and 36 %. Ten percent of infertile men show ASA in their seminal plasma or attached to the surface of spermatozoa, while in approximately 5 % of female infertile partners, ASA occurs in cervical mucus or oviductal fluid. However, these antibodies are also present in approximately 1–2.5 % of fertile men and in 4 % of fertile women, which indicates that not all ASA cause infertility. Serum ASA are mainly of the IgG isotype, while ASA in cervical mucus or seminal plasma belong to the IgA isotype. It has been demonstrated that there is a diversity of ASA bound to the sperm surface, including different Ig classes of ASA, differing localization of the corresponding antigens for ASA, and different biological activities of ASA, in males. Moreover, a relatively high incidence of asthenozoospermia was demonstrated in immunologically infertile males, and a significant effect of sperm-immobilizing antibodies bound to the surface of ejaculated sperm on sperm motility was confirmed.

5.2.2.1.1 Etiology of ASA Formation
There are several hypotheses for ASA formation in men. Theoretically, the blood–testis barrier may be breached by a variety of mechanisms resulting in exposure of immunogenic sperm antigens to the immune system that could initiate an immune response, resulting in an inflammatory reaction and ASA formation. Mechanical obstruction of the genital tract may occur because of congenital abnormalities, surgical intervention, inflammation, and trauma to the epididymis and vas deferens. Several reports suggest that between 50 and 70 % of men after vasectomy subsequently have sera positive for ASA. Frequently, ASA also appears to be of idiopathic origin. ASA in the male may fulfill the criteria of an autoimmune disease.

Production of ASA in women may occur in a variety of ways. Mechanical or chemical disruption of the mucosal layer of the female genital tract may permit exposure to foreign sperm antigens and, ultimately, ASA formation. It is known that after pelvic infection or several uterine or peritoneal inseminations with capacitated spermatozoa, some patients can develop antisperm antibodies.

The prevalence of ASA in nulligravid women with various gynecologic infectious processes was also estimated. Forty-six percent of women diagnosed with PID had sera and cervical mucus positive for ASA compared with an ASA prevalence of 20 % in women who had only a lower genital tract infection. ASA also was detected in 69 % of women with laparoscopically confirmed pelvic adhesive disease or hydrosalpinx but with no prior history of PID.

5.2.2.1.2 ASA and Fertilization
Several studies have shown an inverse relation between the proportion of sperm bound by ASA and the fertilizing capability of sperm. One such study showed that only 14 % of oocytes were fertilized if 70 % or more of sperm were bound by both IgG and IgA antibodies; whereas a fertilization rate of 60 % was observed when less than 70 % of sperm was bound with ASA. Results also imply that different ASA isotypes have different effects on fertilization and some ASA can act synergistically to reduce fertility. ASA of isotypes IgG, IgA, and IgM are all capable of binding to sperm. However, a study showed that IgG ASA on sperm correlated with a reduction in the fertilization rate, whereas IgA and IgM ASA in female serum correlated with a decrease in the fertilization rate.

5.2.2.1.3 Analysis of Cognate Antigens of ASA
In order to understand the relevance of ASA, it is necessary to characterize the cognate antigens of ASA. There are direct tests to detect the presence of ASA on sperm such as the immunobead test, mixed agglutination assay, agglutination tests using donor sperm, and tray agglutination test. These tests only detect the gross binding of antibodies to various locations on sperm and do not examine the antigenic specificities of the ASA. Moreover, ASA may have heterogeneous effects

on sperm functions, obviously depending on their binding sites. They can affect sperm motility, penetration of cervical mucus by spermatozoa, the acrosome reaction, interaction between spermatozoa and zona pellucida, as well as the sperm–egg fusion. However, no proper methods exist which indicate which ASA of an individual man are functionally relevant and which sperm antigens are associated with immunological infertility. The possibility exists that fertilization-related antigens may be the targets of ASA with an inhibitory effect on fertilization. Such antigens consisted of sperm surface antigens including PH-20, PH-30, fertilization antigen-1 (FA-1), sperm agglutination antigen-1 (SAGA-1), and lactate dehydrogenase-C4 (LDH-C4) and acrosomal antigens such as SP-10, all found by immunological methods.

The cognate antigens of agglutinating ASA, which were obtained from sera of infertile women and were mAb raised in the mouse against human sperm proteins. Six sperm proteins have been recognized as target antigens for ASA from fluids of the reproductive tract including YWK-II, BE-20, rSMP-B, BS-63 (nucleoporin-related), BS-17 (calpastatin), and HED-2 (zyxin). Meanwhile, 18 proteins of the sperm membrane were detected as cognate antigens of ASA. Six of these proteins were identified as HSP70 and HSP70-2, disulfide-isomerase-ER60, caspase-3, and two subunits of the proteasome (component C2 and zeta chain).

5.2.2.1.4 Effect of ASA on Sperm Motility and Transport

Since it is likely that ASA only bind to antigens of sperm membranes, it may be speculated that functions of proteins with intra- and extramembranous components p may be altered by ASA and interfere with sperm motility. There is evidence that IgG and IgA ASA inhibit sperm penetration into cervical mucus. The proportion of motile sperm with ASA correlated with the inhibition of sperm penetration in cervical mucus. Moreover, ASA was detected in the cervical mucus from up to 29.6 % of infertile women with immobilizing sperm and prevented passage through the cervical mucus. ASA can also impair

sperm migration from the uterine cavity through the fallopian tubes.

A study examining migration of sperm through cervical mucus indicated that ASA, mainly IgA, directed against the sperm head, along with IgA and IgG ASA directed against the sperm principal piece, severely impaired the ability of sperm to penetrate the cervical mucus. In contrast, the binding of IgG and IgA to the tail tip of sperm did not appear to affect the ability of sperm to penetrate the cervical mucus, providing evidence that cervical mucus aids in the selection of the most fertile sperm of an ejaculate by acting as an immunological filter, preventing the passage of sperm coated with ASA. Impairment of sperm penetration into cervical mucus appears to be a consequence of the activation of the complement cascade by Ig attached to the sperm surface resulting in cell lysis and phagocytosis. This impaired penetrating ability, however, seems to be mediated by the effector region (Fc) portion of the Ig molecules. Interestingly, a 15-kD protein with an amino terminus identical to that of SPLI is found in human cervical mucus, and this inhibits sperm transport. The Ig possesses both an antigen-recognition region (Fab) and an Fc that binds to various leukocytes through specific surface receptors (FcR). Sperm exposed to the Fab portion of IgG of ASA can swim through the cervical mucus, whereas those exposed to intact IgG of ASA cannot.

5.2.2.1.5 Effect of ASA on Capacitation and Acrosome Reaction

Evidence has emerged that ASA might prevent membrane fluidity changes needed for capacitation before fertilization. In addition, sperm incubated with serum containing immobilizing ASA were found to have lower rates of spontaneous and induced acrosome reactions than sperm that were not incubated with serum. Furthermore, ASA can inhibit the ability of sperm to undergo spontaneous capacitation as an antibody raised against a human sperm protein, BS-17, prevented capacitation of human sperm. The effects of ASA on the acrosome reaction have been contradictory. ASA may have a variable effect on the acrosome reaction and capacitation with some ASA adversely altering the ability of sperm to undergo capacitation or acrosome reaction, whereas other ASA do not. A study showed that human follicular fluid contains IgG antibodies capable of inducing the acrosome reaction and inhibiting sperm–ZP binding.

5.2.2.1.6 Effect of ASA on Sperm–Oocyte Binding

There are conflicting results about the ability of ASA to affect sperm–oocyte binding, and it is likely that the antigenic specificity of ASA is important in their effects on fertilization. Some studies reported that binding of head-directed IgG or IgA ASA to sperm reduced sperm binding to human ZP, while other investigators found that ASA did not affect sperm–oocyte binding or that ASA were capable of both stimulating and suppressing sperm–oocyte fusion.

5.2.2.1.7 ASA Treatment

Several strategies have been used in an effort to improve the potentially deleterious effects of ASA-mediated infertility. Methods used to reduce ASA production include condoms and systemic corticosteroid treatment. As repeated or multiple sperm exposure to the female reproductive tract results in ASA formation, condom use decreases sperm exposure, resulting in a theoretical decline in ASA production. This may not be the case, however. Mild inflammatory and immune system suppression with corticosteroids may also provide some couples with limited benefit. In a study of 43 men with ASA-bound sperm, there was a statistically significant decrease in sperm-associated IgG but only little effect on sperm-bound IgA in the steroid versus the placebo group. Furthermore, in spite of a decrease in the antibody titer, there was no statistically significant difference in pregnancy outcome between the two groups. Cyclosporine was also tested in a cohort of ASA-positive men. After treatment, a pregnancy rate of 33 % was observed, but due to the lack of placebo controls, no definite conclusions could be drawn.

There are methods that attempt to remove ASA already bound to sperm which include immunodepletion, sperm washing, and IgA protease treatment. The immunomagnetic separation technique has been tried to separate antibodies bound on the sperm surface but offered only limited success in isolating a sufficient number of ASA-free sperm of good motility. There are mixed reports of simple sperm washing on ASA elution from sperm.

Moreover, several studies have examined the use of assisted reproductive technology (ART) in treatment of ASA, including intrauterine insemination (IUI), intracervical insemination (ICI), IVF, gamete intrafallopian tube transfer (GIFT), subzonal sperm injection (SUZI), and, more recently, intracytoplasmic sperm injection (ICSI). The use of ART in many couples with ASA and unexplained infertility is considered beneficial because it minimizes the impact of these antibodies in impairing gamete recognition and fusion to the oocyte. IUI has been found to be useful for treatment of female and male immunoinfertility by circumventing problems related to sperm transport in the female genital tract, especially sperm passage through the cervical mucus. However, in women having ASA in the cervical mucus, pregnancy rates after IUI were identical to women who did not have ASA if the male partner did not have ASA. However, the pregnancy outcome significantly improved after including ovarian hyperstimulation treatment along with IUI or in some cases of male immunoinfertility. In GIFT procedure, sperm and eggs are mixed in vitro and then transferred to the fallopian tubes for fertilization. In one study, GIFT was performed in 16 immunoinfertile couples that achieved pregnancy rates of 43 % per couple. This study did not include any control group, and the pregnancy rates are comparable with those that are reported after GIFT in patients having other etiologies.

An analysis of data from IVF programs by Chiu and Chamley has provided a great amount of evidence regarding the effects of ASA in serum, semen, and follicular fluid as a possible cause of infertility. These studies generally indicate that couples with ASA have lower pregnancy rates in IVF trials than couples without ASA.

The combined effects of ASA and sperm morphology on fertilization and pregnancy rates in 85 couples with male factor infertility, treated with

38 cycles of IVF and 57 cycles of GIFT, have been analyzed. The ASA-negative group had greater fertilization and pregnancy rates than the ASA-positive group. Interestingly, there are also studies reporting increased rates of IVF outcome including implantation and pregnancy rates in immunoinfertile women compared with women with tubal factor infertility. In the IVF procedure, generally albumin instead of female partner's serum is used as a protein source in the insemination medium that circumvents the antibodies if present in the female partner. Thus, IVF can take care of female but not male immunoinfertility.

ICSI is a method that may allow some couples to avoid fertilization failure secondary to an autoimmune mechanism. Twenty-nine infertile ASA-positive couples were treated with ICSI after 22 of them demonstrated a poor fertilization rate (6 %) during IVF. After ICSI, the fertilization and cleavage rates for the ASA-positive group were similar to the ASA-negative group. It is notable that 46 % of the pregnancies occurring in the ASA-positive group ended in spontaneous pregnancy loss compared with none in the ASA-negative group. A retrospective analysis of 55 ICSI cycles for 32 different couples with high levels of ASA-bound sperm demonstrated a significantly higher fertilization rate between the ASA-positive group undergoing ICSI and an ASA-negative control group undergoing ICSI. Using the ICSI procedure in immunoinfertile men, one can achieve higher fertilization rates than using the IVF procedure; however, the fertilized zygotes show higher rates of degeneration and mortality and decreased embryonic development. However, compared to other methods, ICSI has been the most successful in treating ASA-positive infertility.

By using hybridoma and recombinant DNA technologies as well as various genomic approaches, several sperm antigens have been defined from various laboratories that may be involved in fertilization and fertility. FA-1 and YLP12 have been cloned among at least nine sperm-specific cDNAs. Antibodies to FA-1 antigen inhibit human sperm–ZP interaction and block human sperm capacitation/acrosome reaction by inhibiting tyrosine phosphorylation.

A study was conducted to determine if immunoadsorption with the human sperm FA-1 antigen would remove autoantibodies from the surface of sperm cells of immunoinfertile men and thus increasing their fertilizing capacity. An increased level of antibody-free motile sperm, on an average of 50 and 76 % for IgA and IgG ASA, respectively, was found. The acrosome reaction rates increased significantly and showed improvement in 78 % of the sperm samples after FA-1 adsorption. The IUI of FA-1-treated antibody-free sperm resulted in normal pregnancies and healthy babies, indicating that the antigen treatment does not have a deleterious effect on implantation and embryonic and fetal development.

5.2.2.2 Anti-ovarian Antibodies

Anti-ovarian antibodies (AOAs) form a heterogeneous group of antibodies recognizing several different antigenic targets such as granulosa and thecal cells, zona pellucida, oocyte cytoplasm, corpus luteum, as well as gonadotropins and their receptors. Their involvement in patients with patent premature ovarian failure (POF), a disorder of multicausal etiology leading to infertility in women, is highly likely. POF is defined as secondary amenorrhea with a hypoestrogenic hypergonadotropic serum profile in the menopausal range that finally culminates into partial or total destruction of the primordial follicle pool thereby leading to infertility.

In POF patients, a variety of autoantibodies and possible target antigens have been reported so far, including antibodies binding to mature follicles and corpus luteum, termed steroid cell antibody (SCA). In the ovary, SCA immunostaining was preferentially localized in theca interna cells of antral follicles, but in some cases the granulosa layer and corpus luteum were also stained. Whereas the prevalence of SCAs in POF is 6.5–10 % of patients, it was much higher (87–100 %) in patients with Addison's disease with associated POF. None of these studies showed SCAs to be present in healthy controls, and it is not known whether they could be detected in other ovarian pathologies. Thus, these antibodies seem to be highly specific to anti-adrenal autoimmunity with associated ovarian failure. Moreover, in normally cycling patients with autoimmune endocrine disorders, the appearance of SCAs may be predictive of forthcoming ovarian failure.

The localization of AOAs on cells of the granulosa layer and in oocytes, as well as the expression of FSH and LH receptors in granulosa cells and FSH receptors in the oocyte, is consistent with the hypothesis of gonadotropin receptors being antigenic targets for AOAs. However, different studies on antigonadotropin receptor antibodies suggest that the role of this type of autoantibody in human ovarian diseases remains to be demonstrated.

Only a few studies have demonstrated the existence of antibodies directed against gonadotropins themselves. Anti-FSH antibodies in 92 % and anti-LH antibodies in 65 % of low-responder IVF patients, but not in good responders were detected. POF patients did not present with anti-FSH antibodies, and only 6 % of them had anti-LH antibodies. Patients with endometriosis and polycystic ovary syndrome presented with higher levels of anti-FSH IgA and proposed anti-FSH IgA as a marker for ovarian disorders causing infertility. Most of the research on antigonadotropin antibodies has actually been done to develop contraceptive vaccines in humans, which are discussed below.

Whether the prevalence of anti-ZP antibodies is higher in infertile than fertile women has been examined in numerous studies, but the results are still controversial. In the largest series of infertile women tested, a significantly higher prevalence of serum anti-ZP antibodies in patients with unexplained infertility than in those with infertility of known causes was demonstrated, thus indicating a possible etiological significance of anti-ZP antibodies in some cases of unexplained infertility. Moreover, 66.6 % women with POF belonged to the autoimmune group that ZP was an important antigenic determinant of autoimmune POF and that ovarian autoantibodies circulating in POF patients are specific to ZP.

Only a few studies have been devoted to anti-oocyte antibodies. Studies on human ovarian sections revealed the presence of anti-oocyte antibodies in the serum of 33 % of POF patients, and in another group of patients with ovarian

failure, 46 % had such antibodies detected by ELISA with extracts from unfertilized IVF oocytes.

5.2.2.3 Non-organ-Specific Autoantibodies

The presence of organ-specific autoantibodies to testicular antigens and sperm in men and antibodies to zona pellucida and endometrial antigens in women is considered the possible cause of infertility in a subset of patients with unexplained infertility. However, the presence of other autoantibodies, which are not particularly organ-specific, such as APA, ATA, ANA, or anti-smooth muscle antibodies (SMA), has been increasingly implicated in infertility. Some investigations showed a greater incidence of these antibodies compared to organ-specific antibodies in infertile women as well as an association between their presence and the length of infertility.

In a preliminary study 82.3 % of infertile patients after repeated IVF failure had at least one abnormal result on autoimmune testing but no symptoms of autoimmune disorders. Results of another study on 108 females with reproductive failure versus a control group of 392 women showed that 40.7 % of patients' sera and 14.8 % of control sera contained one or more common autoantibodies, with ANA and SMA most frequently detected.

As mentioned in the section on immunological aspects of early pregnancy loss, APAs, as a heterogeneous group of autoantibodies, are highly associated with reproductive failure. The association of APAs with RPL has led investigators to explore a role for such antibodies in unexplained infertility. The thrombogenic nature of these antibodies has been postulated to interfere with implantation, placentation, and the normal vascular perfusion of the developing embryo. Data on the prevalence of APA in infertile patients must be interpreted based on the numbers of autoantibodies tested, the availability of assay controls, the use of nonstandardized test modalities, patient inclusion criteria, and the variable ranges selected to distinguish normal from abnormal test values. The prevalence of serum APAs in the general population has been reported to be

1–3 %. Clinical criteria include venous or arterial thrombosis, thrombocytopenia, and recurrent fertility failure as well as the presence of serum IgG or IgM anticardiolipin antibodies (aCL) and lupus anticoagulant.

Increased ACA levels in 17 % of infertile patients versus 6 % of the control group were reported. When restricting analysis to fertility patients being treated with IVF, the prevalence of APA was consistently higher (6–38 %) than in control populations consisting of normal parous women (highest prevalence 3.5 %). The consistent observation has been an increased prevalence of APA in the infertile population, especially demonstrated in IVF patients. The essential question has been whether these autoantibodies cause infertility or IVF failure or simply represent serum markers associated with infertility. Similar results have also been obtained from studies on the prevalence of ATA, ANA, or SMA in infertile patients, but it remains difficult to draw conclusions owing to small patient numbers and the lack of control groups. Therefore, the use of APA testing in fertility practice remains unclear based on current data. There is also no compelling evidence that testing for ANA, ATA, or SMA in routine clinical practice is relevant to the diagnosis or treatment of otherwise unexplained infertility.

Women with systemic rheumatic diseases and accompanying reproductive failure have a high prevalence of APAs against cardiolipin and β2-glycoprotein I. The latter antibodies have been shown to have a direct inhibitory effect on the endothelial cells of the female reproductive tract, the early embryo, and the trophoblast in the placenta. Evidence is also accumulating that antiphosphatidylserine antibodies (aPS) are particularly pathogenic to trophoblast. Both animal and in vitro experiments have shown monoclonal and polyclonal aPS and aCL to specifically destroy trophoblast, inhibit syncytium formation, halt hCG production, and limit trophoblast invasion.

Interestingly, 66.7 % of 123 women undergoing IVF had at least one pathological marker in autoimmune testing; a combination of pathological assays was found in 25.2 % patients. Overall, 32.5 % of all patients had a positive titer of APA that is significantly higher than the estimated 2 %

prevalence in a healthy obstetric population. Percentage numbers of patients tested positive for APA range between 15 and 48 %, compared to a percentage in controls of between 0 and 6 %; however, in most studies there were no control groups measured.

The presences of autoantibodies that are not specific to components of the reproductive system in infertile women are viewed by some authors as an epiphenomenon rather than a factor playing a pathogenetic role. In this context, autoantibodies in infertile patients are seen as part of generalized activation of the immune system, because in these patients, in addition to infertility-associated antibodies, other classic autoimmune conditions were observed including monoclonal or polyclonal gammopathies, selective IgA deficiencies, and abnormalities of IgG subclasses. In addition, there is a plausible possibility that reproductive failure, in any of its forms, is the first clinical sign of impending autoimmune disease.

In conclusion, women with reproductive failure and patients with repeated reproductive losses in IVF programs are a highly selected patient group with autoantibody abnormalities. There is a need of immunological diagnostics in the group of patients with unexplained infertility. In the management of reproductive immunology, it has been proposed that it is sufficient to examine antibodies against seven different phospholipids in IgG, IgM, IgA, and sperm and zona pellucida antibodies.

5.2.2.4 NK Cells

An increased blood NK cell cytotoxicity level was associated with recurrent failed implantation after IVF. Interestingly, there were no live births in a group of women with multiple failed IVF cycles and women with a history of RSA whose percentage of blood NK cells was 18.0 % or higher. Risk factors for immunological implantation failure associated with a negative pregnancy test after IVF have included APA, ANA, and ATA, embryotoxic factors detected by an embryotoxicity assay, and elevated levels of circulating NK cells. Seventy percent of women with IVF failure had at least one of these risk factors. More recent studies have focused on elevated CD69 expression on NK cells as being associated with RSA and infertility of unknown etiology. CD69 is a triggering molecule on activated NK cells that is capable of inducing cytotoxicity and stimulating cytokine production. In this study, women with high CD56dimCD16+CD69+ in peripheral blood had reduced implantation rates and higher miscarriage rates.

Taken together, the results of the various investigations suggest that there are alterations in the NK cell population in women with RSA or infertility. However, whether NK cells are increased or decreased depends on whether peripheral blood, endometrium, or first-trimester decidua is analyzed and on the timing of sampling with respect to menstrual cycle or pregnancy. The data fail to distinguish whether the difference in activity and number of NK cells is a cause or an effect of reproductive failure. Further studies are needed to investigate whether the composition or concentration of NK cells is critical in implantation and what might be the options for intervention aimed at NK cells in reproductive failure.

Among women with the combined problems of APA and elevated NK cells who become pregnant with preconception treatment, the live birth rate is about 70 %.

5.2.3   Treatment Options for Immunological Abortion

Heparin plus aspirin, aspirin alone, intravenous immunoglobulin (IVIG) administration, and immunization with allogeneic lymphocytes are the most common treatments in women with immunological RSA. Immunotherapy may be an effective treatment for women with a history of RSA and combined immune abnormalities.

5.2.3.1 Aspirin/Heparin and Steroids
The most common treatment in women with repetitive implantation failure is a combination of low-molecular-weight heparin and aspirin, and several studies have shown the effectiveness of this treatment, also as compared to aspirin alone.

Especially, in women with APA and RSA, this is currently the most recommended treatment. Treatment of APA-positive women with a heparin/aspirin combination significantly improved the birth rate. This therapy may not only be effective but also less costly and logistically simpler to provide than other treatment options. Possible side effects such as decrease in bone density due to heparin have not been seen.

Another treatment option for autoantibody syndromes is prednisolone, which suppresses the inflammatory process and stabilizes the cell. Interestingly, an increasing role of steroids, especially prednisone, in the treatment of recurrent implantation failure, mostly together with heparin, has been proposed over the past years. His experience showed a clear benefit in patients with high autoimmune activity, as shown by high numbers of NK cells or an increased Th1/Th2 ratio. However, there have also been placebo-controlled studies showing that prednisone and aspirin are not effective in promoting live births and even increase the risk of prematurity.

In another study using heparin/aspirin, aspirin alone, steroids, IVIG, and alloimmunization or combined therapy for the treatment of women with RSA, an 80.5 % success rate was observed in immunized women.

More data from placebo-controlled, randomized studies seem to be required.

5.2.3.2 Intravenous Immunoglobulin
For women with RSA due to immunological reasons and failure of the heparin/aspirin therapy, therapy with IVIG remains a safe but still controversial alternative of treatment. It is possible that the use of IVIG may be restricted to patients with RSA unresponsive to conventional treatment with heparin/aspirin. IVIG has also been suggested for use in RSA cases with various serum autoantibodies or a high increase in NK cell numbers, indicating high autoimmune activity.

Several studies have shown a significant benefit of IVIG treatment in women with recurrent miscarriages, while other studies have failed to confirm this beneficial effect. In some trials with IVIG, the lack of a control group made it impossible to evaluate the apparently favorable effect

(768, 1365, 1367). Several placebo-controlled trial studies on IVIG therapy have been published, with more than 300 treated RSA patients. Of these studies, only two showed a possible significant benefit of IVIG treatment in women with recurrent miscarriages, while others failed to confirm this beneficial effect compared to placebo treatment. However, a significant difference in pregnancy success rate between IVIG-treated and IVIG-untreated groups in a study in older women with RSA was reported. A subsequent study with a larger group of women confirmed these positive results. Results from those trials showing a positive effect of IVIG report a live birth rate between 60 and 85 %.

A lack of standardization of IVIG trial design has made study comparison virtually impossible and contributed to the ongoing controversy over IVIG therapy. For example, there have been major differences in patient selection and timing of IVIG regimens. Generally, evaluation of IVIG therapy may be difficult as different authors propose various indications or no exact indication for IVIG and patients from different populations with varying diagnoses are included in the study groups. Trials have also differed in the numbers of previous miscarriages and in the number of patients with RSA after a live birth. Concerning treatment protocols, the trials have shown great diversity with regard to the starting time of treatment, the number of infusions, and the amount of IVIG given. Moreover, additional therapies including aspirin/heparin are often added, and the number of patients included in the studies may be too low to detect any significant effect of IVIG. One review showed that factors associated with successful use of IVIG were an older mean patient age, initiation of IVIG therapy prior to conception, and repeated intervals of IVIG during pregnancy.

The basic effect of IVIG is to neutralize the cytotoxic effect of the maternal immune response against the fetus (Table 5.5). Studies have demonstrated that IVIG suppresses the activity of APA and passively transferred blocking or anti-idiotypic antibodies that inhibit the binding of APA to corresponding antigens.

IVIG exhibits a documented effect in many immunological disorders. Immunomodulation by

Table 5.5 Proposed mechanisms of IVIG

Suppression of lymphocyte activation	Inactivation of complement
Blocking of TCR	Downregulation of NK cell activity
Increase of suppressor T-cell activity	Shift of Th1/Th2 cytokines to Th2

M. Wirth 2006, Personal communication

IVIG is thought to result from passively transferred blocking or anti-idiotypic antibodies, downregulation of B-cell function, inhibition of complement activation, reduction of NK cell activity, and shift of the Th1/Th2 ratio. The last-mentioned analysis showed that in alloimmune abortions, IVIG caused a shift in the Th1/Th2 balance to Th2, while in autoimmune abortions, IVIG possibly drove the Th1/Th2 ratio to a normal balance. A downregulation of peripheral NK cell activity and subsets by massive IVIG treatment of women with RSA was demonstrated. IVIG had no effect on 15 of 17 tested clusters of leukocyte differentiation (CD) markers used but that it downregulated adhesion molecule lymphocyte function-associated antigen-1 (LFA-1) and NK cells. However, there were no statistical differences in the presence of blocking antibodies prior to pregnancy in RSA women included in the IVIG trial compared with women not attending the IVIG trial and controls. Furthermore, they demonstrated that IVIG does not have long-term effect on T- and B-cell subsets in women with RSA.

The fact that IVIG is capable of reducing high concentrations of NK cells in peripheral blood with a short- and long-term efficacy was confirmed in several studies. A positive effect of IVIG on GM-CSF levels was observed, which are usually very low in pregnant RSA patients.

Appropriate patient selection and valid timing of IVIG administration seem to be crucial factors that determine the success of this treatment. IVIG therapy appears to be safe and effective especially for older women with recurrent failure of natural or IVF-induced pregnancy or recurrent aborters with elevated NK cell activity. Monthly administration of low-dose IVIG initiated prior to conception and continuing through the end of the second trimester of pregnancy appears to be the optimal treatment regimen. IVIG has been associated with some undesirable side effects; it is costly and the long-term effects of its use remain to be confirmed. Further experiments should be carried out with large sample sizes for both experimental and placebo treatments and with more exactly defined patient groups and IVIG regimen.

5.2.3.3 Allogeneic Lymphocyte Immunotherapy

The possibility of paternal lymphocyte immunotherapy for women with unexplained RSA has been proposed, a protocol that has become widely performed since then. The idea of third-party lymphocyte immunization for women with RSA relies on observations that renal allograft rejection could be delayed by third-party blood transfusions. Interestingly, another idea was based on paternal lymphocyte immunization with the belief that maternal "blocking antibodies" were necessary for successful pregnancy.

The exact mechanisms of immunotherapy with allogeneic lymphocytes have yet to be elucidated (Table 5.6).

Immunotherapy with leukocytes attempts to block immunological rejection of the fetus by exposing the mother to an overload of self- or third-party antigen. This is thought to mimic the presentation of fetal antigens during pregnancy presumably eliciting maternal immunoglobulin effectors that are believed to be necessary for maintenance of pregnancy. Some investigators suggested that paternal lymphocyte immunotherapy might act as immunogens to enhance the maternal immune response and to induce various humoral antibodies as immunological regulators for maintaining pregnancy. Various studies demonstrated that paternal lymphocyte immunization in women with RSA induced humoral antibodies like APCA, Ab2, and MLR Bf that were correlated with the success of pregnancy. It was further suggested that the humoral antibodies APCA, Ab2, and MLR-Bf produced because of immunotherapy would mask fetal HLA antigens and prevent them from being attacked by the maternal T cells. Initial reports on paternal

Table 5.6 Proposed mechanisms of allogeneic lymphocyte immunotherapy

Induction of humoral antibodies (APCA, Ab2, MLR-Bf)	Increase of PIBF on lymphocytes
Decrease of peripheral NK cells	Increase of PR on lymphocytes
Shift of Th1/Th2 ratio to Th2	

M. Wirth 2006, Personal communication

lymphocyte immunization used the sharing of HLA antigens between spouses as a criterion for immunization. This excess sharing was considered increased in couples with RSA and responsible for the hyporesponsiveness, which was considered to be shown by a lower incidence of APCA, Ab2, and MLR-Bf in RSA couples. The anti-TCR idiotypic antibody that has been reported to be present in the sera of normal pregnant women provides another rationale for immunotherapy. After immunization with paternal lymphocytes, maternal T cells recognizing paternal HLA antigens would expand and serve as immunogens to produce anti-TCR idiotypic antibodies. The anti-TCR idiotypic antibody would then bind specifically to the TCR and suppress the maternal immune response against the fetus, allowing the fetus to escape the maternal immunological attack. Thus, the beneficial effect of this procedure has been attributed to the induction of various humoral antibodies that may block immune rejection of the fetus and help in implantation and fetal growth. In addition, this therapeutic approach also includes a specific and nonspecific T-cell suppression, a shift to Th2-type immunity, and suppression of NK cell activity.

Recently, monocyte functions such as secretion of IL-1α, TNF-α, and IL-6 and cytotoxic activity decreased, whereas IL-10 and TGF-β increased after paternal lymphocyte immunotherapy in women with RSA. In vitro studies showed that a low dose of IL-6 stimulated asymmetric antibody synthesis and a high dose decreased it suggesting that IL-6 regulates the synthesis of asymmetric antibodies in the trophoblast.

Lymphocyte immunization causes an increase in PIBF in women with RSA, which may play a significant role in the maintenance of pregnancy by regulating the Th2 shift. Of interest was the observation that immunization with third-party leukocytes produced equally good results. Thus, some women would abort following immunization with paternal cells but successfully carried pregnancies to term and delivered live babies after immunization with third-party lymphocytes. Such an observation could be interpreted to mean that the husband did not provide an adequate antigenic repertoire for the wife to raise a sufficient immunological response to sustain the pregnancy, a condition that was then fulfilled by the third-party leukocyte donor.

A performed meta-analysis of various randomized and nonrandomized clinical trials for lymphocyte immunization in women with RSA has recently being published. Women with RSA who received paternal lymphocytes were considered as the study group, and those who received autologous lymphocytes, third-party lymphocytes, and normal saline were considered as the control group. Comparing the success rate in pooled data of trials, the success rate was 67 % in women with RSA of the study group who received paternal lymphocyte immunotherapy as compared to 36 % in women with RSA of the control group. These data showed the efficacy of paternal lymphocyte immunotherapy as a therapeutic approach for the treatment of women with RSA. However, despite these promising results, the small sample size and lack of control groups in several studies remain drawbacks. Moreover, women randomized to immunotherapy have tended to be older and have been reported to be at higher risk of RSA than those randomized to control groups. The use of allogeneic lymphocyte immunization using partner or third-party leukocytes in new meta-analyses of the Cochrane databases was found to be associated with an odds ratio of 1.23 (12 trials on 641 women) and 1.39 (3 trials on 156 women), respectively. Both provided no significant effect over placebo in improving the live birth rate, similar to IVIG, with an odds ratio of 0.98. Three authors independently evaluated the randomized, placebo-controlled studies with well-defined treatment criteria and patients. In addition,

lymphocyte immunotherapy has been associated with adverse side effects such as erythrocyte sensitization, thrombocytopenia, and IUGR.

Overall, data on the efficacy of this immunotherapy remain controversial, with several of the published results of randomized allogeneic lymphocyte immunotherapy for women with RSA showing no significant effect. The problem is on the one hand that most of the trials with positive results have been nonrandomized and clinical data have been incomplete. On the other hand, it has been suggested that there are some other factors, such as the number of previous miscarriages, the presence of prior live births, the time of conception after immunization, and the patient's age, which may also influence the outcome of pregnancy.

5.2.3.4 LeukoNorm CytoChemia

The leukocytic ultrafiltrate LeukoNorm CytoChemia (LNCC) has been approved for the treatment of immunologically based RSA and repetitive implantation failure. The treatment outcome of LNCC in patients with multiple failed IVF or ICSI cycles has also being analyzed. Administration of LNCC on five consecutive days from the day of oocyte retrieval significantly improved treatment results with a pregnancy rate of 55 % (40 % clinical pregnancies) as opposed to a rate of 21 % in the nontreatment group. A consecutive multicenter study in Germany with LNCC has shown similar positive results.

5.2.3.5 1α,25-Dihydroxy-vitamin-D$_3$

As 1α,25-Dihydroxy Vitamin D3 (VD3) and its analogs were already known to be effective in the treatment of Th1-immunity-mediated disease, with VD3 as a new immunomodulatory agent for the treatment of women with RSA, another Th1-immunity disease. The mechanism of VD3 activity is not yet fully understood, but it is thought to downregulate the production of Th1 cytokines, such as IL-2, IFN-γ, TNF-α, IL-1, IL-6, and IL-8, as well as increase Th2-associated cytokines in T cells from adults. VD3 also inhibits not only IL-12-generated IFN-γ production but also suppresses IL-4 and IL-13 expression induced by IL-4. As the effects of

VD3 are very similar to immunomodulatory effects of IL-10, it was believed that VD3 could be used as a local immunomodulatory drug for the treatment of RSA. The proposal to use it as an effective immunotherapy in women with RSA needs to be evaluated in well-controlled studies.

5.2.3.6 Dehydrogesterone

Progesterone was recognized early on to be one of the most important steroids required for the maintenance of pregnancy, and so its stereoisomer dydrogesterone became a candidate for the treatment of threatened and habitual abortion. Already in the 1980s, the pregnancy-maintaining effects of dydrogesterone were demonstrated in ovariectomized rats. On PBMCs of women with RSA, dehydrogesterone significantly inhibited the production of the Th1 cytokines IFN-γ and TNF-α and induced an increase in the levels of the Th2 cytokines IL-4 and IL-6 resulting in a substantial shift in the ratio of Th1/Th2 cytokines. The effect of dydrogesterone was blocked by the addition of the progesterone receptor antagonist mifepristone, indicating that dydrogesterone was acting via the progesterone receptor. Dydrogesterone also induced the production of PIBF. Another recent study compared serum cytokine levels in women with threatened abortion to those of healthy pregnant controls and evaluated the impact of dehydrogesterone in the former group. Peripheral cytokine production did not significantly differ between the two groups before and after treatment with dehydrogesterone. The protective effect may therefore be manifested via PIBF rather than controlling cytokine production. In a controlled, randomized clinical trial, 180 women with a history of habitual abortions received either dydrogesterone, hCG, or no treatment until the 12th week of gestation. Dydrogesterone significantly reduced the abortion rate as compared with untreated controls with no increase in obstetric complications. Despite these promising results, there is still a need for more controlled, blinded, and randomized clinical trials in order to draw firm conclusions as to the usefulness of dydrogesterone in women with a history of recurrent miscarriage.

5.3 Immunocontraceptive Approaches

A continuing population explosion and unintended pregnancies continue to pose major public health issues worldwide. The world population currently increases by one billion every 12 years; 95 % of this growth takes place in developing nations. In the USA, half of all pregnancies are said to be unintended, which results in more than one million elective abortions annually. Better education regarding women's health issues and enhanced contraceptive development are necessary to influence this problem. Contraceptive vaccines may provide viable and valuable alternatives to the presently available methods of contraception. This approach involves generating a cellular or humoral immune response against antigens that are critical in the reproductive process. An appropriate antigen is linked to a foreign carrier molecule and when coadministered with an adjuvant causes the immune system to raise neutralizing antibodies. In reversible methods, fertility is regained subsequent to a decline in antibody response, whereas an irreversible block in fertility is evidenced by a failure to regain fertility in spite of undetectable circulatory antibodies.

There are several possible targets for immunological intervention in the female reproductive system. These can be divided into three main categories: contraceptive vaccines targeting gamete production, gamete function, and gamete outcome.

For example, neutralization of gonadotropin-releasing hormone (GnRH) activity in the GnRH/LH/FSH feedback control system by generating a specific antibody response will interfere in the production and maturation of oocytes. At the level of the sperm–egg interaction, possible targets could be surface determinants on the gametes against which an immune response can be elicited. After fertilization, immunological neutralization of hCG by antibodies would result in a failure of blastocyst implantation. An overview is given in Fig. 5.9.

Fig. 5.9 Stages of the reproductive cycle with possible targets for immunological intervention (M. Wirth 2006, Personal communication)

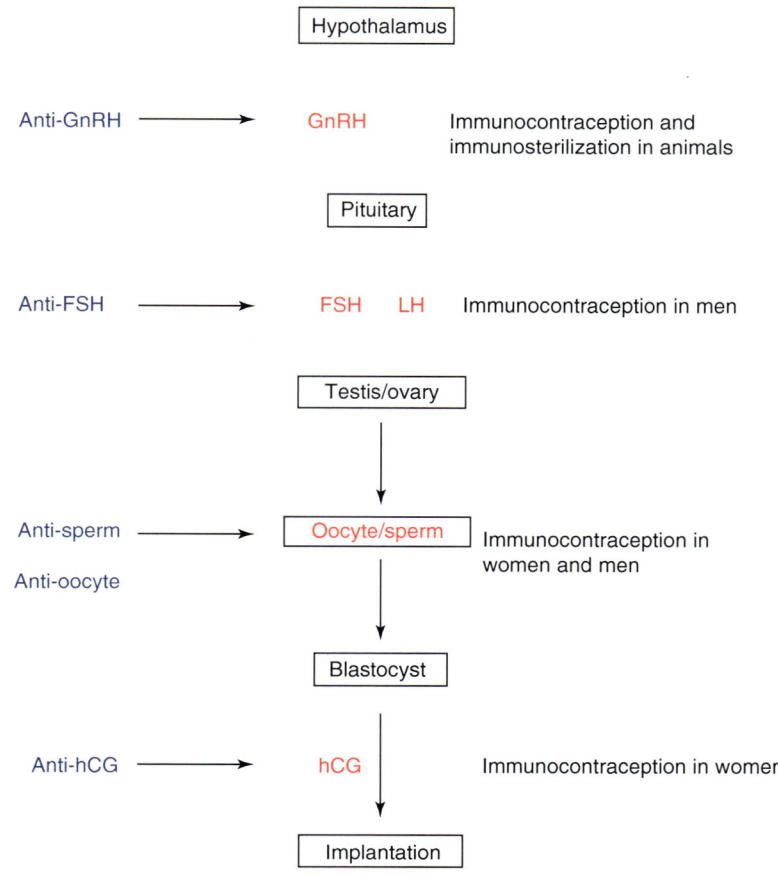

5.3.1 Anti-GnRH Vaccines

GnRH is present in males as well as females; hence, a vaccine against GnRH is usable in both sexes. Furthermore, as its primary structure is largely conserved in mammals, rodents can be employed as a homologous model for testing efficacy and safety.

GnRH by itself is not immunogenic and has to be conjugated to a carrier to mobilize Th cells. Vaccines incorporating GnRH have been developed primarily for use as immunocontraception and immunocastration agents in animals, whereas, in humans, their use is primarily for the treatment of prostate cancer in man and various sex hormone-dependent disorders. For use in human contraception, however, androgen supplementation is required to maintain libido and secondary sex characteristics. Previous studies have already shown that passive or active immunization in order to neutralize GnRH leads to a block of fertility in animals.

Active immunization with a GnRH-based vaccine on white-tailed deer was tested. Treatment led to reduced fawning rates, altered estrus behavior, reduced concentrations of progesterone, and failure to maintain pregnancy following conception. Infertility lasted up to 2 years and was reversible, directly related to the antibody titer. Another application of a GnRH-based vaccine is to perform immunocastration providing an alternative to surgical castration.

A GnRH analog conjugated to Mycobacterium tuberculosis hsp70 has been tested in mice together with two different adjuvants. With either adjuvant, all mice made sufficient antibodies to cause atrophy of the urogenital complex and showed significantly reduced serum levels of testosterone.

Efficiency of a GnRH vaccine in immunocastration of pigs was after worth confirmed.

Enough data have accumulated to conclude that immunosterilizing GnRH-based vaccines can be effectively employed in various animal species without side effects. However, generating antibodies against GnRH may have wide-ranging consequences leading to a block in the secretion of pituitary gonadotropins and may therefore not be acceptable for fertility inhibition in humans. For example, the inhibition of testosterone secretion complicates the potential use of GnRH vaccines in men where androgen supplementation would be required in order to maintain secondary sexual characteristics and libido. The main research field concerning application of anti-GnRH vaccines in humans is not contraception, but the treatment of prostate cancer and other estrogen-dependent conditions.

It should be noted that recombinant vaccines would be substantially cheaper to make on an industrial scale than synthetic vaccines. A multimer recombinant anti-GnRH vaccine had the ability to cause a decline of testosterone to castration level and atrophy of the prostate of rats. Some GnRH vaccines for veterinary use have already been commercialized (VaxstrateTM, ImprovacTM).

5.3.2 Anti-FSH Vaccine

A promising vaccine for males aims to prevent spermatogenesis by immunization against FSH. Successful studies in male bonnet monkeys in which infertility was induced by immunization with ovine FSH are described. Therefore, a phase I clinical trial was carried out using either the ovine FSH αβ-heterodimer or isolated ovine β-chain, purified from sheep pituitary, as the immunogen. FSH-specific antibodies were elicited in all immunized individuals, but, unfortunately, there was no overall reduction in the sperm count in the volunteers due to the antibodies being of fairly low titer. Further trials are intended using recombinant proteins and different doses of the vaccine. One has to remark that it has still not been confirmed that spermatogenesis in humans is dependent on FSH.

5.3.3 Antisperm Vaccines

As discussed in the last chapter, several clinical studies in women have demonstrated that antibodies against sperm are frequently associated with unexplained infertility. Men and women who have infertility attributed to ASA are involuntarily vaccinated models to show how a sperm vaccine will work in humans. Sperm have both auto- and isoantigens, so they can be used for both sexes for contraception. Sperm antigen vaccines are designed to cause agglutination of spermatozoa in the female reproductive tract, and an inability to pass through the cervical mucus. These vaccines may also be applied to males, but it remains a challenging prospect to produce effective neutralizing antibodies in the relevant areas of the male reproductive tract. The intact spermatozoon cannot be used for vaccine development, due to the presence of several antigens on sperm cells that are shared with other somatic cells. Therefore, a sperm antigen suitable for vaccine development must be sperm specific and immunogenic, it must participate in the fertilization process, and its surface expression should be accessible to antibody binding.

Many studies have been performed so far on candidate antigens from male and female gametes in order to demonstrate their ability to induce auto- and/or isoimmune response interfering with fertility. Some of them have been further characterized and complementary DNA (cDNA) encoding these antigens have been cloned and sequenced. Notable among them are the fertilization antigen (FA)-1, sperm protein (SP)-17, testis-specific antigen-1, protein A-kinase anchoring protein, and sperm-associated antigen 9. Active immunization of female animals with some of these antigens, for example, FA-1 and SP-17, has been shown to reduce fertility in vivo.

To date, no single antigen has been shown to cause a 100 % fertility reduction in the mouse model, the maximum reported effect being up to 75 % reduction in fertility of a single antigen; this may be due to the inherent nature of the model and the involvement of multiple antigens in the fertilization cascade. Another reason may be that vaccination with a single antigen has not raised the antibody titer sufficiently to completely block fertility in the local genital tract. However, it is interesting to note that several studies have observed a complete block of fertility in a few mice after immunization with a single antigen. It is possible that these animals develop a high cell-mediated immune response besides an antibody response that also has a deleterious effect on sperm or oocyte function. Immunization with several antigens does cause induction of a cell-mediated immune response and production of cytokines, such as TNF-α and IFN-γ, which have deleterious effects on sperm and embryos. Thus, to enhance the efficacy of a vaccine, it may be important to induce both cell-mediated and humoral immune responses. DNA vaccination may provide a solution, but a DNA vaccination approach has not been examined for a sperm antigen. In other systems, it has already been reported that DNA vaccination favors memory- and cell-mediated responses rather than an effector B-cell response.

In humans, at least four sperm proteins are involved in oocyte ZP binding so that multiple antigens may be involved in the fertilization cascade. Again, vaccination with a single antigen may not raise a high enough antibody titer, especially in the local genital tract, to completely block fertility. At this time, there is no published report examining the contraceptive effect of more than one sperm antigen in a single vaccine formulation in any animal model.

Only a few studies have examined the effect of vaccination based on a sperm antigen on fertility in a nonhuman primate model. Vaccination with testis-specific lactate dehydrogenase (LDH-C4) reduced fertility in female baboons in a study by O'Hearn et al., whereas another study reported no effect on fertility in female monkeys after vaccination with LDH-C4. Recently, male monkeys (*Macaca radiata*) were immunized with an epididymal protein, designated as epididymal protein inhibitor (Eppin). After immunization, 78 % of monkeys developed high antibody titers to Eppin and became infertile, which indicates that antisperm vaccine can theoretically also be used for men.

To conduct phase I and II multicenter clinical trials in a quality-controlled manner, the antigens have to be either recombinant or synthetic molecules. Several synthetic sperm peptides have been investigated for contraception, having caused various degrees of contraceptive effects in animal models. A vaccine prepared by conjugating the synthetic YLP12 peptide with recombinant cholera toxin B subunit (rCTB) was tested in intranasal and intramuscular vaccination of female mice. All vaccinated animals showed a sperm-specific immune response inducing some degree of inhibition of fertility, while the animals with high antibody titers in sera as well as vaginal washings showed a complete block to fertility. Perhaps, monospecific antibodies to sperm antigens may be combined for immunocontraceptive purposes in the form of intravaginal sperm-specific spermicides. A first recombinant miniantibody has been already engineered to the tissue-specific carbohydrate epitope located on the sperm glycoform of the CD52 antigen and shown to agglutinate human sperm cells in a tangled pattern. The S19 mAb was shown to immobilize sperm in the presence of complement, agglutinate sperm, and block sperm interaction with the zona pellucida. The functional findings and the demonstration of male reproductive tract specificity of the S19 epitope on the CD52 glycoprotein serve as further indications that both the S19 mAb and its unique carbohydrate cognate epitope are strong candidates for vaccine development.

5.3.4   Anti-oocyte Zona Pellucida (ZP) Vaccines

Zona pellucida (ZP) as matrix around the oocyte is mainly composed of glycoproteins ZPA, ZPB, and ZPC. It serves as the docking site for species-specific recognition and binding of spermatozoa to the oocyte and protects the growing blastocyst before implantation. Zona glycoproteins have become promising candidate antigens for the development of an immunocontraceptive vaccine.

Antibodies generated against ZP glycoproteins from a given species were shown to react to some extent with the ZP from other species, including humans, and thus permit heterologous immunization. After immunization with porcine ZP, infertility together with follicular atresia and an abnormal hormone profile was observed in female rabbits.

Studies employing different animal models demonstrated that immunization with heat-solubilized porcine ZP led to a block in fertility that was likely to be due to ovarian dystrophy rather than to a block in fertilization. It was suggested that the observed side effects might be due to impurities of other ovarian-associated proteins that may be present in the heat-solubilized ZP preparations. Monkeys immunized with highly purified porcine ZPB and ZPC failed to conceive in the presence of high circulating antibody titers but did not show any adverse effects on ovarian functions. Recombinant proteins may diminish the problems of contaminated ZP glycoproteins isolated from a native source.

Immunization of female baboons with recombinant bonnet monkey ZPB led to a reversible block of fertility. Ovarian histology of the immunized animals revealed the presence of atretic follicles with degenerating oocytes, which may explain failure to conceive.

In addition, the development of live recombinant vectors encoding ZP glycoproteins has been started. Immunization of mice with murine cytomegalovirus as a live recombinant vector expressing mouse ZPC has led to infertility. Another approach is the use of plasmid DNA encoding ZP glycoproteins. Interestingly, immunization of mice with plasmid DNA encoding the partial sequence of rabbit ZPC led to inhibited fertility without any disturbances in folliculogenesis.

A series of experiments demonstrated that the "oophoritogenic" T-cell epitopes present in the zona proteins may be responsible for ovarian dysfunction often observed after immunization with ZP antigens. To circumvent ovarian pathology, synthetic peptides devoid of "oophoritogenic" T-cell epitopes as immunogens have been proposed. However, in vivo studies did not show a consistent reduction in fertility. Another approach may be to employ chimeric recombinant proteins comprising ZP and spermatozoa antigens.

Despite quite promising results, there is a need for long-term active immunization studies before these ZP glycoproteins can be considered for human application.

5.3.5 Anti-hCG Vaccine

The most promising candidate for development of an immunocontraceptive vaccine for females is hCG as it is pregnancy-specific, is synthesized after fertilization, and is judged crucial for the establishment and maintenance of pregnancy at least during the first weeks of gestation. Two fundamentally different strategies have been adopted regarding the development of hCG-based contraceptive vaccines. In one approach, the main consideration was to produce a vaccine that would provide an hCG-specific immune response that did not cross-react with the structurally related LH. The alternative approach considered that such cross-reaction, if it were to occur, would not be harmful, and therefore the prime consideration should be to produce a vaccine capable of eliciting high-titer antibodies.

The efficacy of hCG linked to tetanus toxoid (TT) was tested in various animal studies, with promising results. For this vaccine, the intact β-chain was used and there was no great concern about possible cross-reaction with LH. A multicenter phase I clinical trial on 63 women was conducted which showed the presence of both anti-hCG and anti-TT antibodies. However, antibody titers and the duration of immune response highly varied among immunized women. A more immunogenic vaccine formulation was tested in extensive phase II clinical trials and led to generation of anti-hCG antibody levels high enough to protect against conception in 80 % of immunized women. This vaccine against hCG is the first and only birth control vaccine to go through phase II efficacy trials successfully. It is devoid of side effects, showing no bleeding irregularity, and women keep ovulating normally, produce their own sex hormones, and have regular menstrual cycles. The fact that the luteal phase did not lengthen in vaccinated women provided confirmation that anti-hCG antibodies prevent implantation of the embryo onto the endometrium; interception is therefore before the onset of pregnancy. It should be noted, however, that a birth control vaccine has to be effective in about 90–95 % of recipients in order to be acceptable.

The other vaccine against hCG was developed with support from the WHO Task Force on Vaccines for Fertility Regulation is based on a synthetic peptide of the portion of the β-subunit of the hormone linked to diphtheria toxoid (DT). Potentially contraceptive antibody titers were induced in a phase I clinical study which was followed by a phase II clinical trial that was abandoned due to unacceptable local reactions at the injection site. The immunogenicity of a β-hCG-based DNA vaccine has also been illustrated. The DNA vaccine together with a C3d adjuvant led to a generation of a ninefold higher antibody response compared to β-hCG alone and increased the expression of antigen-specific Th2 humoral immune response in mice.

There is still a need to improve the immunogenicity of the hCG vaccine by incorporating other adjuvants or using other carrier proteins instead of TT. Pilot studies have shown that the conjugation of β-HCG to various peptides not only enhances the quantum of immune responses compared to β-hCG conjugated to TT but also assures antibody responses in mice of different genetic backgrounds. Furthermore, cross-reactivity with LH has to be reduced.

5.3.6   Other Vaccination Strategies

Other potential approaches for the development of immunocontraceptive vaccines include riboflavin carrier protein that is a major transporter of vitamin to the embryo across the placental barrier. Active immunization in animals with this agent significantly reduced fertility.

A pilot project is aimed at the immunological inhibition of syncytial trophoblast fusion as a novel approach to contraception. Fusion-inhibiting recombinant antibodies were generated and used together with autoantibodies from patients with repetitive IVF failure that were shown to inhibit syncytial fusion and are expected to inhibit implantation and to generate anti-idiotypic peptides. These peptides mimic trophoblast epitopes essential for syncytial fusion and are, therefore, considered specific immunogens for the generation of antibodies that will inhibit implantation. Of 300 anti-idiotypic peptides, which were tested for their binding capacity to patient autoantibodies associated with repetitive IVF failure, habitual abortion, and preeclampsia, only three peptides were found to selectively bind to autoantibodies of patients with repetitive IVF failure and were considered safe and efficient enough for evaluation in preclinical and clinical studies required for the development of immune contraceptives.

The application of contraceptive vaccines in humans still needs further investigation and development. The identification and use of novel target candidates that are crucial for gametogenesis, fertilization, and implantation will take more time and effort. Another major challenge will be to increase the immunogenicity of contraceptive vaccines to generate antibody levels in 100 % of the recipients.

Further Reading

Immunology of Pregnancy

Abbas AK, Lichtman AH, Pober JS. Immunologie. Bern/Göttingen/Toronto/Seattle: Verlag Hans Huber; 1996.

Abraham MC, Desjardins M, Filion LG, Garber GE. Inducible immunity to Trichomonas vaginalis in a mouse model of vaginal infection. Infect Immun. 1996;64:3571–5.

Abrahams VM, Mor G. Toll-like receptors and their role in the trophoblast. Placenta. 2005;26:540–7.

Abrahams VM, Bole-Aldo P, Kim YM, Straszewski-Chavez SL, Chaiworapongsa T, Romero R, Mor G. Divergent trophoblast responses to bacterial products mediated by TLRs. J Immunol. 2004;173:4286–96.

Acosta AA, van der Merwe JP, Doncel G, Kruger TF, Sayilgan A, Franken DR, Kolm P. Fertilization efficiency of morphologically abnormal spermatozoa in assisted reproduction is further impaired by antisperm antibodies on the male partner's sperm. Fertil Steril. 1994;62:826–33.

Adachi H, Takakuwa K, Mitsui T, Ishii K, Tamura M, Tanaka K. Results of immunotherapy for patients with unexplained secondary abortions. Clin Immunol. 2003;106:175–80.

Agrawal S, Pandey MK, Mandal S, Mishra L, Agarwal S. Humoral immune response to an allogenic foetus in normal fertile women and recurrent aborters. BMC Pregnancy Childbirth. 2002;2:6.

Alderete JF, Newton E, Dennis C, Neale KA. Antibody in sera of patients infected with Trichomonas vaginalis is to trichomonal proteinases. Genitourin Med. 1991; 67:331–4.

Alderete JF, Newton E, Dennis C, Neale KA. The vagina of women infected with Trichomonas vaginalis has numerous proteinases and antibody to trichomonad proteinases. Genitourin Med. 1991b;67:469–74.

Aldrich CL, Stephenson MD, Karrison T, Odem RR, Branch DW, Scott JR, Schreiber JR, Ober C. HLA-G genotypes and pregnancy outcome in couples with unexplained recurrent miscarriage. Mol Hum Reprod. 2001;7:1167–72.

Allavena P, Giardina G, Bianchi G, Mantovani A. Il-15 is chemotactic for natural killer cells and stimulates their adhesion to vascular endothelium. J Leukoc Biol. 1997;61:729–35.

Allez M, Brimnes J, Dotan I, Mayer L. Expansion of CD8+ T cells with regulatory function after interaction with intestinal ECs. Gastroenterology. 2002;123:1516–26.

Alloub MI, Barr BB, McLaren KM, Smith IW, Bunney MH, Smart GE. Human papillomavirus infection and cervical intraepithelial neoplasia in women with renal allografts. BMJ. 1989;298:153–6.

Aluvihare VR, Kallikourdis M, Betz AG. Regulatory T cells mediate maternal tolerance to the fetus. Nat Immunol. 2004;5:266–71.

Andrews WW, Goldenberg RL, Mercer B, Iams J, Meis P, Moawad A, Das A, Vandorsten JP, Caritis SN, Thurnau G, Miodovnik M, Roberts J, McNellis D. The Preterm Prediction Study: association of second-trime stergenitourinary chlamydia infection with subsequent spontaneous preterm birth. Am J Obstet Gynecol. 2000;183:662–8.

Anton G, Rid J, Mylonas I, Weissenbacher ER. Proinflammatory and antiinflammatory cytokines in the vagina of healthy women and during bacterial vaginosis. 10th annual meeting of the international infectious disease society for obstetrics and gynecology, San Francisco, California; 2005.

Aoki K, Kajiura S, Matsumoto Y, Ogasawara M, Okada S, Yagami Y, Gleicher N. Preconceptional natural-killer-cell activity as a predictor of miscarriage. Lancet. 1995;345:1340–2.

Arck PC. Stress and pregnancy loss: role of immune mediators, hormones and neurotransmitters. Am J Reprod Immunol. 2001;46:117–23.

Arck PC, Meroli FS, Manuel J, Chaouat G, Clark DA. Stress-triggered abortion: inhibition of protective suppression and promotion of tumor necrosis factor-α (TNF-α) release as a mechanism triggering resorptions in mice. Am J Reprod Immunol. 1995;33:74–80.

Arck PC, Ferrick DA, Steele-Norwood D, Egan PJ, Croitoru K, Carding S, Dietl J, Clark DA. Murine T cell determination of pregnancy outcome. II. Distinct Th1 and Th2/3 populations of Vγ1+δ6+ T cells influence success or failure of pregnancy in CBA3DBA/2 matings. Cell Immunol. 1999;196:71–9.

Arck PC, Rose M, Hertwig K, Hagen E, Hildebrandt M, Klapp BF. Stress and immune mediators in miscarriage. Hum Reprod. 2001;16:1505–11.

Arechavaleta-Velasco F, Ogando D, Parry S, Vadillo OF. Production of matrix metalloproteinase-9 in lipopolysaccharide-stimulated human amnion occurs through an autocrine and paracrine proinflammatory cytokine-dependent system. Biol Reprod. 2002;67: 1952–8.

Arici A, MacDonald PC, Casey ML. Modulation of the levels of interleukin-8 messenger ribonucleic acid and interleukin-8 protein synthesis in human endometrial stromal cells by transforming growth factor-beta 1. J Clin Endocrinol Metab. 1996;81:3004–9.

Ashkar AA, Di Santo JP, Croy BA. Interferon gamma contributes to initiation of uterine vascular modification, decidual integrity, and uterine natural killer cell maturation during normal murine pregnancy. J Exp Med. 2000;192:259–70.

Ashkar AA, Black GP, Wei Q, He H, Liang L, Head JR, Croy BA. Assessment of requirements for IL-15 and IFN regulatory factors in uterine NK cell differentiation and function during pregnancy. J Immunol. 2003;171:2937–44.

Askelund K, Liddell HS, Zanderigo AM, Fernando NS, Khong TY, Stone PR, Chamley LW. CD83(+)dendritic cells in the decidua of women with recurrent miscarriage and normal pregnancy. Placenta. 2004; 25:140–5.

Baggia S, Gravett MG, Witkin SS, Haluska GJ, Novy MJ. Interleukin- 1β intra-amniotic infusion induces tumor necrosis factor-α, prostaglandin production, and preterm contractions in pregnant rhesus monkeys. J Soc Gynecol Investig. 1996;3:121–6.

Ban YL, Kong BH, Qu X, Yang QF, Ma YY. BDCA-1+, BDCA-2+ and BDCA-3+ dendritic cells in early human pregnancy decidua. Clin Exp Immunol. 2008;151:399–406.

Barnea ER. Insight into early pregnancy events: the emerging role of the embryo. Am J Reprod Immunol. 2004;51:319–22.

Barrier BF. Immunology of endometriosis. Clin Obstet Gynecol. 2010;53:397–402.

Bartha JL, Comino-Delgado R. Lymphocyte subpopulations in intrauterine growth retardation in women with or without previous pregnancies. Eur J Obstet Gynecol Reprod Biol. 1999;82:23–7.

Bartha JL, Romero-Carmona R, Comino-Delgado R. Inflammatory cytokines in intrauterine growth retardation. Acta Obstet Gynecol Scand. 2003;82: 1099–102.

Bates MD, Quenby S, Takakuwa K, Johnson PM, Vince GS. Aberrant cytokine production by peripheral blood mononuclear cells in recurrent pregnancy loss? Hum Reprod. 2002;17:2439–44.

Bauer S, Pollheimer J, Hartmann J, Husslein P, Aplin JD, Knofler M. Tumor necrosis factor- alpha inhibits trophoblast migration through elevation of plasminogen activator inhibitor-1 in first-trimester villous explant cultures. J Clin Endocrinol Metab. 2004;89:812–22.

Beer AE. Immunopathologic factors contributing to recurrent spontaneous abortions in humans. Am J Reprod Immunol. 1983;4:182–4.

Belardelli F. Role of interferons and other cytokines in the regulation of the immune response. APMIS. 1995; 103:161–79.

Bell SC, Billington WD. Antifetal alloantibody in the pregnant female. Immunol Rev. 1983;75:5–30.

Ben-Hur H, Gurevich P, Berman V, Tchanyshev R, Gurevich E, Zusman I. The secretory immune system as part of the placental barrier in the second trimester of pregnancy in humans. In Vivo. 2001;15:429–35.

Betterle C, Rossi A, Dalla Pria S, Artifoni A, Pedini B, Gavasso S, Caretto A. Premature ovarian failure: auto-immunity and natural history. Clin Endocrinol. 1993;39:35–43.

Blois SM, Alba Soto CD, Tometten M, Klapp BF, Margni RA, Arck PC. Lineage, maturity, and phenotype of uterine murine dendritic cells throughout gestation indicate a protective role in maintaining pregnancy. Biol Reprod. 2004;70:1018–23.

Bluman EM, Bartynski KJ, Avalos BR, Caligiuri MA. Human natural killer cells produce abundant macrophage inflammatory protein-1 alpha in response to monocyte-derived cytokines. J Clin Invest. 1996;97:2722–7.

Blumenstein M, Bowen-Shauver JM, Keelan JA, Mitchell MD. Identification of suppressors of cytokine signaling (SOCS) proteins in human gestational tissue: differential regulation is associated with the onset of labor. J Clin Endocrinol Metab. 2002;87:1094–7.

Bogovic Crnic T, Strbo N, Laskarin G, Cupurdija K, Dorcic D, Juretic K, Dupor J, Sotosek Tokmadzic V, Vlastelic I, Randic LJ, Rukavina RD. Decidual NK cells use Fas/FasL cytolytic pathway. European congress of reproductive immunology, Pilsen, Czech Republic. Am J Reprod Immunol. 2004;51:490.

Boyson JE, Rybalov B, Koopman LA, Exley M, Balk SP, Racke FK, Schatz F, Masch R, Wilson SB, Strominger JL. CD1d and invariant NKT cells at the human maternal-fetal interface. Proc Natl Acad Sci U S A. 2002;99:13741–6.

Briana DD, Liosi S, Gourgiotis D, Boutsikou M, Baka S, Marmarinos A, Hassiakos D, Malamitsi-Puchner A. The potential role of the lectin pathway of complement in the host defence of full-term intrauterine growth restricted neonates at birth. J Matern Fetal Neonatal Med. 2012;25:531–4.

Brown NL, Alvi SA, Elder MG, Bennett PR, Sullivan MH. The regulation of prostaglandin output from term intact fetal membranes by anti-inflammatory cytokines. Immunology. 2000;99:124–33.

Bulla R, Bossi F, Radillo O, De Seta F, Tedesco F. Placental trophoblast and endothelial cells as targets of maternal immune response. Autoimmunity. 2003;36:11–8.

Bulla R, Bossi F, Fischetti F, De Seta F, Tedesco F. The complement system at the fetomaternal interface. Chem Immunol Allergy. 2005;89:149–57.

Bulmer JN, Lash GE. Human uterine natural killer cells: a reappraisal. Mol Immunol. 2005;42:511–21.

Bulmer JN, Sunderland CA. Immunohistological characterization of lymphoid cell populations in the early human placental bed. Immunology. 1984;52:349–57.

Bulmer JN, Morrison L, Smith JC. Expression of class II MHC gene products by macrophages in human utero-placental tissue. Immunology. 1988;63:707–14.

Bulmer JN, Morrison L, Longfellow M, Ritson A, Pace D. Granulated lymphocytes in human endometrium: histochemical and immunohistochemical studies. Hum Reprod. 1991;6:791–8.

Buonocore G, De Filippo M, Gioia D, Picciolini E, Luzzi E, Bocci V, Bracci R. Maternal and neonatal plasma cytokine levels in relation to mode of delivery. Biol Neonate. 1995;68:104–10.

Burch CL, Danaher RJ, Stein DC. Antigenic variation in Neisseria gonorrhoeae: production of multiple lipooligosaccharides. J Bacteriol. 1997;179:982–6.

Burns D, Nourjah P, Wright D, Minkoff H, Landesman S, Rubinstein A, Goedert J, Nugent R. Changes in immune markers during pregnancy and postpartum. J Reprod Immunol. 1999;42:147–65.

Bussen SS, Steck T. Thyroid antibodies and their relation to antithrombin antibodies, anticardiolipin antibodies and lupus anticoagulant in women with recurrent spontaneous abortions (antithyroid, anticardiolipin and antithrombin autoantibodies and lupus anticoagulant in habitual aborters). Eur J Obstet Gynecol Reprod Biol. 1997;74:139–43.

Canadella A, Farber A, Zenclussen AC, Gentile T, Dokmetjian J, Keil A, Blois S, Miranda S, Berod L, Gutierrez G, Markert UR, Margni RA. Interleukin regulation of asymmetric antibody synthesized by isolated placental B cells. Am J Reprod Immunol. 2002a;48:275–82.

Canadella A, Gentile T, Dokmetjian J, Margni RA. Occurrence, properties and function of asymmetric IgG molecules isolated from non-immune human sera. Immunol Invest. 2002b;31:107–20.

Caniggia I, Grisaru-Gravnosky S, Kuliszewsky M, Post M, Lye SJ. Inhibition of TGFβ3 restores the invasive capability of extravillous trophoblast in preeclamptic pregnancies. J Clin Invest. 1999;103:1641–50.

Caramalho I, Lopes-Carvalho T, Ostler D, Zejenay S, Haury M, Demengeot J. Regulatory T cells selectively express Toll-like receptors and are activated by lipopolysaccharide. J Exp Med. 2003;197:403–11.

Carayannopoulos LN, Barks JL, Yokoyama WM, Riley JK. Murine trophoblast cells induce NK cell interferon-gamma production through KLRK1. Biol Reprod. 2010;83:404–14.

Carey JC, Blackwelder WC, Nugent RP, Matteson MA, Rao AV, Eschenbach DA, Lee ML, Retig PJ, Regan JA, Geromanos KL. Antepartum cultures for Ureaplasma urealyticum are not useful in predicting pregnancy outcome. Am J Obstet Gynecol. 1991; 164:728–33.

Carson WE, Giri JG, Lindemann MJ, Linett ML, Ahdieh M, Paxton R, Anderson D, Eisenmann J, Grabstein K, Caligiuri MA. Interleukin (IL) 15 is a novel cytokine that activates human natural killer cells via components of the IL-2 receptor. J Exp Med. 1994; 180:1395–403.

Casey ML, Cox SM, Beutler B, Milewich L, MacDonald PC. Cachectin/tumor necrosis factor- alpha formation in human decidua. Potential role of cytokines in infection-induced preterm labor. J Clin Invest. 1989;83:430–6.

Casey ML, Cox SM, Word RA, MacDonald PC. Cytokines and infection-induced preterm labor. Reprod Fertil Dev. 1990;2:499–509.

Castilla JA, Molina R, Lopez-Nevot MA, Vergara F, Garrido F, Herruzo AJ. Immunosuppressive properties of human follicular fluid. Fertil Steril. 1990;53:271–5.

Caucheteux SM, Kanellopoulos-Langevin C, Ojcius DM. At the innate frontiers between mother and fetus: linking abortion with complement activation. Immunity. 2003;18:169–72.

Chaouat G, Menu E, Wegmann TG. Role of lymphokines of the CSF family and of TNF, gamma interferon and IL-2 in placental growth and fetal survival studied in two murine models of spontaneous resorptions. In: Chaouat G, Mowbray JF, editors. Cellular and molecular biology of the maternal-fetal relationship. Paris: INSERM/John Libbey Eurotext; 1991. p. 91–104.

Chaouat G, Zourbas S, Ostojic S, Lappree-Delage G, Dubanchet S, Ledee N, Martal J. A brief review of recent data on some cytokine expressions at the materno-foetal interface which might challenge the classical Th1/Th2 dichotomy. J Reprod Immunol. 2002;53:241–56.

Chaouat G, Ledee-Bataille N, Dubanchet S, Zourbas S, Sandra O, Martal J. Reproductive immunology 2003: reassessing the Th1/Th2 paradigm? Immunol Lett. 2004;92:207–14.

Chaouat G, Ledee-Bataille N, Dubanchet S. Immunological similarities between implantation and pre-eclampsia. Am J Reprod Immunol. 2005;53:222–9.

Chegini N, Ma C, Roberts M, Williams RS, Ripps BA. Differential expression of interleukin (IL) IL-13 and IL-15 throughout the menstrual cycle in endometrium of normal fertile women and women with recurrent spontaneous abortion. J Reprod Immunol. 2002;56:93–110.

Cheng SJ, Zheng ZQ. Early pregnancy factor in cervical mucus of pregnant women. Am J Reprod Immunol. 2004;51:102–5.

Cheng JG, Rodriguez CI, Stewart CL. Control of uterine receptivity and embryo implantation by steroid hormone regulation of LIF production and LIF receptor activity: towards a molecular understanding of the 'window of implantation'. Rev Endocr Metab Disord. 2002;3:119–26.

Chia KV, Johnson PM. T-lymphocyte subsets in unexplained recurrent spontaneous abortion. Fertil Steril. 1987;48:685–7.

Clark DA, Croitoru K. Th1/Th2,3 imbalance due to cytokine-producing NK, gammadelta T and NK-gammadelta T cells in murine pregnancy decidua in success or failure of pregnancy. Am J Reprod Immunol. 2001;45:257–65.

Clark DA, Arck PC, Chaouat G. Why did your mother reject you? Immunogenetic determinants of the response to environmental selective pressure expressed at uterine level. Am J Reprod Immunol. 1999a;41:5–22.

Clark DA, Ding JW, Chaouat G, Coulam CB, August C, Levy GA. The emerging role of immunoregulation of fibrinogen-related procoagulant Fg12 in the success or spontaneous abortion of early pregnancy in mice and humans. Am J Reprod Immunol. 1999b;42:37–43.

Clark DA, Coulam CB, Daya S, Chaouat G. Unexplained sporadic and recurrent miscarriage in the new millennium: a critical analysis of immune mechanisms and treatments. Hum Reprod Update. 2001a;7:501–11.

Clark DA, Ding JW, Yu G, Phillips J, Levy GA, Gorczynski RM. Fgl2 prothrombinase expression in mouse trophoblast and decidua triggers abortion but may be countered by OX- 2. Mol Hum Reprod. 2001b;7:185–94.

Clark DA, Chaouat G, Gorczynski RM. Thinking outside the box: mechanisms of environmental selective pressures on the outcome of the materno-fetal relationship. Am J Reprod Immunol. 2002;47:275–82.

Colucci F, Boulenouar S, Kieckbusch J, Moffett A. How does variability of immune system genes affect placentation? Placenta. 2011;32:539–45.

Comeglio P, Fedi S, Liotta AA, Cellai AP, Chiarantini E, Prisco D, Mecacci F, Parretti E, Mello G, Abbate R. Blood clotting activation during normal pregnancy. Thromb Res. 1996;84:199–202.

Corwin E, Bozoky I, Pugh L, Johnston N. Interleukin-1beta elevation during the postpartum period. Ann Behav Med. 2003;25:41–7. 257.

Cotch MF, Pastorek JG, Nugent RP, Hillier SL, Gibbs RS, Martin DH, Eschenbach DA, Edelmann R, Carey JC, Regan JA, Krohn MA, Klebanoff MA, Rao AV, Rhoads GG. Trichomonas vaginalis associated with low birth weight and preterm delivery. The Vaginal Infections and Prematurity Study Group. Sex Transm Dis. 1997;24:341–61. 260.

Cotch MF, Hillier SL, Gibbs RS, Eschenbach DA. Epidemiology and outcomes associated with moderate to heavy Candida colonization during pregnancy. Vaginal Infections and Prematurity Study Group. Am J Obstet Gynecol. 1998;178:374–80. 259.

Coulam CB, Goodman C, Roussev RG, Thomason EJ, Beaman KD. Systemic CD56+ cells can predict pregnancy outcome. Am J Reprod Immunol. 1995;33:40–6. 263.

Crocker IP, Baker PN, Fletcher J. Neutrophil function in pregnancy and rheumatoid arthritis. Ann Rheum Dis. 2000;59:555–64.

Croy BA, Esadeg S, Chantakru S, van den Heuvel M, Paffaro VA, He H, Black GP, Ashkar AA, Kiso Y, Zhang J. Update on pathways regulating the activation of uterine natural killer cells, their interactions with decidual spiral arteries and homing of their precursors to the uterus. J Reprod Immunol. 2003a;59:175–91.

Croy BA, He H, Esadeg S, Wei Q, McCartney D, Zhang J, Borzychowski A, Ashkar AA, Black GP, Evans SS, Chantakru S, van den Heuvel M, Paffaro Jr VA, Yamada AT. Uterine natural killer cells: insights into their cellular and molecular biology from mouse modelling. Reproduction. 2003b;126:149–60.

Cunningham DS, Tichenor JR. Decay-accelerating factor protects human trophoblast from complement-mediated attack. Clin Immunol Immunopathol. 1995;74:156–61.

Daher S, De Arruda Geraldes Denardi K, Blotta MH, Mamoni RL, Reck AP, Camano L, Mattar R. Cytokines in recurrent pregnancy loss. J Reprod Immunol. 2004;62:151–7.

Daniel Y, Kupfermine MJ, Baram A, Jaffa AJ, Fait G, Wolman I, Lessing JB. Plasma interleukin-12 is elevated in patients with preeclampsia. Am J Reprod Immunol. 1998;39:376–80.

Daya S, Clark DA. Immunosuppressive factor (or factors) produced by human embryos in vitro. N Engl J Med. 1986;24:1551–2.

De Jong EC, Vieira PL, Kalinski P, Schuitemaker JH, Tanaka Y, Wierenga EA, Yazdanbakhsh M, Kapsenberg ML. Microbial compounds selectively induce Th1 cell-promoting or Th2 cell- promoting dendritic cells in vitro with diverse Th cell-polarizing signals. J Immunol. 2002;168:1704–9.

Dechend R, Müller DN, Wallukat G, Homuth V, Krause M, Dudenhausen J, Luft FC. Activating auto-antibodies against the AT1 receptor in preeclampsia. Autoimmun Rev. 2005;4:61–5.

Dekker GA, Sibai BM. The immunology of preeclampsia. Semin Perinatol. 1999;23:24–33.

Dezzutti C, Guenthner P, Cummins Jr J, Cabrera T, Marshall J, Dillberger A, Lal R. Cervical and prostate primary ECs are not productively infected but sequester human immunodeficiency virus type 1. J Infect Dis. 2001;183:1204–13.

Drake BL, Head JR. Murine trophoblast cells can be killed by lymphokine-activated killer cells. J Immunol. 1989;143:9–14.

Druckmann R, Druckmann MA. Progesterone and the immunology of pregnancy. J Steroid Biochem Mol Biol. 2005;97:389–96.

Dudley DJ, Edwin SS, Van Wagoner J, Augustine NH, Hill HR, Mitchell MD. Regulation of decidual cell chemokine production by group B streptococci and purified bacterial cell wall components. Am J Obstet Gynecol. 1997;177:666–72.

Eastabrook GD, Hu Y, Tan R, Dutz JP, Maccalman CD, von Dadelszen P. Decidual NK cell-derived conditioned medium (dNK-CM) mediates VEGF-C secretion in extravillous cytotrophoblasts. Am J Reprod Immunol. 2012;67:101–11.

Eblen AC, Gercel-Taylor C, Shields LBE, Sanfilippo JS, Nakajima ST, Taylor DD. Alterations in humoral immune responses associated with recurrent pregnancy loss. Fertil Steril. 2000;73:305–13.

Ekerfelt C, Matthiesen L, Berg G, Ernerudh J. Paternal leukocytes selectively increase secretion of IL-4 in peripheral blood during normal pregnancies: demonstrated by a novel one- way MLC measuring cytokine secretion. Am J Reprod Immunol. 1997;38:320–6.

Eley A, Pacey AA, Galdiero M, Galdiero M, Galdiero F. Can Chlamydia trachomatis directly damage your sperm? Lancet Infect Dis. 2005;5:53–7.

Elliot B, Brunham RC, Laga M, Piot P, Ndinya-Achola JO, Maitha G, Cheang M, Plummer FA. Maternal gonococcal infection as a preventable risk factor for low birth weight. J Infect Dis. 1990;161:531–6.

El-Shazly S, Mahseed M, Azizieh F, Al-Harmi JA, Al-Aemi MM. Increased expression of pro- inflammatory cytokines in placentas of women undergoing spontaneous preterm delivery or premature rupture of membranes. Am J Reprod Immunol. 2004;52:45–52.

Emmer PM, Steegers EAP, Kerstens HMJ, Bulten J, Nelen WL, Boer K, Joosten I. Altered phenotype of HLA-G expressing trophoblast and decidual natural killer cells in pathological pregnancies. Hum Reprod. 2002;17:1072–80.

Eneroth E, Remberger M, Vahlne A, Ringden O. Increased serum concentrations of interleukin-2 receptor in the first trimester in women who later developed severe preeclampsia. Acta Obstet Gynecol Scand. 1998;77:591–3.

Eriksson M, Meadows SK, Wira CR, Sentman CL. Unique phenotype of human uterine NK cells and their regulation by endogenous TGF-β. J Leukoc Biol. 2004;76:667–75.

Fan DX, Duan J, Li MQ, Xu B, Li DJ, Jin LP. The decidual gamma-delta T cells up-regulate the biological functions of trophoblasts via IL-10 secretion in early human pregnancy. Clin Immunol. 2011;141:284–92.

Faulk WP, Jarret R, Keane M, Johnson PM, Boackle RJ. Immunological studies of human placentae: complement components in immature and mature chorionic villi. Clin Exp Immunol. 1980;40:299–305.

Faust Z, Laskarin G, Rukavina D, Szekeres-Bartho J. Progesterone-induced blocking factor inhibits degranulation of natural killer cells. Am J Reprod Immunol. 1999;42:71–5.

Feinberg BB. Preeclampsia: the death of Goliath. Am J Reprod Immunol. 2006;55:84–98.

Fernekorn U, Kruse A. Regulation of leukocyte recruitment to the murine maternal/fetal interface. Chem Immunol Allergy. 2005;89:105–17.

Fiddes TM, O'Reilly DB, Cetrulo CL, Miller W, Rudders R, Osband M, Rocklin RE. Phenotypic and functional evaluation of suppressor cells in normal pregnancy and in chronic aborters. Cell Immunol. 1986;97:407–18.

Fidel Jr PL. Immunity in vaginal candidiasis. Curr Opin Infect Dis. 2005;18:107–11.

Franco EL, Harper DM. Vaccination against human papillomavirus infection: a new paradigm in cervical cancer control. Vaccine. 2005;23:2388–94.

Fukushima K, Miyamoto S, Komatsu H, Tsukimori K, Kobayashi H, Seki H, Takeda S, Nakano H. TNFalpha-induced apoptosis and integrin switching in human extravillous trophoblast cell line. Biol Reprod. 2003;68:1771–8.

Gardner L, Moffett A. Dendritic cells in the human decidua. Biol Reprod. 2003;69:1438–46.

Gerber S, Vial Y, Hohlfeld P, Witkin SS. Detection of Ureaplasma urealyticum in second- trimester amniotic fluid by polymerase chain reaction correlates with subsequent preterm labor and delivery. J Infect Dis. 2003;187:518–21.

Gibbs RS, Romero R, Hillier SL, Eschenbach DA, Sweet RL. A review of premature birth and subclinical infection. Am J Obstet Gynecol. 1992;166:1515–28.

Girardi G, Salmon JB. The role of complement in pregnancy and fetal loss. Autoimmunity. 2003;36:19–26.

Girardi G, Berman J, Redecha P, Spruce L, Thurman JM, Kraus D, Hollmann TJ, Casali P, Caroll MC, Wetsel RA, Lambris JD, Holers VM, Salmon JE. Complement C5a receptors and neutrophils mediate fetal injury in the antiphospholipid syndrome. J Clin Invest. 2003;112:1644–54.

Girardi G, Bulla R, Salmon JE, Tedesco F. The complement system in the pathophysiology of pregnancy. Mol Immunol. 2006;43:68–77.

Gorczinsky RM, Hadidi S, Yu G, Clark DA. The same immunoregulatory molecules contribute to successful pregnancy and transplantation. Am J Reprod Immunol. 2002;48:18–26.

Gordon S. Alternative activation of macrophages. Nat Rev Immunol. 2003;3:23–35.

Gorivodsky M, Torchinsky A, Shepshelovich J, Savion S, Fenn A, Carp H, Toder V. CSF-1 expression in the uteroplacental unit of mice with spontaneous and induced pregnancy loss. Clin Exp Immunol. 1999;117:540–9.

Gravett MG, Witkin SS, Novy MJ. A nonhuman primate model for chorioamnionitis and preterm labor. Semin Reprod Endocrinol. 1994;12:246–62.

Groer MW, Davis MW, Smith K, Casey K, Kramer V, Bukovsky E. Immunity, inflammation and infection in post-partum breast and formula feeders. Am J Reprod Immunol. 2005;54:222–31.

Gruber CJ, Huber JC. The role of dehydrogesterone in recurrent (habitual) abortion. J Steroid Biochem Mol Biol. 2005;97:426–30.

Gu Y, Lewis DF, Deere K, Groome LJ, Wang Y. Elevated maternal IL-16 levels, enhanced IL-16 expressions in endothelium and leukocytes, and increased IL-16 production by placental trophoblasts in women with preeclampsia. J Immunol. 2008;181:4418–22.

Gulati S, Bhatnagar S, Raghunandan C, Bhattacharjee J. Interleukin-6 as a predictor of subclinical chorioamnionitis in preterm premature rupture of membranes. Am J Reprod Immunol. 2012;67:235–40.

Guleria I, Pollard JW. The trophoblast is a component of the innate immune system during pregnancy. Nat Med. 2000;6:589–93.

Gutierrez G, Gentile T, Miranda S, Margni RA. Asymmetric antibodies: a protective arm in pregnancy. Chem Immunol Allergy. 2005;89:158–68.

Hammer A, Dohr G. Expression of Fas-ligand in first trimester and term human placental villi. J Reprod Immunol. 2000;46:83–90.

Haq A, Mothi BA, Al-Hussein K, Al-Tufail M, Hollanders J, Jaroudi K, Al-Waili N, Shabani M. Isolation, purification and partial characterization of early pregnancy factor (EPF) from sera of pregnant women. Eur J Med Res. 2001;29:209–14.

Hasegawa I, Tani H, Takakuwa K, Goto S, Yamada K, Kanazawa K. A new lymphocyte serotyping using cytotoxic antibodies from secondary recurrent aborters and its application in cases of recurrent abortion and infertility. Fertil Steril. 1991;55:906–10.

Haviid TV, Hylenius S, Hoegh AM, Kruse C, Christiansen OB. HLA-G polymorphisms in couples with recurrent spontaneous abortions. Tissue Antigens. 2002;60: 122–32.

Heinig J, Wilhelm S, Müller H, Briese V, Bittorf T, Brock J. Determination of cytokine mRNA- expression in term human placenta of patients with gestational hypertension, intrauterine growth retardation and gestational diabetes mellitus using polymerase chain reaction. Zentralb Gynäkol. 2000;122:413–8.

Henessy A, Pilmore HL, Simmons LA, Painter DM. A deficiency of placental IL-10 in preeclampsia. J Immunol. 1999;163:3491–5.

Herz U, Renz H. Fetomaternale Immunität. Neue Konzepte zur Plastizität des Immunsystems während der Schwangerschaft. Gynakologe. 2001;34:494–502.

Heyborne K, Yang-Xin F, Nelson A, Farr A, O'Brien R, Born W. Recognition of trophoblast by γ/δ T cells. J Immunol. 1994;153:2918–26.

Hill JA, Choi BC. Maternal immunological aspects of pregnancy success and failure. J Reprod Fertil Steril Suppl. 2000;55:91–7.

Hill JA, Polgar K, Anderson DJ. T-helper 1-type immunity to trophoblast in women with recurrent spontaneous abortion. JAMA. 1995;273:1933–6.

Hillier SL, Nugent RP, Eschenbach DA, Krohn MA, Gibbs RS, Martin DH, Cotch MF, Edelman R, Pastorek JG, Rao AV, McNellis D, Regan JA, Carey JC, Klebanoff MA. Association between bacterial vaginosis and preterm delivery of a low-birth-weight infant. N Engl J Med. 1995;333:1737–42.

Hirsch E, Muhle RA. Intrauterine bacterial inoculation induces labor in the mouse by mechanisms other than progesterone withdrawal. Biol Reprod. 2002;67: 1337–41.

Holcberg G, Huleihel M, Sapir O, Kats M, Tsadkin M, Furman B, Mazor M, Myatt L. Increased production of tumor necrosis factor-alpha by IUGR human placentae. Eur J Obstet Gynecol Reprod Biol. 2001;94:69–72.

Holland OJ, Linscheid C, Hodes HC, Nauser TL, Gilliam M, Stone P, Chamley LW, Petroff MG. Minor histocompatibility antigens are expressed in syncytiotrophoblast and trophoblast debris: implications for maternal alloreactivity to the fetus. Am J Pathol. 2012;180:256–66.

Holmlund U, Cebers G, Dahlfors AR, Sandstedt B, Bremme K, Ekstrom ES, Scheynius A. Expression and regulation of the pattern recognition receptors Toll-like receptor-2 and Toll- like receptor-4 in the human placenta. Immunology. 2002;107:145–51.

Hsu CD, Meaddough E, Aversa K, Hong SF, Lee IS, Bahodo-Singh RO, Lu LC, Copel JA. Dual roles of amniotic fluid nitric oxide and prostaglandin E2 in preterm labor with intra-amniotic infection. Am J Perinatol. 1998;15:683–7.

Huddlestone H, Schust DJ. Immune interactions at the maternal-fetal interface: a focus on antigen presentation. Am J Reprod Immunol. 2004;51:283–9.

Hunt JS. Cytokine networks in the uteroplacental unit: macrophages as pivotal regulatory cells. J Reprod Immunol. 1989;16:1–17.

Hunt JS. Immunologically relevant cells in the uterus. Biol Reprod. 1994;50:461–6.

Hunt JS, Robertson SA. Uterine macrophages and environmental programming for pregnancy success. J Reprod Immunol. 1996;32:1–25.

Hunt JS, Manning LS, Wood GW. Macrophages in murine uterus are immunosuppressive. Cell Immunol. 1984;85:499–510.

Hunt JS, Vassmer D, Ferguson TA, Miller L. Fas Ligand is positioned in mouse uterus and placenta to prevent trafficking of activated leukocytes between the mother and the conceptus. J Immunol. 1997;158:122–8.

Hwu P, Du MX, Lapointe R, Do M, Taylor MW, Young HA. Indoleamine 2,3-dioxygenase production by human dendritic cells results in the inhibition of T cell proliferation. J Immunol. 2000;164:3596–9.

Hyodo Y, Matsui K, Hayashi N. IL-18 up-regulates perforin-mediated NK activity without increasing perforin messenger RNA expression by binding to constitutively expressed IL-18 receptor. J Immunol. 1999;162:1662–8.

Ida A, Tsuji Y, Murakana J, Kanazawa R, Nakata Y, Adachi S, Okamura H, Koyama K. IL-18 in pregnancy; the elevation of IL-18 in maternal peripheral blood during labor and complicated pregnancies. J Reprod Immunol. 2000;47:65–74.

Ingman WV, Robertson SA. Defining the actions of transforming growth factor beta in reproduction. Bioessays. 2002;24:904–14.

Ito K, Tanaka T, Tsutsumi N, Obata F, Kashiwagi N. Possible mechanisms of immunotherapy for maintaining pregnancy in recurrent spontaneous aborters: analysis of anti-idiotypic antibodies directed against autologous T-cell receptors. Hum Reprod. 1999;14:650–5.

Ito M, Nakashima A, Hidaka T, Okabe M, Bac ND, Ina S, Yoneda S, Shiozaki A, Sumi S, Tsuneyama K, Nikaido T, Saito S. A role for IL-17 in induction of an inflammation at the fetomaternal interface in preterm labour. J Reprod Immunol. 2010;84:75–85.

Jablonowska B, Palfi M, Ernerudh J, Kjellberg S, Selbing A. Blocking antibodies in blood from patients with recurrent spontaneous abortion in relation to pregnancy outcome and intravenous immunoglobulin treatment. Am J Reprod Immunol. 2001;45:226–31.

Jablonowska B, Palfi M, Matthiesen L, Selbing A, Kjellberg S, Ernerudh J. T and B lymphocyte subsets in patients with unexplained recurrent spontaneous abortion: IVIG versus placebo treatment. Am J Reprod Immunol. 2002;48:312–8.

Jacobson B, Holst RM, Mattsby-Baltzer I, Nikolaitchouk N, Wennerholm UB, Hagberg H. Interleukin-18 in cervical mucus and amniotic fluid: relationship to microbial invasion of the amniotic fluid, intra-amniotic inflammation and preterm delivery. BJOG. 2003;110:598–603.

Janeway Jr CA, Travers P. Immunologie. 2nd ed. Heidelberg/Berlin/Oxford: Spektrum Akademischer Verlag; 1997.

Jauniaux E, Gulbis B, Schandene L, Collette J, Hustin J. Distribution of interleukin-6 in maternal and embryonic tissues during the first trimester. Mol Hum Reprod. 1996;2:239–43.

Jensen F, Wallukat G, Herse F, Budner O, El-Mousleh T, Costa SD, Dechend R, Zenclussen AC. CD19+CD5+ cells as indicators of preeclampsia. Hypertension. 2012;59:861–8.

Joachim R, Zenclussen AC, Polgar B, Douglas AJ, Fest S, Knackstedt M, Klapp BF, Arck PC. The progesterone derivative dydrogesterone abrogates murine stress-triggered abortion by inducing a Th2 biased local immune response. Steroids. 2003;68:931–40.

Johansson M, Bromfield JJ, Jasper MJ, Robertson SA. Semen activates the female immune response during early pregnancy in mice. Immunology. 2004;112:290–300.

Jokhi PP, King A, Sharkey AM, Smith SK, Loke YW. Screening for cytokine messenger ribonucleic acids in purified human decidual lymphocyte populations by the reverse- transcriptase polymerase chain reaction. J Immunol. 1994;153:4427–35.

Juretic K, Strbo N, Bogovic Crncic T, Laskarin G, Rukavina D. An insight into the dendritic cells at the maternal-fetal interface. Am J Reprod Immunol. 2004;52:350–5.

Kalinka J, Sobala W, Wasiela M, Brzezinska-Blaszczyk E. Decreased proinflammatory cytokines in cervicovaginal fluid, as measured in midgestation, are associated with preterm delivery. Am J Reprod Immunol. 2005;54:70–6.

Kalish RB, Vardhana S, Gupta M, Chasen ST, Perni SC, Witkin SS. Interleukin-1 receptor antagonist gene polymorphism and multifetal pregnancy outcome. Am J Obstet Gynecol. 2003;189:911–4.

Kalish RB, Vardhana S, Gupta M, Perni SC, Chasen ST, Witkin SS. Polymorphisms in the tumor necrosis factor-a gene at position −308 and the inducible 70 kDa heat shock protein gene at position +1267 in multifetal pregnancies and preterm premature rupture of fetal membranes. Am J Obstet Gynecol. 2004a;191:1368–74.

Kalish RB, Vardhana S, Gupta M, Perni SC, Witkin SS. Interleukin-4 and −10 gene polymorphisms and spontaneous preterm birth in multifetal gestations. Am J Obstet Gynecol. 2004b;190:702–6.

Kämmerer U. Antigen presenting cells in the decidua. Chem Immunol Allergy. 2005;89:96–104.

Kämmerer U, Schoppet M, McLellen AD, Kapp M, Huppertz HI, Kampgen E, Dietl J. Human decidua contains potent immunostimulatory CD83(+) dendritic cells. Am J Pathol. 2000;157:159–69.

Kämmerer U, Eggert AO, Kapp M, McLellan AD, Geijtenbeek TB, Dietl J, van Kooyk Y, Kampgen E. Unique appearance of proliferating antigen-presenting cells expressing DC-SIGN (CD209) in the deciduas of early human pregnancy. Am J Pathol. 2003; 162:887–96.

Katano K, Aoki A, Sasa H, Ogasawara M, Matsuura E, Yagami Y. Beta 2-glycoprotein I- dependent anticardiolipin antibodies as a predictor of adverse pregnancy outcomes in healthy pregnant women. Hum Reprod. 1996;11:509–12.

Kayisli UA, Mahutte NG, Arici A. Uterine chemokines in reproductive physiology and pathology. Am J Reprod Immunol. 2002;47:213–21.

Keelan JA, Blumenstein M, Helliwell RJA, Sato TA, Marvin KW, Mitchell MD. Cytokines, prostaglandins and parturition-a review. Placenta. 2003;24(Suppl):S33–46.

Kelemen K, Bognar I, Paal M, Szekeres-Bartho J. A progesterone-induced protein increases the synthesis of asymmetric antibodies. Cell Immunol. 1996; 167:129–34.

Kelly RW. Inflammatory mediators and cervical ripening. J Reprod Immunol. 2002;57:217–24.

Kelly KA, Gray HL, Walker JC, Rank RG, Wormley FL, Fidel Jr PL. Chlamydia trachomatis infection does not enhance local cellular immunity against concurrent Candida vaginal infection. Infec Immun. 2001;69:3451–4.

Kemp B, Schmitz S, Krusche CA, Rath W, von Rango U. Dendritic cells are equally distributed in intrauterine and tubal ectopic pregnancies. Fertil Steril. 2011;95: 28–32.

Kigozi GG, Brahmbhatt H, Wabwire-Mangen F, Waver MJ, Serwadda D, Sewankambo N, Gray RH. Treatment of Trichomonas in pregnancy and adverse outcomes of pregnancy: a subanalysis of a randomized trial in Rakai, Uganda. Am J Obstet Gynecol. 2003;189:1398–400.

Kim YM, Romero R, Oh SY, Kim CJ, Kilburn BA, Armant DR, Nien JK, Gomez R, Mazor M, Saito S, Abrahams VM, Mor G. Toll-like receptor 4: a potential link between "danger signals", the innate immune system, and preeclampsia? Am J Obstet Gynecol. 2005;193:1137–43.

Kim MG, Shim JY, Pak JH, Jung BK, Won HS, Lee PR, Kim A. Progesterone modulates the expression of interleukin-6 in cultured term human uterine cervical fibroblasts. Am J Reprod Immunol. 2012;67:369–75.

King J, Flenady V. Prophylactic antibiotics for inhibiting preterm labor with intact membranes. Cochrane Database Syst Rev. 2003(1);CD002255.

King A, Burrows T, Verma S, Hiby S, Loke YW. Human uterine lymphocytes. Hum Reprod Update. 1998;4: 480–5.

King A, Allan DS, Bowen M, Powis AJ, Joseph S, Verma S, Hiby SE, McMichael AJ, Loke YW, Braud VM. HLA-E is expressed on trophoblast and interacts with CD94/NKG2 receptors on decidual NK cells. Eur J Immunol. 2000a;30:1623–31.

King A, Burrows T, Hiby S, Joseph S, Bowen JM, Verma S, Burrows TD, Loke YW. Surface expression of HLA-C antigen by human extravillous trophoblast. Placenta. 2000b;21:376–87.

King A, Hiby S, Gardner L, Joseph S, Bowen JM, Verma S, Burrows T, Loke YW. Recognition of trophoblast HLA class I molecules by decidual NK cell receptors- a review. Placenta. 2000c;21(Suppl):S81–5.

Kitaya K, Yasuda J, Yagi I, Tada Y, Fushiki S, Honjo H. IL-15 expression at human endometrium and decidua. Biol Reprod. 2000;63:683–7.

Kitzmiller JL, Bernischke K. Immunofluorescent study of placental bed vessels in pre- eclampsia of pregnancy. Am J Obstet Gynecol. 1973;115:248–51.

Klebanoff MA, Regan JA, Rao AV, Nugent RP, Blackwelder WC, Eschenbach DA, Pastorek 2nd JG, Williams S, Gibbs RS, Carey JC. Outcome of the Vaginal Infections and Prematurity Study: results of a clinical trial of erythromycin among pregnant women colonized with group B streptococci. Am J Obstet Gynecol. 1995;172:1540–5.

Klebanoff MA, Carey J, Hauth JC, Hillier SL, Nugent RP, Thom EA, Ernest JM, Heine RP, Wapner RJ, Trout W, Moawad A, Leveno KJ, Miodovnik M, Siai BM, Van Dorsten JP, Dombrowski MP, O'Sullivan MJ, Varner M, Langer O, McNellis D, Roberts JM, National Institute of Child Health and Human Development Network of Maternal-Fetal Medicine Units. Failure of metronidazole to prevent preterm delivery among pregnant women with asymptomatic Trichomonas vaginalis infection. N Engl J Med. 2001;345:487–93.

Klein LL, Gibbs RS. Infection and preterm birth. Obstet Gynecol Clin North Am. 2005;32:397–410.

Knackstedt M, Ding JW, Arck PC, Hertwig K, Coulam CB, August C, Lea R, Dudenhausen JW, Gorczynski RM, Levey GA, Clark DA. Activation of a novel prothrombinase, fg12 as a basis for pregnancy complication in spontaneous abortion and pre-eclampsia. Am J Reprod Immunol. 2001;46:196–210.

Koch CA, Platt JL. Natural mechanisms for evading graft rejection: the fetus as an allograft. Springer Semin Immunopathol. 2003;25:95–117.

Kokawa K, Shikone T, Nakano R. Apoptosis in human chorionic villi and deciduas during normal embryonic development and spontaneous abortion in first trimester. Placenta. 1998;19:21–6.

Komlos L, Zamir R, Joshua H, Halbracht I. Common HLA antigens in couples with repeated abortions. Clin Immunol Immunopathol. 1977;7:330–5.

Kruse A, Greif M, Moriabadi NF, Marx L, Toyka KV, Riekmann P. Variations in cytokine mRNA expression during normal human pregnancy. Clin Exp Immunol. 2000;119:317–22.

Kumazaki K, Nakayama M, Yanagihara I, Suehara N, Wada Y. Immunohistochemical distribution of Toll-like receptor 4 in term and preterm human placentas from normal and complicated pregnancy including chorioamnionitis. Hum Pathol. 2004;35:47–54.

Kusakabe K, Okada T, Sasaki F, Kiso Y. Cell death of uterine natural killer cells in murine placenta during placentation and preterm periods. J Vet Med Sci. 1999;61:1093–100.

Kutteh WH, Rote NS, Silver R. Antiphospholipid antibodies and reproduction: the antiphospholipid antibody syndrome. Am J Reprod Immunol. 1999; 41:133–52.

Kwak JYH, Beaman KD, Gilman-Sachs A, Ruiz JE, Schewitz D, Beer AE. Up-regulated expression of CD56+, CD56+/CD16+, and CD19+ cells in peripheral blood lymphocytes in pregnant women with recurrent pregnancy loss. Am J Reprod Immunol. 1995;34:93–9.

Kwak-Kim J, Gilman-Sachs A. Clinical implication of natural killer cells and reproduction. Am J Reprod Immunol. 2008;59:388–400.

Lachapelle MH, Miron P, Hennings R. Endometrial T and NK cells in patients with recurrent spontaneous abortion. Altered profile and pregnancy outcome. J Immunol. 1995;156:4027–34.

Lachapelle M, Miron P, Hemmings R, Roy DC. Endometrial T, B and NK cells in patients with recurrent spontaneous abortion. J Immunol. 1996;156: 4027–34.

Laird SM, Tuckerman EM, Cork BA, Linjawi S, Blakemore AIF, Li TC. A review of immune cells and molecules in women with recurrent miscarriage. Hum Reprod Update. 2003;9:163–74.

Lamont RF, Sawant SR. Infection in the prediction and antibiotics in the prevention of spontaneous preterm labor and preterm birth. Minerva Ginecol. 2005;57: 423–33.

Lamont RF, Duncan SLB, Mandal D, Bassett P. Intravaginal clindamycin cream to reduce preterm birth in women with abnormal genital tract flora. Obstet Gynecol. 2003;101:516–22.

Laskarin G, Strbo N, Sotosek V, Rukavina D, Faust Z, Szekeres-Bartho J, Podack ER. Progesterone directly and indirectly affects perforin expression in cytolytic cells. Am J Reprod Immunol. 1999;45:312–20.

Laskarin G, Tokmadzic V, Strbo N, Bogovic T, Szekeres-Bartho J, Randic L, Podack ER, Rukavina D. Progesterone induced blocking factor (PIBF) mediates progesterone induced suppression of decidual lymphocyte cytotoxicity. Am J Reprod Immunol. 2002; 48:201–9.

Laskarin G, Strbo N, Bogovic Crnic T, Juretic K, Ledee Bataille N, Chaouat G, Rukavina D. Physiological role of IL-15 and IL-18 at the maternal-fetal interface. Chem Immunol Allergy. 2005;89:10–25.

Lass A, Weiser W, Munafo A, Loumaye E. Leukemia inhibitory factor in human reproduction. Fertil Steril. 2001;76:1091–6.

Le Bouteiller P, Blaschitz A. The functionality of HLA-G is emerging. Immunol Rev. 1999;167:233–44.

Le Bouteiller P, Legrand-Abravanel F, Solier C. Soluble HLA-G1 at the materno-foetal interface-a review. Placenta. 2003a;24(Suppl):S10–5.

Le Bouteiller P, Pizzato N, Barakonyi A, Solier C. HLA-G, pre-eclampsia, immunity and vascular events. J Reprod Immunol. 2003b;59:219–34.

Lea RG, Underwood J, Flanders KC, Hirte H, Banwatt D, Finotto S, Ohno I, Daya S, Harley C, Michel M. A subset of patients with recurrent spontaneous abortion is deficient in transforming growth factor

beta-2-producing "suppressor cells" in uterine tissue near the placental attachment site. Am J Reprod Immunol. 1995;34:52–64.

Lee J, Choi BC, Cho C, Hill JA, Baek KH, Kim JW. Trophoblast apoptosis is increased in women with evidence of Th1 immunity. Fertil Steril. 2005;83: 1047–9.

Lee CL, Chiu PC, Lam KK, Siu SO, Chu IK, Koistinen R, Koistinen H, Seppala M, Lee KF, Yeung WS. Differential actions of glycodelin-A on Th-1 and Th-2 cells: a paracrine mechanism that could produce the Th-2 dominant environment during pregnancy. Hum Reprod. 2011a;26:517–26.

Lee SY, Buhimschi IA, Dulay AT, Ali UA, Zhao G, Abdel-Razeq SS, Bahtiyar MO, Thung SF, Funai EF, Buhimschi CS. IL-6 trans-signaling system in intra-amniotic inflammation, preterm birth, and preterm premature rupture of the membranes. J Immunol. 2011b;186:3226–36.

Leitich H, Bodner-Adler B, Brunbauer M, Kaider A, Egarter C, Husslein P. Bacterial vaginosis as a risk factor for preterm delivery: a meta-analysis. Am J Obstet Gynecol. 2003a;189:139–47.

Leitich H, Brunbauer M, Bodner-Adler B, Kaider A, Egarter C, Husslein P. Antibiotic treatment of bacterial vaginosis in pregnancy: a meta-analysis. Am J Obstet Gynecol. 2003b;188:752–8.

Lessin DL, Hunt JS, King CR, Wood GW. Antigen expression by cells near the maternal-fetal interface. Am J Reprod Immunol Microbiol. 1988;16:1–7.

Lewis DF, Canzoneri BJ, Wang Y. Maternal circulating TNF-alpha levels are highly correlated with IL-10 levels, but not IL-6 and IL-8 levels, in women with pre-eclampsia. Am J Reprod Immunol. 2009;62:269–74.

Li DK, Wi S. Changing paternity and the risk of pre-eclampsia/ eclampsia in the subsequent pregnancy. Am J Epidemiol. 2000;151:57–62.

Librach CL, Feigenbaum SL, Bass KE, Cui TY, Verastas N, Sadovsky Y, Quigley JP, French DL, Fisher SJ. Interleukin-1β regulates human cytotrophoblast metalloproteinase activity and invasion in vitro. J Biol Chem. 1994;269:17125–31.

Lim K, Bass K, Zhou Y, Chun S, McMaster M, Janatpour M. Human cytotrophoblast differentiation is abnormal in preeclampsia. Am J Pathol. 1997;151:1809–18.

Lockwood CJ. Predicting premature delivery-no easy task. N Engl J Med. 2002;346:282–4.

Loke YW, King A. Immunology of implantation. Baillieres Best Pract Res Clin Obstet Gynaecol. 2000;14:827–37.

Loke YW, King A, Burrows TD. Decidua in human implantation. Hum Reprod. 1995;10:14–21.

Lord GM, Matarese G, Howard JK, Baker RJ, Bloom SR, Lechler RI. Leptin modulates the T- cell immune response and reverse starvation-induced immunosuppression. Nature. 1998;394:897–901.

Lorincz AT, Reid R, Jenson AB, Greenberg MD, Lancaster W, Kurman RJ. Human papillomavirus infection of the cervix: relative risk associations of 15 common anogenital types. Obstet Gynecol. 1992;79:328–37.

Lumley J. Defining the problem: the epidemiology of pre-term birth. BJOG. 2003;110(Suppl):S3–7.

Luppi P, McKnight C, Mathie T, Faas S, Rudert WA, Stewart-Akers AM, Trucco M, DeLoia JA. Evidence for superantigen involvement in preeclampsia. Am J Reprod Immunol. 2000;43:187–96.

Luppi P, Haluszczak C, Trucco M, Deloia JA. Normal pregnancy is associated with peripheral leukocyte activation. Am J Reprod Immunol. 2002;47:72–81.

Lutz MB, Schuler G. Immature, semi-mature and fully mature dendritic cells: which signals induce tolerance or immunity? Trends Immunol. 2002;23:445–9.

Lyall F, Simpson H, Bulmer JN, Barber A, Robson SC. Transforming growth factor-beta expression in human placenta and placental bed in third trimester normal pregnancy, preeclampsia, and fetal growth restriction. Am J Pathol. 2001;159:1827–38.

MacKenzie CR, Gonzalez RG, Kniep E, Roch S, Daubener W. Cytokine mediated regulation of interferon-gamma-induced IDO activation. Adv Exp Med Biol. 1999;467:533–9.

MacLean MA, Wilson R, Jenkins C, Miller H, Walker JJ. Interleukin-2 receptor concentrations in pregnant women with a history of recurrent miscarriage. Hum Reprod. 2002;7:221–7.

Macones GA, Parry S, Elkousy M, Clothier B, Ural SH, Strauss JF. A polymorphism in the promoter region of TNF and bacterial vaginosis: preliminary evidence of gene-environment interaction in the etiology of spontaneous preterm birth. Am J Obstet Gynecol. 2004;190:1504–8.

Makhseed M, Raghupathy R, Azizieh F, Farhat R, Hassan N, Bandar A. Circulating cytokines and CD30 in normal human pregnancy and recurrent spontaneous abortions. Hum Reprod. 2000;15:2011–7.

Makrigiannakis A, Karamouti M, Drakakis P, Loutradis D, Antsaklis A. Fetomaternal immunotolerance. Am J Reprod Immunol. 2008;60:482–96.

Margni RA, Malan BI. Paradoxical behaviour of asymmetric IgG antibodies. Immunol Rev. 1998;163:77–87.

Martin DH, Eschenbach DA, Cotch MF, Nugent RP, Rao AV, Klebanoff MA, Lou Y, Rettig PJ, Gibbs RS, Pastorek 2nd JG, Regan JA, Kaslow RA. Double-blind placebo-controlled treatment trial of Chlamydia trachomatis endocervical infections in pregnant women. Infect Dis Obstet Gynecol. 1997;5:10–7.

Marzi M, Vigano A, Trabattoni D, Villa ML, Salvaggio A, Clerici E, Clerici M. Characterization of type 1 and type 2 cytokine production profile in physiologic and pathologic human pregnancy. Clin Exp Immunol. 1996;106:127–33.

Matthiesen L, Berg G, Ernerudh J, Skogh T. Lymphocyte subsets and autoantibodies in pregnancies complicated by placental disorders. Am J Reprod Immunol. 1995;33:31–9.

Matthiesen L, Ekerfelt C, Berg G, Ernerudh J. Increased numbers of circulating interferon- gamma and interleukin-4 secreting cells during normal pregnancy. Am J Reprod Immunol. 1998;39:362–7.

Matthiesen L, Berg G, Ernerudh J, Ekerfelt C, Jonsson Y, Sharma S. Immunology of preeclampsia. Chem Immunol Allergy. 2005;89:49–61.

Mattsby-Baltzer I, Hosseini N. The IL-6 response in human cervix epithelial and monocytic cell lines stimulated by bacteria associated with bacterial vaginosis and Escherichia coli. Int J STD AIDS. 1997;8 Suppl 1:34.

Maxion HK, Kelly KA. Chemokine expression patterns differ within anatomically distinct regions of the genital tract during Chlamydia trachomatis infection. Infect Immun. 2002;70:1538–46.

McDonald H, Brocklehurst P, Parsons J. Antibiotics for treating bacterial vaginosis in pregnancy. Cochrane Database Syst Rev. 2005;1:CD000262.

McIntire RH, Hunt JS. Antigen presenting cells and HLA-G-a review. Placenta. 2005;26(Suppl):S104–10.

Medawar PB. Some immunological and endocrinological problems raised by the evolution of viviparity in vertebrates. Symp Soc Exp Biol. 1953;7:320–38.

Chaouat G, Robillard PY, Dekker G. Fourth International Workshop on immunology of preeclampsia, Dec. 2004, Reunion, France. J Reprod Immunol. 2005;67: 103-111.

Meis PJ, Klebanoff M, Thom E, Dombrowski MP, Sibai B, Moawad AH, Spong CY, Hauth JC, Miodovnik M, Varner MW, Leveno KJ, Caritis SN, Iams JD, Wapner RJ, Conway D, O'Sullivan MJ, Carpenter M, Mercer B, Ramin SM, Thorp JM, Peaceman AM. Prevention of recurrent preterm delivery by 17α-hydroxyprogesterone caproate. N Engl J Med. 2003;348:2379–85.

Mellor AL, Munn DH. Extinguishing maternal immune responses during pregnancy: implications for immunosuppression. Semin Immunol. 2001;13:213–8.

Miller L, Hunt JS. Sex steroid hormones and macrophage function. Life Sci. 1996;59:1–14.

Milns NR, Gardner ID. Maternal T cells and human pregnancy outcome. J Reprod Immunol. 1989;15:175–8.

Minagawa M, Narita J, Tada T, Maruyama S, Shimizu T, Bannai M, Oya H, Hatakeyama K, Abo T. Mechanisms underlying immunologic states during pregnancy: possible association of the sympathetic nervous system. Cell Immunol. 1999;196:1–13.

Mincheva-Nilsson L, Baranov V, Yeung M, Hammarstrom S, Hammarstrom ML. Immunomorphologic studies in human decidua-associated lymphoid cells in normal early pregnancy. J Immunol. 1994;152:2020–32.

Minkoff H, Grunebaum AN, Schwarz RH, Feldman J, Cummings M, Crombleholme W, Clark L, Pringle G, McCormack WM. Risk factors for prematurity and premature rupture of membranes: a prospective study of the vaginal flora in pregnancy. Am J Obstet Gynecol. 1984;150:965–72.

Miyazaki S, Tsuda H, Sakai M, Hori S, Sasaki Y, Futatani T, Miyawaki T, Saito S. Predominance of Th2-promoting dendritic cells in early human pregnancy decidua. J Leukoc Biol. 2003;74:514–22.

Mizuno M, Aoki K, Kimbara T. Functions of macrophages in human decidual tissue in early pregnancy. Am J Reprod Immunol. 1994;31:180–8.

Moffett A, Loke YW. The immunological paradox of pregnancy: a reappraisal. Placenta. 2004;25:1–8.

Moffett-King A. Natural killer cells and pregnancy. Nat Rev Immunol. 2002;2:656–63.

Molnar M, Romero R, Hertelendy F. Interleukin-1 and tumor necrosis factor stimulate arachidonic acid release and phospholipids metabolism in human myometrial cells. Am J Obstet Gynecol. 1993;169:825–9.

Molnar M, Rigo JJ, Romero R, Hertelendy F. Oxytocin activates mitogen-activated protein kinase and up-regulates cyclooxygenase-2 and prostaglandin production in human myometrial cells. Am J Obstet Gynecol. 1999;181:42–9.

Monzon-Bordonaba F, Vadillo-Ortega F, Feinberg RF. Modulation of trophoblast function by tumor necrosis factor-α: a role in pregnancy establishment and maintenance. Am J Obstet Gynecol. 2002;187:1574–80.

Mor G, Abrahams VM. Potential role of macrophages as immunoregulators of pregnancy. Reprod Biol Endocrinol. 2003;1:119–27.

Mor G, Cardenas I. The immune system in pregnancy: a unique complexity. Am J Reprod Immunol. 2010;63:425–33.

Morales PJ, Pace JL, Platt JS, Phillips TA, Morgan K, Fazleabas AT, Hunt JS. Placental cell expression of HLA-G2 isoforms is limited to the invasive trophoblast phenotype. J Immunol. 2003;171:6215–24.

Morton H. Early pregnancy factor: an extracellular chaperonin 10 homologue. Immunol Cell Biol. 1998; 76:483–96.

Morton H, Hegh V, Clunie GJA. Studies of the rosette inhibition test in pregnant mice: evidence of immunosuppression? Proc R Soc Lond B Biol Sci. 1976;193:413–9.

Munn DH, Zhou M, Attwood JT, Bondarev I, Conway SJ, Marshall B, Brown C, Mellor AL. Prevention of allogeneic fetal rejection by tryptophan catabolism. Science. 1998;281:1191–3.

Muranaka J, Tsuji Y, Hasegawa A, Ida A, Nakata Y, Kanazawa R, Koyama K. Interleukin-18 as an important new cytokine in pregnancy. Am J Reprod Immunol. 1998;40:278.

Murphy S, Fast L, Sharma S. IL-10, uterine NK cells, inflammation, and pregnancy. Am J Reprod Immunol. 2004;51:434.

Naccasha N, Gervasi MT, Chaiworapongsa T, Berman S, Yoon BH, Maymon E, Romero R. Phenotypic and metabolic characteristics of monocytes and granulocytes in normal pregnancy and maternal infection. Am J Obstet Gynecol. 2001;185:1118–23.

Nakanishi K, Yoshimoto T, Tsutsui H, Okamura H. Interleukin-18 is a unique cytokine that stimulates both Th1 and Th2 responses depending on its cytokine milieu. Cytokine Growth Factor Rev. 2001;12: 53–72.

Nenadic DB, Pavlovic MD. Cervical fluid cytokines in pregnant women: relation to vaginal wet mount findings and polymorphonuclear leukocyte counts. Eur J Obstet Gynecol Reprod Biol. 2008;140:165–70.

Novy MJ, Duffy L, Axthelm MK, Cook MJ, Haluska GJ, Witkin S, Gerber S, Gravett MG, Sadowsky D, Cassell GH. Experimental primate model for Ureaplasma chorioamnionitis and preterm labor. J Soc Gynecol Investig. 2001;8(Suppl):48A.

Ntrivalas EI, Kwak-Kim J, Gilman-Sachs A, Chung-Bang H, Ng SC, Beaman KD, Mantouvalos HP, Beer AE. Status of peripheral blood natural killer cells in women with recurrent spontaneous abortions and infertility of unknown etiology. Hum Reprod. 2001;16:855–61.

Ntrivalas EI, Bowser CR, Kwak-Kim J, Beaman KD, Gilman-Sachs A. Expression of killer immunoglobulin-like receptors on peripheral blood NK cell subsets of women with recurrent spontaneous abortions or implantation failures. Am J Reprod Immunol. 2005;53:215–21.

O'Neill C. The role of paf in embryo physiology. Hum Reprod Update. 2005;11:215–28.

Ober C, Hyslop T, Elias S, Weikamp LR, Hauck WW. Human leucocyte antigen matching and fetal loss. Result of a 10 year prospective study. Hum Reprod. 1998;13:33–8.

Ogasawara MS, Aoki K, Aoyama T, Katano K, Iinuma Y, Ozaki Y, Suzumori K. Elevation of transforming growth factor-beta1 is associated with recurrent miscarriage. J Clin Immunol. 2000;20:453–7.

Ohshima K, Nakashima M, Sonoda K, Kikuchi M, Watanabe T. Expression of RCAS1 and FasL in human trophoblast and uterine glands during pregnancy: the possible role in immune privilege. Clin Exp Immunol. 2001;123:481–6.

Okamura H, Tsutsui H, Kashiwamura SI, Yoshimoto T, Nakanishi K. Interleukin 18: a novel cytokine that augments innate and acquired immunity. Adv Immunol. 1998;70:281–311.

Olivares EG, Montes MJ, Oliver CJ, Galindo JA, Ruiz C. Cultured human decidual stromal cells express B7-1 (CD80) and B7-2 (CD86) and stimulate allogeneic T cells. Biol Reprod. 1997;57:609–15.

Omu AE, Al-Quattan F, Diejomaoh ME, Al-Yamata M. Differential levels of T helper cytokines in preeclampsia: pregnancy, labor and puerperium. Acta Obstet Gynecol Scand. 1999;78:675–80.

Orgad S, Loewenthal R, Gazit E, Sadetzki S, Novikov I, Carp H. The prognostic value of anti- paternal antibodies and leukocyte immunizations on the proportion of live births in couples with consecutive recurrent miscarriages. Hum Reprod. 1999;14:2974–9.

Osmann I, Young A, Ledingham MA, Thomson AJ, Jordan F, Greer IA, Norman JE. Leukocyte density and pro-inflammatory cytokine expression in human fetal membranes, decidua, cervix, and myometrium before and during labor at term. Mol Hum Reprod. 2003;9:41–5.

Ostojic S, Dubanchet S, Chaouat G, Abdelkarim M, Truyens C, Caron F. Demonstration of the presence of IL-16, IL-17 and IL-18 at the murine fetomaternal interface during murine pregnancy. Am J Reprod Immunol. 2003;49:101–12.

Pampfer S, Cordi S, Cikos S, Picry B, Vanderheyden I, Hertogh RD. Activation of nuclear factor-kappaB and induction of apoptosis by tumor necrosis factor-alpha in the mouse uterine epithelial WEG-1 cell line. Biol Reprod. 2000;63:879–86.

Pandey MK, Agrawal S. Prevalence of anti-idiotypic antibodies in pregnancy v/s recurrent spontaneous (RSA) women. Obstet Gynae Today. 2003;7:574–8.

Pandey MK, Agrawal S. Induction of MLR-Bf and protection of fetal loss: a current double blind randomized trial of paternal lymphocyte immunization for women with recurrent spontaneous abortion. Int Immunopharmacol. 2004;4:289–98.

Pandey MK, Saxena V, Agrawal S. Characterization of mixed lymphocyte reaction blocking antibodies (MLR-Bf) in human pregnancy. BMC Pregnancy Childbirth. 2003;3:2.

Pandey MK, Rani R, Agrawal S. An update in recurrent spontaneous abortion. Arch Gynecol Obstet. 2005;272:95–108.

Par G, Geli J, Kozma N, Varga P, Szekeres-Bartho J. Progesterone regulates IL-12 expression in pregnancy lymphocytes by inhibiting phospholipase A2. Am J Reprod Immunol. 2003;49:1–5.

Pasare C, Medzhitov R. Toll pathway-dependent blockade of CD4+CD25+ T cell-mediated suppression by dendritic cells. Science. 2003;299:1033–6.

Patel FA, Clifton VL, Chwalisz K, Challis JR. Steroid regulation of prostaglandin dehydrogenase activity and expression in human term placenta and choriodecidua in relation to labor. J Clin Endocrinol Metab. 1999;84:291–9.

Paulesu L, Bocci V, King A, Loke YW. Immunocytochemical localization of interferons in human trophoblast populations. J Biol Regul Homeost Agents. 1991;5:81–5.

Peltier MR. Immunology of term and preterm labor. Reprod Biol Endocrinol. 2003;1:122–33.

Perni SC, Vardhana S, Tuttle SL, Kalish RB, Chasen ST, Witkin SS. Fetal interleukin-1 receptor antagonist gene polymorphism, intra-amniotic interleukin-1β levels, and a history of spontaneous abortion. Am J Obstet Gynecol. 2004;191:1318–23.

Perni SC, Kalish RB, Hutson JM, Karasahin E, Bongiovanni AM, Ratushny V, Chasen ST, Witkin SS. Differential expression of immune system-related components in midtrimester amniotic fluid from singleton and twin pregnancies. Am J Obstet Gynecol. 2005;193:942–6.

Perricone R, De Carolis C, Giacomelli R, Guarino MD, De Sanctis G, Fontana L. GM-CSF and pregnancy: evidence of significantly reduced blood concentrations in unexplained recurrent abortion efficiently reverted by intravenous immunoglobulin treatment. Am J Reprod Immunol. 2003;50:232–7.

Perricone R, Di Muzio G, Perricone C, Giacomelli R, De Nardo D, Fontana L, De Carolis C. High levels of peripheral blood NK cells in women suffering from recurrent spontaneous abortion are reverted from high-dose intravenous immunoglobulins. Am J Reprod Immunol. 2006;55:232–9.

Piao HL, Tao Y, Zhu R, Wang SC, Tang CL, Fu Q, Du MR, Li DJ. The CXCL12/CXCR4 axis is involved in the maintenance of Th2 bias at the maternal/fetal interface in early human pregnancy. Cell Mol Immunol. 2012;9:423–30.

Piccinni MP. T cells in pregnancy. Chem Immunol Allergy. 2005;89:3–9.

Piccinni MP, Giudizi MG, Biagiotti R, Beloni L, Giannarini L, Sapognaro S, Parronchi P, Manetti R, Livi C, Romagnani S, Maggi E. Progesterone favors the development of human T helper cells producing Th2-type cytokines and promotes both IL-4 production and membrane CD30 expression in established Th1 cell clones. J Immunol. 1995;155:128–33.

Piccinni MP, Beloni L, Livi C, Maggi E, Scarselli GF, Romagnani S. Defective production of both leukaemia inhibitory factor and type 2 T-helper cytokines by decidual T cells in unexplained recurrent abortions. Nat Med. 1998;4:1020–4.

Piccinni MP, Scaletti C, Maggi E, Romagnani S. Role of hormone-controlled Th1- and Th2-type cytokines in successful pregnancy. J Neuroimmunol. 2000;109:30–3.

Piccinni MP, Scaletti C, Mavilia C, Lavzzeri E, Romagnani P, Natali I, Pellegrini S, Livi C, Romagnani S, Maggi E. Production of IL-4 and leukemia inhibitory factor by T cells of the cumulus oopherus: a favorable microenvironment for pre-implantation embryo development. Eur J Immunol. 2001;31:2431–7.

Pillay K, Coutsoudis A, Agadzi-Naqvi AK, Kuhn L, Coovadia HM, Janoff EN. Secretory leukocyte protease inhibitor in vaginal fluids and perinatal human immunodeficiency virus type 1 transmission. J Infect Dis. 2001;183:653–6.

Pöhlmann TG, Busch S, Mussil B, Winzer H, Weinert J, Mebes I, Schaumann A, Fitzgerald JS, Markert UR. The possible role of the JAK/STAT pathway in lymphocytes at the fetomaternal interface. Chem Immunol Allergy. 2005;89:26–35.

Polanczyk MJ, Carson BD, Subramanian S, Afentoulls M, Vandenbark AA, Ziegler SF, Offner H. Estrogen drives expansion of the CD4+CD25+ regulatory T cell compartment. J Immunol. 2004;173:2227–30.

Pollard JW, Hunt JS, Wiktor-Jedrzejczak W. A pregnancy defect in the osteopetrotic (op/op) mouse demonstrates the requirement for CSF-1 in female fertility. Dev Biol. 1991;148:273–8.

Pollard JK, Thai D, Mitchell MD. Evidence for a common mechanism of action of interleukin-1β, tumor necrosis factor-α, and epidermal growth factor on prostaglandin production in human chorion cells. Am J Reprod Immunol. 1993;30:146–53.

Pollard JK, Thai D, Mitchell MD. Mechanism of cytokine stimulation of prostaglandin biosynthesis in human decidua. J Soc Gynecol Investig. 1994;1:31–6.

Prll J, Bensussan A, Goffin F, Foidart JM, Berrebi A, Le Bouteiller P. Tubal versus uterine placentation: similar HLA-G expressing extravillous cytotrophoblast invasion but different maternal leukocyte recruitment. Tissue Antigens. 2000;56:479–91.

Quack KC, Vassiliadou N, Pudney J, Anderson DJ, Hill JA. Leukocyte activation in the decidua of chromosomally normal and abnormal fetuses from women with recurrent abortion. Hum Reprod. 2001; 16:949–55.

Quenby S, Bates M, Doig T, Brewster J, Lewis-Jones DI, Johnson PM, Vince G. Pre- implantation endometrial leukocytes in women with recurrent miscarriage. Hum Reprod. 1999;14:2386–91.

Quenby S, Vince G, Farquharson R, Aplin J. Recurrent miscarriage: a defect in nature's quality control? Hum Reprod. 2002;17:1959–63.

Quinn KA, Morton H. Effect of anti-EPF monoclonal antibodies on the in vivo growth of transplanted murine tumors. Cancer Immunol Immunother. 1992;34:265–71.

Rabot M, Tabiasco J, Polgar B, Aguerre-Girr M, Berrebi A, Bensussan A, Strbo N, Rukavina D, Le Bouteillier P. HLA class I/NK cell receptor interaction in early human decidua basalis: possible functional consequences. Chem Immunol Allergy. 2005;89: 72–83.

Raghupathy R, Makhseed M, Azizieh F, Hassan N, Al-Azemi M, Al-Shamali E. Maternal Th1- and Th2-type reactivity to placental antigens in normal human pregnancy and unexplained recurrent spontaneous abortions. Cell Immunol. 1999;196:122–30.

Raghupathy R, Makhseed M, Azizieh F, Omu A, Gupta M, Farhat R. Cytokine production by maternal lymphocytes during normal pregnancy and in unexplained recurrent spontaneous abortion. Hum Reprod. 2000;15:713–8.

Raghupathy R, Mutawa EA, Makhseed M, Azizieh F, Szekeres-Bartho J. Modulation of cytokine production by dehydrogesterone in lymphocytes from women with recurrent miscarriage. BJOG. 2005;112: 1096–101.

Ralph SG, Rutherford AJ, Wilson JD. Influence of bacterial vaginosis on conception and miscarriage in the first trimester: cohort study. Br Med J. 1999;319:220–3.

Ratts VS, Tao XJ, Webster CB, Swanson PE, Smith SD, Brownbill P, Krajewski S, Reed JC, Tilly JL, Nelson DM. Expression of BCL-2, BAX and BAK in the trophoblast layer of the term human placenta: a unique model of apoptosis within a syncytium. Placenta. 2000;21:361–6.

Redman CW, Sargent IL. Preeclampsia and the systemic inflammatory response. Semin Nephrol. 2004;24: 565–70.

Reimer T, Koczan D, Gerber B, Richter D, Theisen HJ, Friese K. Microarray analysis of differentially expressed genes in placental tissue of preeclampsia: up-regulation of obesity related genes. Mol Hum Reprod. 2002;8:674–80.

Reisenberger K, Egarter C, Knofler M, Schiebel I, Gregor H, Hirschl AM, Heinze G, Husslein P. Cytokine and prostaglandin production by amnion cells in response to the addition of different bacteria. Am J Obstet Gynecol. 1998;178:50–3.

Reister F, Frank HG, Kingdom JC, Heyl W, Kaufmann P, Rath W, Huppertz B. Macrophage- induced apoptosis limits endovascular trophoblast invasion in the uterine wall of preeclamptic women. Lab Invest. 2001;81: 1143–52.

Richani K, Soto E, Romero R, Espinoza J, Chaiworapongsa T, Nien JK, Edwin S, Kim YM, Hong JS, Mazor M. Normal pregnancy is characterized by systemic activation of the complement system. J Matern Fetal Neonatal Med. 2005;17:239–45.

Rieger L, Kämmerer U, Hofmann J, Sutterlin M, Dietl J. Choriocarcinoma cells modulate the cytokine production of decidual large granular lymphocytes in coculture. Am J Reprod Immunol. 2001;46:137–43.

Riley SC, Leask R, Denison FC, Wisely K, Calder AA, Howe DC. Secretion of tissue inhibitors of matrix metalloproteinases by human fetal membranes, decidua and placenta at parturition. J Endocrinol. 1999;162:351–9.

Rivera DL, Olister SM, Liu X, Thompson JH, Zhang XJ, Pennline K, Azuero R, Clark DA, Miller MJ. Interleukin-10 attenuates experimental fetal growth restriction and demise. FASEB J. 1998; 12:189–97.

Roberts JM, Cooper DW. Pathogenesis and genetics of preeclampsia. Lancet. 2001;357:53–6.

Robertson SA. Immune regulation of conception and embryo implantation-all about quality control? J Reprod Immunol. 2010;85:51–7.

Robillard PY, Hulsey TC. Association of pregnancy-induced hypertension, pre-eclampsia, and eclampsia with duration of sexual cohabitation before conception. Lancet. 1996;347:619.

Robillard PY, Dekker GA, Hulsey TC. Revisiting the epidemiological standard of preeclampsia. Primigravidity or primipaternity? Eur J Obstet Gynecol Reprod Biol. 1999;84:37–41.

Robillard PY, Hulsey TC, Dekker GA, Chaouat G. Preeclampsia and human reproduction. An essay of a long term reflection. J Reprod Immunol. 2003;59: 93–100.

Rodgers WH, Matrisian LM, Guidice LC, Dsupin B, Cannon P, Svitek C, Gorstein F, Osteen KG. Patterns of matrix metalloproteinase expression in cycling endometrium imply different functions and regulation by steroid hormones. J Clin Invest. 1994;94: 946–53.

Roh CR, Oh WJ, Yoon BK, Lee JH. Up-regulation of matrix metalloproteinase-9 in human myometrium during labor: a cytokine-mediated process in uterine smooth muscle cells. Mol Hum Reprod. 2000;6: 96–102.

Romero R, Mazor M, Tartakovsky B. Systemic administration of interleukin-1 induces preterm parturition in mice. Am J Obstet Gynecol. 1991;165:969–71.

Romero R, Chaiworapongsa T, Kuivaniemi H, Tromp G. Bacterial vaginosis, the inflammatory response and the risk of preterm birth: a role for genetic epidemiology in the prevention of preterm birth. Am J Obstet Gynecol. 2004;190:1509–19.

Ross MG. Inflammatory mediators weaken the amniotic membrane barrier through disruption of tight junctions. J Physiol. 2011;589:5.

Rouas-Freiss N, LeMaoult J, Moreau P, Dausset J, Carosella ED. HLA-G in transplantation: a relevant molecule for inhibition of graft rejection? Am J Transplant. 2003;3:11–6.

Roussev RG, Stern JJ, Kaider BD. Anti-endothelial cell antibodies: another cause for pregnancy loss? Am J Reprod Immunol. 1998;39:89–95.

Russell P. Inflammatory lesions of the human placenta. I. Clinical significance of acute chorioamnionitis. Am J Diagn Gynecol Obstet. 1979;1:127–37.

Russwurm GP, Mackler AM, Fagoaga OR, Brown WS, Sakala EP, Yellon SM, Nehlsen- Cannarella SL. Soluble human leukocyte antigens, interleukin-6 and interferon-γ during pregnancy. Am J Reprod Immunol. 1998;38:256–62.

Sacks GP, Tudena K, Sargent IL, Redman CWG. Normal pregnancy and preeclampsia both produce inflammatory changes in peripheral blood leukocytes akin to those of sepsis. Am J Obstet Gynecol. 1998;179:80–6.

Sacks G, Sargent I, Redman C. An innate view of human pregnancy. Immunol Today. 1999;20:114–8.

Sadowsky DW, Duffy LB, Axthelm MK, Cook MJ, Witkin SS, Gravett MG, Cassell GH, Novy MJ. Experimental primate model for Mycoplasma hominis chorioamnionitis and preterm labor. J Soc Gynecol Investig. 2002;8(Suppl):A206.

Sadowsky DW, Novy MJ, Witkin SS, Gravett MG. Dexamethasone or interleukin-10 blocks interleukin-1β-induced uterine contractions in pregnant rhesus monkeys. Am J Obstet Gynecol. 2003;188:252–63.

Saito S, Sakai M. Th1/Th2 balance in preeclampsia. J Reprod Immunol. 2003;59:161–73.

Saito S, Nishikawa K, Morii T, Enomoto M, Narita N, Motoyoshi K, Ichijo M. Cytokine production by CD16-CD56 natural killer cells in the human early pregnancy decidua. Int Immunol. 1993;5:559–63.

Saito S, Umekage H, Sakamoto Y, Sakai M, Tanebe K, Sasaki Y, Morikawa H. Increased T- helper-1-type immunity and decreased T helper- 2-type immunity in patients with preeclampsia. Am J Reprod Immunol. 1999;41:297–306.

Saito S, Sasaki Y, Sakai M. CD4+CD25 regulatory T cells in human pregnancy. J Reprod Immunol. 2005;65: 111–20.

Saito S, Nakashima A, Myojo-Higuma S, Shiozaki A. The balance between cytotoxic NK cells and regulatory NK cells in human pregnancy. J Reprod Immunol. 2008;77:14–22.

Saito S, Nakashima A, Shima T, Ito M. Th1/Th2/Th17 and regulatory T-cell paradigm in pregnancy. Am J Reprod Immunol. 2010;63:601–10.

Sakaguchi S. Naturally arising CD4+ regulatory T cells for immunologic self-tolerance and negative control of immune responses. Annu Rev Immunol. 2004;22: 531–62.

Sakai M, Tanebe K, Sasaki Y, Momma K, Yoneda S, Saito S. Evaluation of the tocolytic effect of a selective cyclooxygenase-2 inhibitor in a mouse model of lipopolysaccharide-induced preterm delivery. Mol Hum Reprod. 2001;7:595–602.

Sakai M, Ogawa K, Shiozaki A, Yoneda S, Sasaki Y, Nagata K, Saito S. Serum granulysin is a marker for Th1 type immunity in pre-eclampsia. Clin Exp Immunol. 2004;136:114–9.

Sakata K, Sakata A, Kong L, Dang H, Talal N. Role of Fas/FasL interaction in physiology and pathology: the good and the bad. Clin Immunol Immunopathol. 1998;87:1–7.

Sasaki Y, Miyazaki S, Sakai M, Saito S. CD4+CD25+ regulatory T cells are increased in the human early pregnancy decidua and have immunosuppressive activity. Am J Reprod Immunol. 2003;49:356.

Sasaki Y, Sakai M, Miyazaki S, Higuma S, Shiozaki A, Saito S. Decidual and peripheral blood CD4+CD25+ regulatory T cells in early pregnancy subjects and spontaneous abortion cases. Mol Hum Reprod. 2004;10:347–53.

Scharfe-Nugent A, Corr SC, Carpenter SB, Keogh L, Doyle B, Martin C, Fitzgerald KA, Daly S, O'Leary JJ, O'Neill LA TLR9 provokes inflammation in response to fetal DNA: mechanism for fetal loss in preterm birth and preeclampsia. J Immunol. 2012;188: 5706–12.

Schober L, Radnai D, Schmitt E, Mahnke K, Sohn C, Steinborn A. Term and preterm labor: decreased suppressive activity and changes in composition of the regulatory T-cell pool. Immunol Cell Biol. 2012;90:935–44.

Sedlmayr P, Blaschitz A, Wintersteiger R, Semlitsch M, Hammer A, MacKenzie CR, Walcher W, Reich O, Takikawa O, Dohr G. Localization of indoleamine 2,3-dioxygenase in human female reproductive organs and the placenta. Mol Hum Reprod. 2002;8: 385–91.

Selvaggi L, Lucivero G, Iannone A, dell'Osso A, Loverro G, Antonaci S, Bonomo L, Bettochi S. Analysis of mononuclear cell subsets in pregnancies with intra-uterine growth retardation. Evidence of chronic B-lymphocyte activation. J Perinat Med. 1983;11: 213–7.

Sennstrom MB, Ekman G, Westergren-Thorsson G, Malmstrom A, Bystrom B, Endresen U, Mlambo N, Norman M, Stabi B, Brauner A. Human cervical ripening, an inflammatory process mediated by cytokines. Mol Hum Reprod. 2000;6:375–81.

Shao L, Jacobs AR, Johnson VV, Mayer L. Activation of CD8+ regulatory T cells by human placental trophoblasts. J Immunol. 2005;174:7539–47.

Sharkey AM, King A, Clark DE, Burrows TD, Jokhi PP, Charnock-Jones DS, Loke YW, Smith SK. Localization of leukaemia inhibitory factor and its receptor in human placenta throughout pregnancy. Biol Reprod. 1999;60:335–64.

Shimaoka Y, Hidaka Y, Tada H, Nakamura T, Mitsuda N, Morimoto Y, Murata Y, Amino N. Changes in cytokine production during and after normal pregnancy. Am J Reprod Immunol. 2000;44:143–7.

Silver HM, Sperling RS, St Clair PJ, Gibbs RS. Evidence relating bacterial vaginosis to intraamniotic infection. Am J Obstet Gynecol. 1989;161:808–12.

Simhan HN, Caritis SN, Krohn MA, Martinez de Tejada B, Landers DV, Hillier SL. Decreased cervical proinflammatory cytokines permit subsequent upper genital tract infection during pregnancy. Am J Obstet Gynecol. 2003;189:560–7.

Simon C, Moreno C, Remohi J, Pellicer A. Cytokines and embryo implantation. J Reprod Immunol. 1998;39:117–31.

Sindram-Trujillo AP, Scherjon SA, van Hulst-van Miert PP, Kanhai HHH, Roelen DL, Class FHJ. Comparison of decidual leukocytes following spontaneous vaginal delivery and elective cesarean section in uncomplicated human term pregnancy. J Reprod Immunol. 2003a;62:125–37.

Sindram-Trujillo AP, Scherjon SA, van Hulst-van Miert PP, van Schip JJ, Kanhai HH, Roelen DL, Claas FH. Differential distribution of NK cells in decidua basalis compared with decidua parietalis after uncomplicated human term pregnancy. Hum Immunol. 2003b;64:921–9.

Sinha D, Wlls M, Faulk WP. Immunological studies of human placentae: complement components in pre-eclamptic chorionic villi. Clin Exp Immunol. 1984;56:175–84.

Skinner GR, Turyk ME, Benson CA, Wilbanks GD, Heseltine P, Galpin J, Kaufman R, Goldberg L, Hartley CE, Buchan A. The efficacy and safety of Skinner herpes simplex vaccine towards modulation of herpes genitalis; report of a prospective, double-blind placebo- controlled trial. Med Microbiol Immunol. 1997;186:31–6.

Smith SC, Baker PN, Symonds EM. Placental apoptosis in normal human pregnancy. Am J Obstet Gynecol. 1997;177:57–65.

Somerset DA, Zheng Y, Kilby MD, Sansom DM, Drayson MT. Normal human pregnancy is associated with an elevation in the immune suppressive CD25+CD4+ regulatory T-cell subset. Immunology. 2004;112:38–43.

Southcombe J, Tannetta D, Redman C, Sargent I. The immunomodulatory role of syncytiotrophoblast microvesicles. PLoS One. 2011;6:e20245.

Stallmach T, Hebisch G, Orban P, Lu X. Aberrant positioning of trophoblast and lymphocytes in the feto-maternal interface with pre-eclampsia. Virchows Arch. 1999;434:207–11.

Steiborn A, Geisse M, Kaufmann M. Expression of cytokine receptors in the placenta in term and preterm labor. Placenta. 1998;19:165–70.

Steinborn A, Schmitt E, Kisielewicz A, Rechenberg S, Seissler N, Mahnke K, Schaier M, Zeier M, Sohn C. Pregnancy-associated diseases are characterized by the composition of the systemic regulatory T cell (Treg) pool with distinct subsets of Tregs. Clin Exp Immunol. 2012;167:84–98.

Stewart CL, Kaspar P, Brunet LJ, Bhatt H, Gadi I, Kontgen F, Abbondanzo SJ. Blastocyst implantation depends on maternal expression of leukemia inhibitory factor. Nature. 1992;359:76–9.

Stewart-Akers AM, Krasnow JS, Brekosky J, DeLoia JA. Endometrial leukocytes are altered numerically and functionally in women with implantation defects. Am J Reprod Immunol. 1998;39:1–11.

Stray-Pedersen B, Stray-Pedersen S. Etiologic factors and subsequent reproductive performance in 195 couples with a prior history of habitual abortion. Am J Obstet Gynecol. 1984;148:140–6.

Subit M, Gantt P, Broce M, Seybold DJ, Randall G. Endometriosis-associated infertility: double intrauterine insemination improves fecundity in patients positive for antiendometrial antibodies. Am J Reprod Immunol. 2011;66:100–7.

Szekeres-Bartho J. Immunological relationship between the mother and the foetus. Int Rev Immunol. 2002;21:471–95.

Szekeres-Bartho J, Barakonyi A, Polgar B, Par G, Faust ZS, Palkovics T, Szereday L. The role of γ/δ T cells in progesterone mediated immunomodulation during pregnancy: a review. Am J Reprod Immunol. 1999;42:44–8.

Szekeres-Bartho J, Polgar B, Kelemen K, Par G, Szereday L. Progesterone-mediated immunomodulation and anti-abortive effects: the role of the progesterone-induced blocking factor. Poster presentation. 10th World Congress on the Menopause, Berlin; 10–14 June 2002.

Szekeres-Bartho J, Polgar B, Kozma N, Miko E, Par G, Szereday L, Barakonyi A, Palkovics T, Papp O, Varga P. Progesterone-dependent immunomodulation. Chem Immunol Allergy. 2005;89:118–25.

Szereday L, Varga P, Szekeres-Bartho J. Cytokine production in pregnancy. Am J Reprod Immunol. 1997;38:418–21.

Tachi C, Tachi S, Knyszynski A, Lindner HR. Possible involvement of macrophages in embryo- maternal relationships during ovum implantation in the rat. J Exp Zool. 1981;217:81–92.

Tamura M, Takakuwa K, Arakawa M, Yasuda M, Kazama Y, Tanaka K. Relationship between MLR blocking antibodies and the outcome of the third pregnancy in patients with two consecutive spontaneous abortions. J Perinat Med. 1998;26:49–53.

Taylor RN. Preeclampsia. In: Glasser SR, Aplin JD, Giudice LC, Tabibzadeh S, editors. The endometrium. New York: Taylor & Francis; 2002. p. 604–25.

Taylor RN, Lebovic DI, Hornung D, Mueller MD. Endocrine and paracrine regulation of endometrial angiogenesis. Ann N Y Acad Sci. 2001;943:109–21.

Tedesco F, Radillo O, Candussi G, Nazzaro A, Mollnes TE, Pecorari D. Immunohistochemical detection of terminal complement complex and S protein in normal and pre-eclamptic placentae. Clin Exp Immunol. 1990;80:236–40.

Tedesco F, Pausa M, Nardon E, Narchi G, Bulla R, Livi C, Guaschino S, Meroni PL. Prevalence and biological effects of anti-trophoblast and anti-endothelial cell antibodies in patients with recurrent spontaneous abortions. Am J Reprod Immunol. 1997;38:205–11.

Terranova PF, Hunter VJ, Roby KF, Hunt JS. Tumor necrosis factor-α in the female reproductive tract. Proc Soc Exp Biol Med. 1995;209:325–42.

Terrone DA, Rinehart BK, Granger JP, Barrilleaux PS, Martin Jr JN, Bennett WA. Interleukin- 10 administration and bacterial endotoxin-induced preterm birth in a rat model. Obstet Gynecol. 2001;98:476–80.

Tiller H, Killie MK, Husebekk A, Skogen B, Ni H, Kjeldsen-Kragh J, Oian P. Platelet antibodies and fetal growth: maternal antibodies against fetal platelet antigen 1a are strongly associated with reduced birthweight in boys. Acta Obstet Gynecol Scand. 2012;91:79–86.

Todd HM, Dundoo VL, Gerber WR, Cwiak CA, Baldassare JJ, Hertelendy F. Effect of cytokines on prostaglandin E2 and prostacyclin production in primary cultures of human myometrial cells. J Matern Fetal Med. 1996;5:161–7.

Toder V, Fein A, Carp H, Torchinsky A. TNF-α in pregnancy loss and embryo maldevelopment: a mediator of detrimental stimuli or a protector of the fetoplacental unit? J Assist Reprod Genet. 2003;20:73–81.

Tomazin R, van Schoot NE, Goldsmith K, Jugovic K, Sempe P, Früh K, Johnson DC. Herpes simplex virus type 2 ICP47 inhibits human TAP but not mouse TAP. J Virol. 1998;72:2560–3.

Torchinsky A, Gongadze M, Orenstein H, Savion S, Fein A, Toder V. TNF-alpha acts to prevent occurrence of malformed fetuses in diabetic mice. Diabetologica. 2004;47:32–139.

Torchinsky A, Markert UR, Toder V. TNF-α-mediated stress-induced early pregnancy loss: a possible role of leukaemia inhibitory factor. Chem Immunol Allergy. 2005;89:62–71.

Tramont EC. Inhibition of adherence of Neisseria gonorrhoeae by human genital secretions. J Clin Invest. 1977;59:117–24.

Trundley A, Moffett A. Human uterine leukocytes and pregnancy. Tissue Antigens. 2004;63:1–12.

Ugwumadu A, Manyonda I, Reid F, Hay P. Effect of early oral clindamycin on late miscarriage and preterm delivery in asymptomatic women with abnormal vaginal flora and bacterial vaginosis: a randomised controlled trial. Lancet. 2003;361:983–8.

Uzumcu M, Coskun S, Jaroudi K, Hollanders MG. Effect of human chorionic gonadotropin on cytokine production from human endometrial cells in vitro. Am J Reprod Immunol. 1998;40:83–8.

Van der Meer A, Lukassen HGM, van Lierop MJC, Wijnands F, Mosselman S, Braat DDM, Joosten I. Membrane-bound HLA-G activates proliferation and interferon-γ production by uterine natural killer cells. Mol Hum Reprod. 2004;10:189–95.

Van Voorhis WC, Barrett LK, Sweeney YT, Kuo CC, Patton DL. Repeated Chlamydia trachomatis infection of Macaca nemestrina fallopian tubes produces a Th1-like cytokine response associated with fibrosis and scarring. Infect Immun. 1997;65:2175–82.

Vanderpuye OA, Labarrere CA, McIntyre JA. The complement system in reproduction. Fertil Immunol. 1992;27:145–55.

Varla-Leftherioti M. The significance of the women's repertoire of natural killer cell receptors in the maintenance of pregnancy. Chem Immunol Allergy. 2005; 89:84–95.

Vassiliadis S, Ranella A, Papadimitriou L, Makrygiannakis A, Athanassakis I. Serum levels of pro- and anti-inflammatory cytokines in non-pregnant women, during pregnancy, labor and abortion. Mediators Inflamm. 1998;7:69–72.

Vassiliadou N, Bulmer JN. Immunohistochemical evidence for increased numbers of "classic" CD57+ natural killer cells in the endometrium of women suffering spontaneous early pregnancy loss. Hum Reprod. 1996;11:1569–74.

Vassiliadou N, Bulmer JN. Characterization of endometrial T lymphocyte subpopulations in spontaneous early loss. Hum Reprod. 1998;13:44–7.

Verma S, Hiby SE, Loke YW, King A. Human decidual natural killer cells express the receptor for and respond to the cytokine interleukin 15. Biol Reprod. 2000;62:959–68.

Vinatier D, Dufour P, Cosson M, Houpeau JL. Antiphospholipid syndrome and recurrent miscarriages. Eur J Obstet Gynecol Reprod Biol. 2001; 96:37–50.

Vince GS, Starkey PM, Austgulen R, Kwiatkowski D, Redman CWG. Interleukin-6, tumor necrosis factor and soluble tumor necrosis factor receptors in preeclampsia. Br J Obstet Gynaecol. 1995;102:20–5.

Voisin G, Chaouat G. Demonstration, nature and properties of maternal antibodies fixed on placenta and directed against paternal alloantigens. J Reprod Fertil. 1974;21:89–103.

von Landenberg P, Matthias T, Zaech J, Schultz M, Lorber M, Blank M, Shoenfeld Y. Antiprothrombin antibodies are associated with pregnancy loss in patients with the antiphospholipid syndrome. Am J Reprod Immunol. 2003;49:51–6.

Vrachnis N, Malamas FM, Sifakis S, Tsikouras P, Iliodromiti Z. Immune aspects and myometrial actions of progesterone and CRH in labor. Clin Dev Immunol. 2012;2012:937618.

Walker JJ. Antioxidants and inflammatory cell responses in preeclampsia. Semin Reprod Endocrinol. 1998; 16:47–55.

Wallace K, Richards S, Dhillon P, Weimer A, Edholm ES, Bengten E, Wilson M, Martin Jr JN, LaMarca B. CD4+ T-helper cells stimulated in response to placental ischemia mediate hypertension during pregnancy. Hypertension. 2011;57:949–55.

Walther T, Wallukat G, Jank A, Bartel S, Schultheiss HP, Faber R, Stepan H. Angiotensin II type 1 receptor agonistic antibodies reflect fundamental alterations in the uteroplacental vasculature. Hypertension. 2005;46: 1275–9.

Wang Y, Lewis DF, Adair CD, Gu Y, Mason L, Kipikasa JH. Digibind attenuates cytokine TNFalpha-induced endothelial inflammatory response: potential benefit role of digibind in preeclampsia. J Perinatol. 2009;29: 195–200.

Wang B, Koga K, Osuga Y, Cardenas I, Izumi G, Takamura M, Hirata T, Yoshino O, Hirota Y, Harada M, Mor G, Taketani Y. Toll-like receptor-3 ligation-induced indoleamine 2, 3-dioxygenase expression in human trophoblasts. Endocrinology. 2011;152:4984–92.

Watanabe M, Iwatani Y, Kaneda T, Hidaka Y, Mitsuda N, Morimoto Y, Amino N. Changes in T, B, and NK lymphocyte subsets during and after normal pregnancy. Am J Reprod Immunol. 1997;37:368–77.

Watari M, Watari H, DiSanto ME, Chacko S, Shi GP, Strauss JF. Proinflammatory cytokines induce expression of matrix-metabolizing enzymes in human cervical smooth muscle cells. Am J Pathol. 1999;154: 1755–62.

Weber C, Arck PC, Mazurek B, Klapp BF. Impact of a relaxation training on psychometric and immunologic parameters in tinnitus sufferers. J Psychosom Res. 2002;52:29–33.

Wegmann TG, Lin H, Guilbert L, Mosmann TR. Bidirectional cytokine interactions in the maternal-fetal relationship: is successful pregnancy a TH2 phenomenon? Immunol Today. 1993;14:353–6.

Wells M, Bennett J, Bulmer JN, Jackson P, Holgate CS. Complement component deposition in uteroplacental (spiral) arteries in normal human pregnancy. J Reprod Immunol. 1987;12:125–35.

Wicherek L, Basta P, Sikora J, Galazka K, Rytlewski K, Grabiec M, Lazar A, Kalinka J. RCAS1 decidual immunoreactivity in severe pre-eclampsia: immune cell presence and activity. Am J Reprod Immunol. 2007;58:358–66.

Wilcox AJ, Weinberg CR, O'Connor JF, Baird DD, Schalaterer JP, Canfield RE, Armstong EG, Nisula BC. Incidence of early loss of pregnancy. N Engl J Med. 1988;319:189–94.

Wilczinsky JR. Th1/Th2 cytokines balance-yin and yang of reproductive immunology. Eur J Obstet Gynecol Reprod Biol. 2005;122:136–43.

Wilczynski JR, Tchorzewski H, Banasik M, Glowacka E, Wieczorek A, Lewkowicz P, Malinowski A, Szpakowski M, Wilczynski J. Lymphocyte subset distribution and cytokine secretion in third trimester decidua in normal pregnancy and preeclampsia. Eur J Obstet Gynecol Reprod Biol. 2003;1:8–15.

Wilczynski JR, Radwan P, Tchorzewski H, Banasik M. Immunotherapy of patients with recurrent spontaneous miscarriage and idiopathic infertility: does the immunization-dependent Th2 cytokine overbalance really matter? Arch Immunol Ther Exp (Warsz). 2012;60:151–60.

Wilson R, McInnes I, Leung B, McKillop JH, Walker JJ. Altered interleukin 12 and nitric oxide levels in recurrent miscarriage. Eur J Obstet Gynecol Reprod Biol. 1997;75:211–4.

Wilson R, Moor J, Jenkins C, Miller H, Walker JJ, McLean MA, Norman J, McInnes IB. Abnormal first trimester serum interleukin 18 levels are associated with a poor outcome in women with a history of recurrent miscarriage. Am J Reprod Immunol. 2004;51: 156–9.

Witkin SS, Vardhana S, Yih M, Doh K, Bongiovanni AM, Gerber S. Polymorphism in intron 2 of the fetal interleukin-1 receptor antagonist genotype influences midtrimester amniotic fluid concentrations of interleukin-1b and interleukin-1 receptor antagonist and pregnancy outcome. Am J Obstet Gynecol. 2003;189:1413–7.

Witkin SS, Linhares IM, Bongiovanni AM, Herway C, Skupski D. Unique alterations in infection-induced immune activation during pregnancy. BJOG. 2011;118:145–53.

Witkin SS, Chervenak J, Bongiovanni AM, Herway C, Linhares IM, Skupski D. Influence of mid-trimester amniotic fluid on endogenous and lipopolysaccharide-mediated responses of mononuclear lymphoid cells. Am J Reprod Immunol. 2012;67:28–33.

Wuu YD, Pampfer S, Becquet P, Vanderheyden I, Lee KH, De Hertogh R. Tumor necrosis factor α decreases the viability of mouse blastocysts in vitro and in vivo. Biol Reprod. 1999;60:479–83.

Xie F, Hu Y, Turvey SE, Magee LA, Brunham RM, Choi KC, Krajden M, Leung PC, Money DM, Patrick DM, Thomas E, von Dadelszen P. Toll-like receptors 2 and 4 and the cryopyrin inflammasome in normal pregnancy and pre-eclampsia. BJOG. 2010;117:99–108.

Xu C, Mao D, Holers VM, Palanca B, Cheng AM, Molina H. A critical role for murine complement regulator crry in fetomaternal tolerance. Science. 2000;287: 498–501.

Xu P, Alfaidy N, Challis JR. Expression of matrix metalloproteinase (MMP)-2 and MMP-9 in human placenta and fetal membranes in relation to preterm and term labor. J Clin Endocrinol Metab. 2002;87:1353–61.

Yahata T, Kurabayashi T, Honda A, Takakiuwa K, Tanaka K, Abo T. Decrease in the proportion of granulated CD56+ T-cells in patients with a history of recurrent abortion. J Reprod Immunol. 1998;38:63–73.

Yamada H, Atsumi T, Kato EH, Shimada S, Morikawa M, Minakami H. Prevalence of diverse antiphospholipid antibodies in women with recurrent spontaneous abortion. Fertil Steril. 2003;80:1276–8.

Yamada H, Shimada S, Kato EH, Morikawa M, Iwabushi K, Kishi R, Onoe K, Minakami H. Decrease in a specific killer cell immunoglobulin-like receptor on peripheral natural killer cells in women with recurrent spontaneous abortion of unexplained etiology. Am J Reprod Immunol. 2004;51:241–7.

Yamamoto T, Takahashi Y, Kase N, Mori H. Role of decidual natural killer cells in patients with missed abortion: differences between cases with normal and abnormal chromosome. Clin Exp Immunol. 1999;116:449–52.

Yang D, Chertov O, Bykovskaia SN, Chen Q, Buffo MJ, Shogan J, Anderson M, Schröder JM, Wang JM, Howard OMZ, Oppenheim JJ. β-defensins: linking innate and adaptive immunity through dendritic and T cell CCR6. Science. 1999;286:525–8.

Yang Y, Huang CT, Huang X, Pardoll DM. Persistent Toll-like receptor signals are required for reversal of regulatory T cell-mediated CD8 tolerance. Nat Immunol. 2004;5:508–15.

Yang Z, Kong B, Mosser DM, Zhang X. TLRs, macrophages, and NK cells: our understandings of their functions in uterus and ovary. Int Immunopharmacol. 2011;11:1442–50.

Yoshimura T, Inaba M, Sugiura K, Nakajima T, Ito T, Nakamura K, Kanzaki H, Ikehara S. Analyses of dendritic cell subsets in pregnancy. Am J Reprod Immunol. 2003;50:137–45.

Young A, Thomson AJ, Ledingham MA, Jordan F, Greer IA, Norman JE. Immunolocalization of proinflammatory cytokines in myometrium, cervix, and fetal membranes during human parturition at term. Biol Reprod. 2002;66:445–9.

Young SL, Lyddon TD, Jorgensson RL, Misfeldt ML. Expression of Toll-like receptors in human endometrial ECs and cell lines. Am J Reprod Immunol. 2004;52:67–73.

Zarember KA, Godowski PJ. Tissue expression of human Toll-like receptors and differential regulation of Toll-like receptor mRNAs in leukocytes in response to microbes, their products, and cytokines. J Immunol. 2002;168:554–61.

Zhao HB, Wang C, Li RX, Tang CL, Li MQ, Du MR, Hou XF, Li DJ. E-cadherin, as a negative regulator of invasive behavior of human trophoblast cells, is downregulated by cyclosporin A via epidermal growth factor/extracellular signal-regulated protein kinase signaling pathway. Biol Reprod. 2010;83:370–6.

Zheng ZQ, Qin ZH. Detection of early pregnancy factor-like activity in human amniotic fluid. Am J Reprod Immunol Microbiol. 1990;22:9–11.

Zhou HM, Ramachandran S, Kim JG, Raynor DB, Rock JA, Parthasarathy S. Implications in the management of pregnancy: II. Low levels of gene expression but enhanced uptake and accumulation of umbilical cord glycodelin. Fertil Steril. 2000;73:843–7.

Zhou X, Zhang GY, Wang J, Lu SL, Cao J, Sun LZ. A novel bridge between oxidative stress and immunity: the interaction between hydrogen peroxide and human leukocyte antigen G in placental trophoblasts during preeclampsia. Am J Obstet Gynecol. 2012;206:447. e7–16.

Immunological Infertility

Abrahams VM, Bole-Aldo P, Kim YM, Straszewski-Chavez SL, Chaiworapongsa T, Romero R, Mor G. Divergent trophoblast responses to bacterial products mediated by TLRs. J Immunol. 2004;173:4286–96.

Abrahams VM, Aldo PB, Murphy SP, Visintin I, Koga K, Wilson G, Romero R, Sharma S, Mor G. TLR6 modulates first trimester trophoblast responses to peptidoglycan. J Immunol. 2008;180:6035–43.

Acosta AA, van der Merwe JP, Doncel G, Kruger TF, Sayilgan A, Franken DR, Kolm P. Fertilization efficiency of morphologically abnormal spermatozoa in assisted reproduction is further impaired by antisperm antibodies on the male partner's sperm. Fertil Steril. 1994;62:826–33.

Adeghe AJ. Effect of washing on sperm surface autoantibodies. Br J Urol. 1987;60:360–3.

Ahmed A, Li XF, Shams M, Gregory J, Rollason T, Barnes NM, Newton JR. Localization of the angiotensin II and its receptor subtype expression in human endometrium and identification of a novel high-affinity angiotensin II binding site. J Clin Invest. 1995; 96:848–57.

Akira S. Mammalian Toll-like receptors. Curr Opin Immunol. 2003;15:5–11.

Akira S, Takeda K. Toll-like receptor signaling. Nat Rev Immunol. 2004;4:499–511.

Akiyama M, Okabe H, Takakura K, Fujiyama Y, Noda Y. Expression of macrophage inflammatory protein-1 alpha (MIP-1alpha) in human endometrium throughout the menstrual cycle. Br J Obstet Gynaecol. 1999; 106:725–30.

Akoum A, Jolicoeur C, Boucher A. Estradiol amplifies interleukin-1-induced monocyte chemotactic protein-1 expression by ectopic endometrial cells of women with endometriosis. J Clin Endocrinol Metab. 2000;85:896–904.

Alderete JF, Newton E, Dennis C, Neale KA. Antibody in sera of patients infected with Trichomonas vaginalis is to trichomonal proteinases. Genitourin Med. 1991;67:331–4.

Al-Harthi L, Spear GT, Hashemi FB, Landay A, Sha BE, Roebuck KA. A human immunodeficiency virus (HIV)-inducing factor from the female genital tract activates HIV-1 gene expression through the kappaB enhancer. J Infect Dis. 1998;178:1343–51.

Allison JL, Schust DJ. Recurrent first trimester pregnancy loss: revised definitions and novel causes. Curr Opin Endocrinol Diabetes Obes. 2009;16:446–50.

Alloub MI, Barr BB, McLaren KM, Smith IW, Bunney MH, Smart GE. Human papillomavirus infection and cervical intraepithelial neoplasia in women with renal allografts. BMJ. 1989;298:153–6.

Aoki K, Kajiura S, Matsumoto Y, Ogasawara M, Okada S, Yagami Y, Gleicher N. Preconceptional natural-killer-cell activity as a predictor of miscarriage. Lancet. 1995;345:1340–2.

Backos M, Rai R, Thomas E, Murphy M, Dore C, Regan L. Bone density changes in pregnant women treated with heparin: a prospective, longitudinal study. Hum Reprod. 1999;14:2876–80.

Barrier BF. Immunology of endometriosis. Clin Obstet Gynecol. 2010;53:397–402.

Beer AE. Immunopathologic factors contributing to recurrent spontaneous abortions in humans. Am J Reprod Immunol. 1983;4:182–4.

Beer AE, Semprini AE, Zhu XY, Quebbeman JF. Pregnancy outcome in human couples with recurrent spontaneous abortions: HLA antigen profiles; HLA antigen sharing; female serum MLR blocking factors; and paternal leukocyte immunization. Exp Clin Immunogenet. 1985;2:137–53.

Beer AE, Kwak JYH, Ruiz JE. Immunophenotypic profiles of peripheral blood lymphocytes in women with recurrent pregnancy losses and infertile women with multiple failed in vitro fertilization cycles. Am J Reprod Immunol. 1996;35:376–82.

Benki S, Mostad SB, Richardson BA, Mandaliya K, Kreiss JK, Overbaugh J. Cyclic shedding of HIV-1 RNA in cervical secretions during the menstrual cycle. J Infect Dis. 2004;189:2192–201.

Benoff S, Cooper GW, Hurley I, Mandel FS, Rosenfeld DL. Antisperm antibody binding to human sperm inhibits capacitation induced changes in the levels of plasma membrane sterols. Am J Reprod Immunol. 1993;30:113–30.

Betterle C, Rossi A, Dalla Pria S, Artifoni A, Pedini B, Gavasso S, Caretto A. Premature ovarian failure: autoimmunity and natural history. Clin Endocrinol. 1993;39:35–43.

Bianchi A, Dosquet C, Henry S, Couderc MC, Ferchal F, Scieux C. Chlamydia trachomatis growth stimulates interleukin-8 production by human monocytic U-937 cells. Infect Immun. 1997;65:2434–6.

Blumenstein M, Bowen-Shauver JM, Keelan JA, Mitchell MD. Identification of suppressors of cytokine signaling (SOCS) proteins in human gestational tissue: differential regulation is associated with the onset of labor. J Clin Endocrinol Metab. 2002;87:1094–7.

Bohring C, Krause W. Characterization of spermatozoa surface antigens by antisperm antibodies and its influence on acrosomal exocytosis. Am J Reprod Immunol. 2003a;50:411–9.

Bohring C, Krause W. Immune infertility: towards a better understanding of sperm (auto)- immunity. The value of proteomic analysis. Hum Reprod Update. 2003b;18:915–24.

Bohring C, Krause W. The role of antisperm antibodies during fertilization and for immunological infertility. Chem Immunol Allergy. 2005;88:15–26.

Bohring C, Skrzypek J, Krause W. Influence of antisperm antibodies on the acrosome reaction as determined by flow cytometry. Fertil Steril. 2001;76:275–80.

Bouloux PM, Wass JA, Parslow JM, Hendry WF, Besser GM. Effect of cyclosporine A in male autoimmune infertility. Fertil Steril. 1986;46:81–5.

Boulton IC, Gray-Owen SD. Neisserial binding to CEACAM1 arrests the activation and proliferation of CD4+ T lymphocytes. Nat Immunol. 2002;3:229–36.

Bronson RA, Fusi F, Cooper GW, Phillips DM. Antisperm antibodies induce polyspermy by promoting adherence of human sperm to zona-free hamster eggs. Hum Reprod. 1990;5:690–6.

Brown NL, Alvi SA, Elder MG, Bennett PR, Sullivan MH. The regulation of prostaglandin output from term intact fetal membranes by anti-inflammatory cytokines. Immunology. 2000;99:124–33.

Bubanovic I. 1alpha, 25-dihydroxy-vitamin-D3 as new immunotherapy in treatment of recurrent spontaneous abortion. Med Hypotheses. 2004;63:250–3.

Bulmer JN, Morrison L, Longfellow M, Ritson A, Pace D. Granulated lymphocytes in human endometrium: histochemical and immunohistochemical studies. Hum Reprod. 1991;6:791–8.

Buve A, Weiss H, Laga M, Van Dyck E, Musonda R, Zekeng L, Kahindo M, Anagonou S, Morison L, Robinson NJ, Hayes RJ. The Study Group on Heterogeneity of HIV Epidemics in African Cities. The epidemiology of trichomoniasis in women in four African cities. AIDS. 2001;15 Suppl 4:S89–96.

Calleja-Agius J, Muttukrishna S, Pizzey AR, Jauniaux E. Pro- and antiinflammatory cytokines in threatened miscarriages. Am J Obstet Gynecol. 2011;205:83 e88–16.

Casey ML, Cox SM, Beutler B, Milewich L, MacDonald PC. Cachectin/tumor necrosis factor- alpha formation in human decidua. Potential role of cytokines in infection-induced preterm labor. J Clin Invest. 1989;83:430–6.

Chang TH, Jih MH, Wu TC. Relationship of sperm antibodies in women and men to human in vitro fertilization, cleavage, and pregnancy rate. Am J Reprod Immunol. 1993;30:108–12.

Chaouat G, Lankar D. Vaccination against spontaneous abortion in mice by preimmunization with an anti-idiotypic antibody. Am J Reprod Immunol Microbiol. 1988;16:146–50.

Check JH. The use of heparin for preventing miscarriage. Am J Reprod Immunol. 2012;67:326–33.

Check JH, Bollendorf A, Katsoff D, Kozak J. The frequency of antisperm antibodies in the cervical mucus of women with poor postcoital tests and their effect on pregnancy rates. Am J Reprod Immunol. 1994;32:38–42.

Check JH, Arwitz M, Gross J, Peymer M, Szekeres-Bartho J. Lymphocyte immunotherapy (LI) increases serum levels of progesterone induced blocking factor (PIBF). Am J Reprod Immunol. 1997;37:17–20.

Chernyshov VP, Tumanova LE, Sudoma IA, Bannikov VI. Th1 and Th2 in human IVF pregnancy with allogenic fetus. Am J Reprod Immunol. 2008;59:352–8.

Chiu WWC, Chamley LW. Clinical associations and mechanisms of action of antisperm antibodies. Fertil Steril. 2004;83:529–35.

Choudhury SR, Knapp LA. Human reproductive failure I: immunological factors. Hum Reprod Update. 2000;7:113–34.

Christiansen OB. Intravenous immunoglobulin in the prevention of recurrent spontaneous abortion. The European experience. Am J Reprod Immunol. 1998;39:77–81.

Christiansen OB, Mathieson O, Husth M, Rasmussen KL, Ingerslev HJ, Lauritsen JG, Grunnet N. Placebo-controlled trial of treatment of unexplained secondary recurrent spontaneous abortions and recurrent late spontaneous abortions with i.v. immunoglobulin. Hum Reprod. 1995;10:2690–5.

Christiansen OB, Pedersen B, Rosgaard A, Husth M. A randomized, double-blind, placebo- controlled trial of intravenous immunoglobulin in the prevention of recurrent miscarriage. Evidence for a therapeutic effect in women with secondary miscarriage. Hum Reprod Update. 2002;17:809–16.

Coddington CC, Demochowski R, Oehninger S, Auman JR, Hodgen GD. Hemizona assay: evaluation of fertility potential in patients with vasectomy reversal. Arch Androl. 1997;38:143–50.

Colucci F, Boulenouar S, Kieckbusch J, Moffett A. How does variability of immune system genes affect placentation? Placenta. 2011;32:539–45.

Coulam CB, Roussev RG. Correlation of NK cell activation and inhibition markers with NK cytoxicity among women experiencing immunologic implantation failure after in vitro fertilization and embryo transfer. J Assist Reprod Genet. 2003;20:58–62. 264.

Coulam CB, Adamson SC, Annegers JF. Incidence of premature ovarian failure. Obstet Gynecol. 1986;67: 604–6. 262.

Crosignani PG, Rubin BL. Male infertility update. The ESHRE Capri Workshop Group. Hum Reprod. 1998;13:2025–32.

Cunningham DS, Fulgham DL, Rayl DL, Hansen KA, Alexander NJ. Antisperm antibodies to sperm surface antigens in women with genital tract infection. Am J Obstet Gynecol. 1991;164:791–6.

Dai Z, Nasr Reel M, Deng S, Diggs L, Larsen CP, Rothstein DM, Lakkis FG. Impaired recall of CD8 memory T cells in immunologically privileged tissue. J Immunol. 2005;174:1165–70.

Daitoh T, Kamada M, Yamano S, Murayama S, Kobayashi T, Maegawa M. High implantation rate and consequently high pregnancy rate by in vitro fertilization-embryo transfer treatment in infertile women with antisperm antibody. Fertil Steril. 1995;63:87–91.

Dal Pra C, Chen S, Furmaniak J, Smith BR, Pedini B, Moscon A, Zanchetta R, Betterle C. Autoantibodies to steroidogenic enzymes in patients with premature ovarian failure with and without Addison's disease. Eur J Endocrinol. 2003;148:565–70.

Damewood MD, Zacur HA, Hoffman GJ, Rock JA. Circulating antiovarian antibodies in premature ovarian failure. Obstet Gynecol. 1986;68:850–4.

Davidson EJ, Kitchener HC, Stern PL. The use of vaccines in the prevention and treatment of cervical cancer. Clin Oncol. 2002;14:193–200.

De Almeida M, Gazagne I, Jeulin C, Herry M, Belaisch-Allart J, Frydman R, Jouannet P, Testart J. In-vitro processing of sperm with autoantibodies and in-vitro fertilization results. Hum Reprod. 1989;4:49–53.

Defranco EA, Jacobs TS, Plunkett J, Chaudhari BP, Huettner PC, Muglia LJ. Placental pathologic aberrations in cases of familial idiopathic spontaneous preterm birth. Placenta. 2011;32:386–90.

Diekman AB, Norton EJ, Klotz KL, Westbrook YA, Shibahara H, Naaby-Hansen S, Flickinger CJ, Herr JC. N-linked glycan of a sperm CD52 glycoprotein associated with human infertility. FASEB J. 1999;13:1301–13.

El Demiry MI, Hargreave TB, Busuttil A, Elton R, James K, Chisholm GD. Immunocompetent cells in human testis in health and disease. Fertil Steril. 1987;48: 470–9.

Eley A, Pacey AA, Galdiero M, Galdiero M, Galdiero F. Can Chlamydia trachomatis directly damage your sperm? Lancet Infect Dis. 2005;5:53–7.

El-Roeiy A, Gleicher N. Definition of normal autoantibody levels in an apparently healthy population. Obstet Gynecol. 1988;72:596–602.

El-Zibdeh MY. Dehydrogesterone in the reduction of recurrent spontaneous abortion. J Steroid Biochem Mol Biol. 2005;97:431–4.

Fernekorn U, Kruse A. Regulation of leukocyte recruitment to the murine maternal/fetal interface. Chem Immunol Allergy. 2005;89:105–17.

Filippini A, Riccioli A, Padula F, Lauretti P, D'Alessio A, De Cesaris P, Gandini L, Lenzi A, Ziparo E. Control and impairment of immune privilege in the testis and in semen. Hum Reprod Update. 2001;7:444–9.

Foresta C, Varotto A, Caretto A. Immunomagnetic method to select human sperm without sperm surface-bound autoantibodies in male autoimmune infertility. Arch Androl. 1990;24:221–5.

Forsum U, Holst E, Larsson PG, Vasquez A, Jakobsson T, Mattsby-Baltzer I. Bacterial vaginosis-a microbiological and immunological enigma. APMIS. 2005;113:81–90.

Fukui A, Fujii S, Yamaguchi E, Kimura H, Sato S, Saito Y. Natural killer cell subpopulations and cytotoxicity for infertile patients undergoing in vitro fertilization. Am J Reprod Immunol. 1999;41:413–22.

Gafter U, Sredni B, Segal J, Kalechman Y. Suppressed cell-mediated immunity and monocyte and natural killer cell activity following allogeneic immunization of women with spontaneous recurrent abortion. J Clin Immunol. 1997;17:408–19.

Geva E, Amit A, Lerner-Geva L, Azem F, Yovel I, Lessing JB. Autoimmune disorders: another possible cause for in-vitro fertilization and embryo transfer failure. Hum Reprod. 1995;10:2560–3.

Geva E, Lessing JB, Lerner-Geva L, Azem F, Yovel I, Amit A. The presence of antithyroid antibodies in euthyroid patients with unexplained infertility and tubal obstruction. Am J Reprod Immunol. 1997;37: 184–6.

Gleicher N. Autoantibodies in infertility: current opinion. Hum Reprod Update. 1998;4:169–76.

Gleicher N. Reproductive failure prior to the onset of clinical autoimmune disease. Rheumatology. 1999;38:485–7.

Gleicher N, Pratt D, Dudkiewicz A. What do we really know about autoantibody abnormalities and reproductive failure: a critical review. Autoimmunity. 1993;16:115–40.

Goldberg E, VandeBerg JL, Mahony MC, Doncel GF. Immune response of male baboons to testis-specific LDH-C4. Contraception. 2001;64:93–8.

Gonzales GF, Muñoz G, Sánchez R, Henkel R, Gallegos-Avila G, Diaz-Gutierrez O, Vigil P, Vásquez F, Kortebani G, Mazzolli A, Bustos-Obregon B. Update on the impact of Chlamydia trachomatis infection on male infertility. Andrologia. 2004;36:1–23.

Graphou O, Chioti A, Pantazi A, Tsukoura C, Kontopoulou V, Guorgiadou E, Balafoutas C, Koussoulakos S, Margaritis LH, Varla-Leftherioti M. Effect of intravenous immunoglobulin treatment on the Th1/Th2 balance in women with recurrent spontaneous abortions. Am J Reprod Immunol. 2003;49:21–9.

Gruber CJ, Huber JC. The role of dehydrogesterone in recurrent (habitual) abortion. J Steroid Biochem Mol Biol. 2005;97:426–30.

Gupta S, Goldberg JM, Aziz N, Goldberg E, Krajcir N, Agarwal A. Pathogenic mechanisms in endometriosis-associated infertility. Fertil Steril. 2008;90:247–57.

Haas Jr GG, Manganiello P. A double-blind, placebo-controlled study of the use of methylprednisolone in infertile men with sperm-associated immunoglobulins. Fertil Steril. 1987;47:295–301.

Haller K, Mathieu C, Rull K, Matt K, Bene MC, Uibo R. IgG, IgA and IgM antibodies against FSH: serological markers of pathogenic autoimmunity or of normal immunoregulation? Am J Reprod Immunol. 2005;54:262–9.

Hamatani T, Tanabe K, Kamei K, Sakai N, Yamamoto Y, Yoshimura Y. A monoclonal antibody to human SP-10 inhibits in vitro the binding of human sperm to hamster oolemma but not human zona pellucida. Biol Reprod. 2000;62:1201–8.

Han CS, Mulla MJ, Brosens JJ, Chamley LW, Paidas MJ, Lockwood CJ, Abrahams VM. Aspirin and heparin effect on basal and antiphospholipid antibody modulation of trophoblast function. Obstet Gynecol. 2011;118:1021–8.

Head JR, Neaves WB, Billingham RE. Immune privilege in the testis. I. Basic parameters of allograft survival. Transplantation. 1983;36:423–31.

Hedger MP. Testicular leukocytes: what are they doing? Rev Reprod. 1997;2:38–47.

Hedger MP. Macrophages and the immune responsiveness of the testis. J Reprod Immunol. 2002;57:19–34.

Hedger MP, Meinhardt A. Cytokines and the immune-testicular axis. J Reprod Immunol. 2003;58:1–26.

Heidenreich A, Bonfig R, Wilbert DM, Strohmaier WL, Engelmann UH. Risk factors for antisperm antibodies in infertile men. Am J Reprod Immunol. 1994;31:69–76.

Helmerhorst FM, Finken MJ, Erwich JJ. Antisperm antibodies: detection assays for antisperm antibodies: what do they test? Hum Reprod. 1999;14:1669–71.

Hirano M, Kamada M, Maegawa M, Gima H, Aono T. Binding of human secretory leukocyte protease inhibitor in uterine cervical mucus to immunoglobulins: pathophysiology in immunologic infertility and local immune defense. Fertil Steril. 1999;71:1108–14.

Hjort H. Do autoantibodies to sperm reduce fecundity? A mini review in historical perspective. Am J Reprod Immunol. 1998;40:215–22.

Ito K, Tanaka T, Tsutsumi N, Obata F, Kashiwagi N. Possible mechanisms of immunotherapy for maintaining pregnancy in recurrent spontaneous aborters: analysis of anti-idiotypic antibodies directed against autologous T-cell receptors. Hum Reprod. 1999;14:650–5.

Jablonowska B, Selbing A, Palfi M, Ernerudh J, Kjellberg S, Lindton B. Prevention of recurrent spontaneous abortion by intravenous immunoglobulin: a double-blind, placebo-controlled study. Hum Reprod. 1999;14:838–41.

Jablonowska B, Palfi M, Ernerudh J, Kjellberg S, Selbing A. Blocking antibodies in blood from patients with recurrent spontaneous abortion in relation to pregnancy outcome and intravenous immunoglobulin treatment. Am J Reprod Immunol. 2001;45:226–31.

Jablonowska B, Palfi M, Matthiesen L, Selbing A, Kjellberg S, Ernerudh J. T and B lymphocyte subsets in patients with unexplained recurrent spontaneous abortion: IVIG versus placebo treatment. Am J Reprod Immunol. 2002;48:312–8.

Jager S, Kremer J, Kuiken J, Mulder I. The significance of the Fc part of antispermatozoal antibodies for the shaking phenomenon in the sperm-cervical mucus contact test. Fertil Steril. 1981;36:792–7.

Jerzak M, Rechberger T, Baranowski W, Semczuk M. Immunotherapy as an effective treatment of recurrent spontaneous abortion-own experience. Ginekol Pol. 2003;74:1107–11.

Jung WW, Chun T, Sul D, Hwang KW, Kang HS, Lee DJ, Han IK. Strategies against human papillomavirus infection and cervical cancer. J Microbiol. 2004;42:255–66.

Kaider AS, Kaider BD, Janowicz PB, Roussev RG. Immunodiagnostic evaluation in women with reproductive failure. Am J Reprod Immunol. 1999;42:335–46.

Kalinka J, Radwan M. The impact of dehydrogesterone supplementation on serum cytokine profile in women with threatened abortion. Am J Reprod Immunol. 2006;55:115–21.

Kallen CB, Arici A. Immune testing in infertility practice: truth or deception? Curr Opin Obstet Gynecol. 2003;15:225–31.

Kamada M, Daitoh T, Mori K, Maeda N, Hirano K, Irahara M, Aono T, Mori T. Etiological implication of autoantibodies to zona pellucida in human female infertility. Am J Reprod Immunol. 1992;28:104–9.

Kaplan P, Naz RK. The fertilization antigen-1 does not have proteolytic/acrosin activity, but its monoclonal antibody inhibits sperm capacitation and acrosome reaction. Fertil Steril. 1992;58:396–402.

Keck C, Gerber-Schafer C, Clad A, Wilhelm C, Breckwoldt M. Seminal tract infections: impact on male fertility and treatment options. Hum Reprod Update. 1998;4:891–903.

Kelkar RL, Meherji PK, Kadam SS, Gupta SK, Nandedkar TD. Circulation of auto-antibodies against zona pellucida and thyroid microsomal antigen in women with premature ovarian failure. J Reprod Immunol. 2005;66:53–67.

Kern S, Robertson SA, Mau VJ, Maddocks S. Cytokine secretion by macrophages in the rat testis. Biol Reprod. 1995;53:1407–16.

Koide SS, Wang L, Kamada M. Antisperm antibodies associated with infertility: properties and encoding genes of target antigens. Proc Soc Exp Biol Med. 2000;224:123–32.

Krause W. Leitlinie immunologische Infertilität. J Dtsch Dermatol Ges. 2005;3:650–5.

Krause W, Bohring C. Male infertility and genital chlamydial infection: victim or perpetrator? Andrologia. 2003;35:209–16.

Kwak JYH, Beaman KD, Gilman-Sachs A, Ruiz JE, Schewitz D, Beer AE. Up-regulated expression of CD56+, CD56+/CD16+, and CD19+ cells in peripheral blood lymphocytes in pregnant women with recurrent pregnancy loss. Am J Reprod Immunol. 1995;34:93–9.

Kwak JYH, Kwak FMY, Ainbinder SW, Ruiz AM, Beer AE. Elevated peripheral blood natural killer cells are effectively downregulated by immunoglobulin G infusion in women with recurrent spontaneous abortions. Am J Reprod Immunol. 1996;35:363–9.

Kwak JYH, Gilman-Sachs A, Moretti M, Beaman KD, Beer AE. Natural killer cell cytotoxicity and paternal lymphocyte immunization in women with recurrent spontaneous abortions. Am J Reprod Immunol. 1998;40:352–8.

Kwak-Kim J, Gilman-Sachs A. Clinical implication of natural killer cells and reproduction. Am J Reprod Immunol. 2008;59:388–400.

Lahteenmaki A, Reima I, Hovatta O. Treatment of severe male immunological infertility by intracytoplasmic sperm injection. Hum Reprod. 1995;10:2824–8.

Laird SM, Tuckerman EM, Cork BA, Linjawi S, Blakemore AIF, Li TC. A review of immune cells and molecules in women with recurrent miscarriage. Hum Reprod Update. 2003;9:163–74.

Laisk T, Peters M, Saare M, Haller-Kikkatalo K, Karro H, Salumets A. Association of CCR5, TLR2, TLR4 and MBL genetic variations with genital tract infections and tubal factor infertility. J Reprod Immunol. 2010;87:74–81.

Laskin CA, Bombardier C, Hannah ME, Mandel FP, Ritchie JW, Farewell V, Farine D, Spitzer K, Fielding L, Soloninka CA, Yeung M. Prednisone and aspirin in women with autoantibodies and unexplained recurrent fetal loss. N Engl J Med. 1997;337:148–53.

Li MQ, Tang CL, Du MR, Fan DX, Zhao HB, Xu B, Li DJ. CXCL12 controls over-invasion of trophoblasts via upregulating CD82 expression in DSCs at maternal-fetal interface of human early pregnancy in a paracrine manner. Int J Clin Exp Pathol. 2011;4:276–86.

Li LP, Fang YC, Dong GF, Lin Y, Saito S. Depletion of invariant NKT cells reduces inflammation-induced preterm delivery in mice. J Immunol. 2012;188:4681–9.

Lin QD, Qiu LH. Pathogenesis, diagnosis, and treatment of recurrent spontaneous abortion with immune type. Front Med China. 2010;4:275–9.

Luborsky J. Ovarian autoimmune disease and ovarian autoantibodies. J Womens Health Gend Based Med. 2002;11:585–99.

Macdonald GJ. Maintenance of pregnancy in ovariectomized rats with steroid analogs and the reproductive ability of the progeny. Biol Reprod. 1982;27:261–7.

Mahony MC, Blackmore PF, Bronson RA, Alexander NJ. Inhibition of human sperm-zona pellucida tight binding in the presence of antisperm antibody positive polyclonal patient sera. J Reprod Immunol. 1991;19:287–301.

Marin-Briggiler CI, Vazquez-Levin MH, Gonzalez-Echeverria F, Blaquier JA, Miranda PV, Tezon JG. Effect of antisperm antibodies present in follicular fluid upon acrosome reaction and sperm-zona pellucida interaction. Am J Reprod Immunol. 2003;50:209–19.

Masuko-Hongo K, Hayashi K, Yonamine K, Tokuyama M, Nishioka K, Kato T. Disappearance of clonally expanded T cells after allogeneic leukocyte immunotherapy in peripheral blood of patients with habitual abortion. Hum Immunol. 2001;62:1111–21.

Mazumdar S, Levine AS. Antisperm antibodies: etiology, pathogenesis, diagnosis and treatment. Fertil Steril. 1998;70:799–810.

McIntyre JA. Antiphospholipid antibodies in implantation failure. Am J Reprod Immunol. 2003;49:221–9.

Meng YH, Shao J, Li H, Hou YL, Tang CL, Du MR, Li MQ, Li DJ. CsA improves the trophoblasts invasiveness through strengthening the cross-talk of trophoblasts and decidual stromal cells mediated by CXCL12 and CD82 in early pregnancy. Int J Clin Exp Pathol. 2012;5:299–307.

Menge AC, Beitner O. Interrelationships among semen characteristics, antisperm antibodies, and cervical mucus penetration assays in infertile human couples. Fertil Steril. 1989;51:486–92.

Menge AC, Ohl DA, Christman GM, Naz RK. Fertilization antigen (FA-1) removes antisperm autoantibodies from sperm of infertile men resulting in increased rates of acrosome reaction. Fertil Steril. 1999;71:256–60.

Mettler L, Bachmann J, Schmutzler A. High prevalence of markers for immunological disorders in IVF patients. Int J Gynaecol Obstet. 2004;86:59–60.

Meyer WR, Lavy G, DeCherney AH, Visintin I, Economy K, Luborsky JL. Evidence of gonadal and gonadotropin antibodies in women with a suboptimal ovarian response to exogenous gonadotropin. Obstet Gynecol. 1990;75:795–9.

Monga M, Roberts JA. Sperm agglutination by bacteria: receptor-specific interactions. J Androl. 1994;15:151–6.

Monnier-Barbarino P, Forges T, Faure GC, Bene MC. Gonadal antibodies interfering with female reproduction. Best Pract Res Clin Endocrinol Metab. 2005;19:135–48.

Morikawa M, Yamada H, Kato EH, Shimada S, Kishi T, Yamada T, Kobashi G, Fujimoto S. Massive intravenous immunoglobulin treatment in women with four or more recurrent spontaneous abortions of unexplained etiology: down-regulation of NK cell activity and subsets. Am J Reprod Immunol. 2001;46:399–404.

Myles DG, Primakoff P. Sperm proteins that serve as receptors for the zona pellucida and their posttesticular modification. Ann N Y Acad Sci. 1991;637:486–91.

Myles DG, Kimmel LH, Blobel CP, White JM, Primakoff P. Identification of a binding site in the disintegrin domain of fertilin required for sperm-egg fusion. Proc Natl Acad Sci U S A. 1994;91:4195–8.

Myogo K, Yamano S, Nakagawa K, Kamada M, Maegawa M, Irahara M, Aono T. Sperm- immobilizing antibodies block capacitation in human spermatozoa. Arch Androl. 2001;47:135–42.

Nagy ZP, Verheyen G, Liu J, Joris H, Janssenseillen C, Wisanto A, Devroey P, Van Steirteghem AC. Results of 55 intracytoplasmic sperm injection cycles in the treatment of male- immunological infertility. Hum Reprod. 1995;10:1775–80.

Nakashima A, Shima T, Inada K, Ito M, Saito S. The balance of the immune system between T cells and NK cells in miscarriage. Am J Reprod Immunol. 2012;67:304–10.

Naz RK. Molecular and immunological characteristics of sperm antigens involved in egg binding. J Reprod Immunol. 2002;53:13–23.

Naz RK. Modalities for treatment of antisperm antibodies mediated infertility: novel perspectives. Am J Reprod Immunol. 2004;51:390–7.

Negishi Y, Wakabayashi A, Shimizu M, Ichikawa T, Kumagai Y, Takeshita T, Takahashi H. Disruption of maternal immune balance maintained by innate DC subsets results in spontaneous pregnancy loss in mice. Immunobiology. 2012;217:951–61.

Norton MT, Fortner KA, Oppenheimer KH, Bonney EA. Evidence that CD8 T-cell homeostasis and function remain intact during murine pregnancy. Immunology. 2010;131:426–37.

Novotny SR, Wallace K, Heath J, Moseley J, Dhillon P, Weimer A, Wallukat G, Herse F, Wenzel K, Martin Jr JN, Dechend R, Lamarca B. Activating autoantibodies to the angiotensin II type I receptor play an important role in mediating hypertension in response to adoptive transfer of CD4+ T lymphocytes from placental ischemic rats. Am J Physiol Regul Integr Comp Physiol. 2012;302:R1197–201.

Omu AE, Makhseed M, Mohammed AT, Munim RA. Characteristics of men and women with circulating antisperm antibodies in a combined infertility clinic in Kuwait. Arch Androl. 1997;39:55–64.

Omwandho CA, Tinneberg HR, Tumbo-Oeri AG, Roberts TK, Falconer J. Recurrent pregnancy losses and the role of immunotherapy. Arch Gynecol Obstet. 2000;264:3–12.

Orgad S, Loewenthal R, Gazit E, Sadetzki S, Novikov I, Carp H. The prognostic value of anti- paternal antibodies and leukocyte immunizations on the proportion of live births in couples with consecutive recurrent miscarriages. Hum Reprod. 1999;14:2974–9.

Ozcimen EE, Kiyici H, Uckuyu A, Yanik FF. Are CD57+ natural killer cells really important in early pregnancy failure? Arch Gynecol Obstet. 2009;279:493–7.

Pandey MK, Agrawal S. Induction of MLR-Bf and protection of fetal loss: a current double blind randomized trial of paternal lymphocyte immunization for women with recurrent spontaneous abortion. Int Immunopharmacol. 2004;4:289–98.

Pandey MK, Saxena V, Agrawal S. Characterization of mixed lymphocyte reaction blocking antibodies (MLR-Bf) in human pregnancy. BMC Pregnancy Childbirth. 2003;3:2.

Pandey MK, Thakur S, Agrawal S. Lymphocyte immunotherapy and its probable mechanism in the maintenance of pregnancy in women with recurrent spontaneous abortion. Arch Gynecol Obstet. 2004;269:161–72.

Pandey MK, Rani R, Agrawal S. An update in recurrent spontaneous abortion. Arch Gynecol Obstet. 2005;272:95–108.

Park DW, Lee HJ, Park CW, Hong SR, Kwak-Kim J, Yang KM. Peripheral blood NK cells reflect changes in decidual NK cells in women with recurrent miscarriages. Am J Reprod Immunol. 2010;63:173–80.

Pelletier RM, Byers SW. The blood-testis barrier and Sertoli cell junctions: structural considerations. Microsc Res Tech. 1992;20:3–33.

Perricone R, De Carolis C, Giacomelli R, Guarino MD, De Sanctis G, Fontana L. GM-CSF and pregnancy: evidence of significantly reduced blood concentrations in unexplained recurrent abortion efficiently reverted by intravenous immunoglobulin treatment. Am J Reprod Immunol. 2003;50:232–7.

Perricone R, Di Muzio G, Perricone C, Giacomelli R, De Nardo D, Fontana L, De Carolis C High levels of peripheral blood NK cells in women suffering from recurrent spontaneous abortion are reverted from high-dose intravenous immunoglobulins. Am J Reprod Immunol. 2006;55:232–9.

Pichler J, Gerstmayr M, Szepfalusi Z, Urbanek R, Peterlik M, Willheim M. 1 alpha, 25(OH)2D3 inhibits not only Th1 but also Th2 differentiation in human cord blood T cells. Pediatr Res. 2002;52:12–8.

Porter T, Lacoursiere Y, Scott J. Immunotherapy for recurrent miscarriage. Cochrane Database Syst Rev. 2006;19:CD000112.

Putowski L, Darmochwal-Kolarz D, Rolinski J, Oleszczuk J, Jakowicki J. The immunological profile of infertile women after repeated IVF failure (preliminary study). Eur J Obstet Gynecol Reprod Biol. 2004;10:192–6.

Raghupathy R, Mutawa EA, Makhseed M, Azizieh F, Szekeres-Bartho J. Modulation of cytokine production by dehydrogesterone in lymphocytes from women with recurrent miscarriage. BJOG. 2005;112:1096–101.

Rai R, Cohen H, Dave M, Regan L. Randomised controlled trial of aspirin and aspirin plus heparin in pregnant women with recurrent miscarriage associated with phospholipid antibodies (or antiphospholipid antibodies). BMJ. 1997;314:253–7.

Reimand K, Talja I, Metsküla K, Kadastik Ü, Matt K, Uibo R. Autoantibody studies of female patients with reproductive failure. J Reprod Immunol. 2001;51:167–76.

Rigal D, Vermot-Desroches C, Heitz S, Bernaud J, Alfonsi F, Monier JC. Effects of intravenous immunoglobulins (IVIG) on peripheral blood B, NK, and T cell subpopulation in women with recurrent spontaneous abortions: specific effects on LFA-1 and CD56 molecules. Clin Immunol Immunopathol. 1994;71:309–14.

Robertson SA. Immune regulation of conception and embryo implantation-all about quality control? J Reprod Immunol. 2010;85:51–7.

Robertson SA, Guerin LR, Moldenhauer LM, Hayball JD. Activating T regulatory cells for tolerance in early pregnancy – the contribution of seminal fluid. J Reprod Immunol. 2009;83:109–16.

Rogenhofer N, Ochsenkuhn R, von Schonfeldt V, Assef RB, Thaler CJ. Antitrophoblast antibodies are associated with recurrent miscarriages. Fertil Steril. 2012;97:361–6.

Sainio-Pöllänen S, Saari T, Simell O, Pöllänen P. CD-28-CD80/CD86 interactions in testicular immunoregulation. J Reprod Immunol. 1996;31:145–63.

Saito S, Nakashima A, Shima T. Future directions of studies for recurrent miscarriage associated with immune etiologies. J Reprod Immunol. 2011;90:91–5.

Sanocka D, Fraczek M, Jedrzejczak P, Szumala-Kakol A, Kurpisz M. Male genital tract infection: an influence on leukocytes and bacteria on semen. J Reprod Immunol. 2004;62:111–24.

Sanocka-Maciejewska D, Ciupinska M, Kurpisz M. Bacterial infection and semen quality. J Reprod Immunol. 2005;67:51–6.

Scharfe-Nugent A, Corr SC, Carpenter SB, Keogh L, Doyle B, Martin C, Fitzgerald KA, Daly S, O'Leary JJ, O'Neill LA. TLR9 provokes inflammation in response to fetal DNA: mechanism for fetal loss in preterm birth and preeclampsia. J Immunol. 2012;188:5706–12.

Schuppe HC. Testikuläre Entzündungsreaktionen bei Fertilitätsstörungen des Mannes. Habilitationsschrift Justus-Liebig-Universität Giessen, 2002.

Schuppe HC, Meinhardt A. Immune privilege and inflammation of the testis. Chem Immunol Allergy. 2005;88:1–14.

Sher G, Matzner W, Feinman M, Maassarani G, Zouves C, Chong P, Ching W. The selective use of heparin/aspirin therapy alone, or in combination with intravenous immunoglobulin G, in the management of anti-phospholipid antibody-positive women undergoing in vitro fertilization. Am J Reprod Immunol. 1998;40:74–82.

Shibahara H, Shigeta M, Toji H, Koyama K. Sperm immobilizing antibodies interfere with sperm migration from the uterine cavity through the fallopian tubes. Am J Reprod Immunol. 1995;34:120–4.

Shibahara H, Hirano Y, Takamizawa S, Sato I. Effect of sperm-immobilizing antibodies bound to the surface of ejaculated human spermatozoa on sperm motility in immunologically infertile men. Fertil Steril. 2003a;79:641–2.

Shibahara H, Shiraishi Y, Hirano Y, Suzuki T, Takamizawa S, Suzuki M. Diversity of the inhibitory effects on fertilization by anti-sperm antibodies bound to the surface of ejaculated human sperm. Hum Reprod. 2003b;18:1469–73.

Shibahara H, Shiraishi Y, Suzuki M. Diagnosis and treatment of immunologically infertile males with anti-sperm antibodies. Reprod Med Biol. 2005;4:133–41.

Simon A, Laufer N. Repeated implantation failure: clinical approach. Fertil Steril. 2012;97:1039–43.

Smith ML, Schust DJ. Endocrinology and recurrent early pregnancy loss. Semin Reprod Med. 2011;29:482–90.

Stephenson MD, Dreher K, Houlihan E, Wu V. Prevention of unexplained recurrent spontaneous abortion using intravenous immunoglobulin: a prospective, randomized, double- blinded, placebo-controlled trial. Am J Reprod Immunol. 1998;39:82–8.

Stricker RB, Winger EE. Update on treatment of immunologic abortion with low-dose intravenous immunoglobulin. Am J Reprod Immunol. 2005;54:390–6.

Stricker RB, Steinleitner A, Bookoff CN, Weckstein LN, Winger EE. Successful treatment of immunologic abortion with low-dose intravenous immunoglobulin. Fertil Steril. 2000;73:536–40.

Stricker RB, Steinleitner A, Winger EE. Intravenous immunoglobulin therapy for immunologic abortion. Clin Appl Immunol Rev. 2002;2:187–99.

Subit M, Gantt P, Broce M, Seybold DJ, Randall G. Endometriosis-associated infertility: double intrauterine insemination improves fecundity in patients positive for antiendometrial antibodies. Am J Reprod Immunol. 2011;66:100–7.

Szarka A, Rigo Jr J, Lazar L, Beko G, Molvarec A. Circulating cytokines, chemokines and adhesion molecules in normal pregnancy and preeclampsia determined by multiplex suspension array. BMC Immunol. 2010;11:59.

Taylor C, Faulk WP. Prevention of recurrent abortion with leucocyte transfusions. Lancet. 1981;2:68–70.

Taylor PV, Campbell JM, Scott JS. Presence of autoantibodies in women with unexplained infertility. Am J Obstet Gynecol. 1989;161:377–9.

The German RSA/IVIG Group. Intravenous immunoglobulin in the prevention of recurrent miscarriage. Br J Obstet Gynaecol. 1994;101:1072–7.

Thum MY, Bhaskaran S, Abdalla HI, Ford B, Sumar N, Shehata H, Bansal AS. An increase in the absolute count of CD56dimCD16+CD69+ NK cells in the peripheral blood is associated with a poorer IVF treatment and pregnancy outcome. Hum Reprod. 2004;19:2395–400.

Tincani A, Branch W, Levy RA, Piette JC, Carp H, Rai RS, Khamashta M, Shoenfeld Y. Treatment of pregnant patients with antiphospholipid syndrome. Lupus. 2003;12:524–9.

Ulcova-Gallova Z. Antiphospholipid antibodies and reproductive failure. Chem Immunol Allergy. 2005;88:139–49.

Van der Merwe JP, Kruger TF, Windt ML, Hulme VA, Menkveld R. Treatment of male sperm autoimmunity by using the gamete intrafallopian transfer procedure with washed spermatozoa. Fertil Steril. 1990;53:682–7.

Van Voorhis BJ, Stovall DW. Autoantibodies and infertility: a review of the literature. J Reprod Immunol. 1997;33:239–56.

Vissenberg R, Goddijn M. Is there a role for assisted reproductive technology in recurrent miscarriage? Semin Reprod Med. 2011;29:548–56.

Wallace K, Richards S, Dhillon P, Weimer A, Edholm ES, Bengten E, Wilson M, Martin Jr JN, LaMarca B. CD4+ T-helper cells stimulated in response to placental ischemia mediate hypertension during pregnancy. Hypertension. 2011;57:949–55.

Wei SG, Wang LF, Miao SY, Zong SD, Koide SS. Fertility studies with antisperm antibodies. Arch Androl. 1994;32:251–62.

Windt ML, Menkveld R, Kruger TF, Van Der Merwe JP, Van Zyl JA. Effect of sperm washing and swim-up on antibodies bound to sperm membrane: use of immunobead/sperm cervical mucus contact tests. Arch Androl. 1989;22:55–9.

Witkin SS. Circulating antibodies to Chlamydia trachomatis in women: relationship to antisperm and antichlamydial antibodies in semen of male partners. Hum Reprod. 1996;11:1635–7.

Witkin SS. Immunological aspects of genital chlamydia infections. Best Pract Res Clin Obstet Gynaecol. 2002;16:865–74.

Witkin SS, Viti D, David SS, Stangel J, Rosenwaks Z. Relation between antisperm antibodies and the rate of fertilization of human oocytes in vitro. J Assist Reprod Genet. 1992;9:9–13.

Würfel W. Immuntherapie bei wiederholten Aborten and ART-Versagern. München: Medifact- publishing; 2003.

Würfel W, Fiedler K, Krüsmann G, Smolka B, von Hertwig I. Verbesserung der Behandlungsergebnisse durch LeukoNorm CytoChemia® bei Patientinnen mit mehrfachen frustranen IVF- und ICSI-Behandlungszyklen. Zentralbl Gynakol. 2001;123:361–5.

Yamada H, Kishida T, Kobayashi N, Kato H, Hoshi N, Fujimoto S. Massive immunoglobulin treatment in women with four or more recurrent spontaneous primary abortions of unexplained etiology. Hum Reprod. 1998;13:2620–3.

Yamada H, Atsumi T, Kato EH, Shimada S, Morikawa M, Minakami H. Prevalence of diverse antiphospholipid antibodies in women with recurrent spontaneous abortion. Fertil Steril. 2003;80:1276–8.

Yamada H, Atsumi T, Kobashi G, Ota C, Kato EH, Tsuruga N, Ohta K, Yasuda S, Koike T, Minakami H. Antiphospholipid antibodies increase the risk of pregnancy-induced hypertension and adverse pregnancy outcomes. J Reprod Immunol. 2009;79:188–95.

Yang H, Qiu L, Di W, Zhao A, Chen G, Hu K, Lin Q. Proportional change of CD4+CD25+ regulatory T cells after lymphocyte therapy in unexplained recurrent spontaneous abortion patients. Fertil Steril. 2009;92:301–5.

Zenclussen AC, Kortebani G, Mazzolli A, Margni R, Malan BI. Interleukin-6 and soluble interleukin-6 receptor serum levels in recurrent spontaneous abortion women immunized with paternal white cells. Am J Reprod Immunol. 2000;44:22–9.

Immunocontraceptive Approaches

Abbas AK, Lichtman AH, Pober JS. Immunologie. Bern/Göttingen/Toronto/Seattle: Verlag Hans Huber; 1996.

Adiga PR, Subramanian S, Rao J, Kumar M. Prospects of riboflavin carrier protein (RCP) as an antifertility vaccine in male and female mammals. Hum Reprod Update. 1997;3:325–34.

Ahmed A, Li XF, Shams M, Gregory J, Rollason T, Barnes NM, Newton JR. Localization of the angiotensin II and its receptor subtype expression in human endometrium and identification of a novel high-affinity angiotensin II binding site. J Clin Invest. 1995;96:848–57.

Bagavant H, Thillai-Koothan P, Sharma MG, Talwar GP, Gupta SK. Antifertility effects of porcine zona pellucida-3 immunization using permissible adjuvants in female bonnet monkeys (Macaca radiata): reversibility, effect on follicular development and hormonal profiles. J Reprod Fertil. 1994;102:17–25.

Davidson EJ, Kitchener HC, Stern PL. The use of vaccines in the prevention and treatment of cervical cancer. Clin Oncol. 2002;14:193–200.

Domagala A, Kurpisz M. Identification of sperm immunoreactive antigens for immunocontraceptive purposes: a review. Reprod Biol Endocrinol. 2004;2:11–8.

Domagała A, Kurpisz M. CD52 antigen-a review. Med Sci Monit. 2001;7:325–31.

Dunshea FR, Colantoni C, Howard K, McCauley I, Jackson P, Long KA, Lopaticki S, Nugent EA, Simons JA, Walker J, Hennessy DP. Vaccination of boars with a GnRH vaccine (Improvac) eliminates boar taint and increases growth performance. J Anim Sci. 2001;79:2524–35.

Ferro VA. Current advances in antifertility vaccines for fertility control and noncontraceptive applications. Expert Rev Vaccines. 2002;1:443–52.

Frank HG, Bose P, Albieri-Borges A, Borges M, Greindl A, Neulen J, Pötgens AJG, Kaufmann P. Evaluation of fusogenic trophoblast surface epitopes as targets for immune contraception. Contraception. 2005;71:282–93.

Grow DR, Ahmed S. New contraceptive methods. Obstet Gynecol Clin North Am. 2000;27:901–16.

Gupta A, Pal R, Ahlawat S, Bhatia P, Singh O. Enhanced immunogenicity of a contraceptive vaccine using diverse synthetic carriers with permissible adjuvant. Vaccine. 2001;19:3384–9.

Gupta SK, Chakravarty S, Kadunganattil S. Immunocontraceptive approaches in females. Chem Immunol Allergy. 2005;88:98–108.

Hannesdottir SG, Han X, Lund T, Singh M, Van der Zee R, Roitt IM, Delves PJ. Changes in the reproductive system of male mice immunized with a GnRH-analogue conjugated to mycobacterial hsp70. Reproduction. 2004;128:365–71.

Hardy CM, Mobbs KJ. Expression of recombinant mouse sperm protein sp56 and assessment of its potential for use as an antigen in an immunocontraceptive vaccine. Mol Reprod Dev. 1999;52:216–24.

Laylor R, Porakishvili N, de Souza JB, Playfair JHL, Delves PJ, Lund T. DNA vaccination favours memory rather than effector B cell response. Clin Exp Immunol. 1999;117:106–12.

Lea IA, van Lierop MJ, Widgren EE, Grootenhuis A, Wen Y, van Duin M, O'Rand MG. A chimeric sperm peptide induces antibodies and strain-specific reversible infertility in mice. Biol Reprod. 1998;59:527–36.

Lea IA, Widgren EE, O'Rand MG. Analysis of recombinant mouse zona pellucida protein-2 (ZP- 2) constructs for immunocontraception. Vaccine. 2002;20:1515–23.

Lemons AR, Naz RK. Contraceptive vaccines targeting factors involved in establishment of pregnancy. Am J Reprod Immunol. 2011;66:13–25.

Lloyd ML, Shellam GR, Papadimitriou JM, Lawson MA. Immunocontraception is induced in BALB/c mice inoculated with murine cytomegalovirus expressing mouse zona pellucida 3. Biol Reprod. 2003;68:2024–32.

Lou AM, Garza KM, Hunt D, Tung KS. Antigen mimicry in autoimmune disease sharing of amino acid residues critical for pathogenic T cell activation. J Clin Invest. 1993;92:2111–23.

Miki K, Willis WD, Brown PR, Golding EH, Fulcher KD, Eddy EM. Targeted disruption of the Akap4 gene causes defects in sperm flagellum and motility. Dev Biol. 2002;248:331–42.

Miller LA, Johns BE, Killians GJ. Immunocontraception of white-tailed deer with GnRH vaccine. Am J Reprod Immunol. 2000;44:266–74.

Moudgal NR, Ravindranath N, Murthy GS, Dighe RR, Aravindan GR, Martin F. Long-term contraceptive efficacy of vaccine of ovine follicle-stimulating hormone in male bonnet monkeys (Macaca radiata). J Reprod Fertil. 1992;96:91–102.

Moudgal NR, Jeyakumar M, Krishnamurthy HN, Sridhar S, Krishnamurthy H, Martin F. Development of male contraceptive vaccine: a perspective. Hum Reprod Update. 1997;3:335–46.

Naz RK. Vaccine for contraception targeting sperm. Immunol Rev. 1999;171:193–202.

Naz RK. Antisperm vaccine for contraception. Am J Reprod Immunol. 2005;54:378–83.

Naz RK. Effect of fertilization antigen (FA-1) DNA vaccine on fertility of female mice. Mol Reprod Dev. 2006a;73:1473–9.

Naz RK. Effect of sperm DNA vaccine on fertility of female mice. Mol Reprod Dev. 2006b;73:918–28.

Naz RK. Immunocontraceptive effect of Izumo and enhancement by combination vaccination. Mol Reprod Dev. 2008;75:336–44.

Naz RK. Development of genetically engineered human sperm immunocontraceptives. J Reprod Immunol. 2009a;83:145–50.

Naz RK. Status of contraceptive vaccines. Am J Reprod Immunol. 2009b;61:11–8.

Naz RK. Antisperm contraceptive vaccines: where we are and where we are going? Am J Reprod Immunol. 2011;66:5–12.

Naz RK, Ahmad K. Molecular identities of human sperm proteins that bind human zona pellucida: nature of sperm-zona interaction, tyrosine kinase activity and involvement of FA-1. Mol Reprod Dev. 1994;39:397–408.

Naz RK, Chauhan SC. Human sperm-specific peptide vaccine that causes long-term reversible contraception. Biol Reprod. 2002;67:674–80.

Naz RK, Mehta K. Cell mediated immune responses to sperm antigens: effects of murine sperm and embryos. Biol Reprod. 1989;41:533–42.

Naz RK, Subhash CC, Leema PR. Expression of alpha and gamma-interferon receptors in sperm cell. Mol Reprod Dev. 2000;56:189–97.

Naz RK, Gupta SK, Gupta JC, Vyas HK, Talwar GP. Recent advances in contraceptive vaccine development: a mini-review. Hum Reprod. 2005;20: 3271–83.

Norton EJ, Diekman AB, Westbrook VA, Flickinger CK, Herr JC. RASA, a recombinant single- chain variable fragment (scFV) antibody directed against the human sperm surface: implications for the novel contraceptives. Hum Reprod. 2001;16:1854–60.

Norton EJ, Diekman AB, Westbrook VA, Mullins DW, Klotz KL, Gilmer LL, Thomas TS, Wright DC, Brisker J, Engelhard VH, Flickinger CJ, Herr JC. A male genital tract-specific carbohydrate epitope on human CD52: implications for immunocontraception. Tissue Antigens. 2002;60:354–64.

O'Hearn PA, Liang ZG, Bambra CS, Goldberg E. Colinear synthesis of an antigen-specific B- cell epitope with a 'promiscuous' tetanus toxin T-cell epitope: a synthetic peptide immunocontraceptive. Vaccine. 1997;15:1761–6.

O'Rand MG, Widgren EE, Sivashanmugam P, Richardson RT, Hall SH, French FS, Vande Voort CA, Ramachandra SG, Ramesh V, Jagannadha RA. Reversible immunocontraception in male monkeys immunized with Eppin. Science. 2004;306:1189–90.

Paterson M, Wilson MR, Jennings ZA, van Duin M, Aitkin RJ. Design and evaluation of a ZP3 peptide vaccine in a homologous primate model. Mol Hum Reprod. 1999;5:342–52.

Robertson SA. Immune regulation of conception and embryo implantation-all about quality control? J Reprod Immunol. 2010;85:51–7.

Sairam MR, Krishnamurthy H. The role of follicle-stimulating hormone in spermatogenesis: lessons from knockout animal models. Arch Med Res. 2001;32:601–8.

Samuel AS, Naz RK. Isolation of human single chain variable fragment antibodies against specific sperm antigens for immunocontraceptive development. Hum Reprod. 2008;23:1324–37.

Santhanam R, Naz RK. Novel human testis-specific cDNA: molecular cloning, expression and immunobiological effects of the recombinant protein. Mol Reprod Dev. 2001;60:1–12.

Shankar S, Mohapatra B, Verma S, Selvi R, Jagdish N, Suri A. Isolation and characterization of a haploid germ cell specific sperm associated antigen 9 (SPAG9) from the baboon. Mol Reprod Dev. 2004;69:186–93.

Stevens VC. Progress in the development of human chorionic gonadotropin antifertility vaccines. Am J Reprod Immunol. 1996;35:148–55.

Talwar GP. Vaccines and passive immunological approaches for the control of fertility and hormone-dependent cancers. Immunol Rev. 1999;171:173–92.

Talwar GP, Sharma NC, Dubey SK, Salahuddin M, Das C, Ramakrishnan S, Kumar S, Hingorani V.

Isoimmunization against human chorionic gonadotropin with conjugates of processed β-subunit of the hormone and tetanus toxoid. Proc Natl Acad Sci U S A. 1976;73:218–22.

Talwar GP, Gupta SK, Singh V, Sahal D, Iyer KS, Singh O. Bioeffective monoclonal antibody against the decapeptide gonadotropin-releasing hormone: reacting determinant and action on ovulation and estrus suppression. Proc Natl Acad Sci U S A. 1985;82: 1228–31.

Talwar GP, Singh O, Pal R, Chatterjee N, Sahai P, Dhall K, Kaur J, Das SK, Suri S, Buckshee K, Saraya L, Saxena BB. A vaccine that prevents pregnancy in women. Proc Natl Acad Sci U S A. 1994;91:8532–6.

Talwar GP, Raina K, Gupta JC, Ray R, Wadhwa S, Ali MM. A recombinant luteinising- hormone-releasing-hormone immunogen bioeffective in causing prostatic atrophy. Vaccine. 2004;22:3713–21.

Tollner TL, Overstreet JW, Branciforte D, Primakoff PD. Immunization of female Cynomolgus macaques with a synthetic epitope of sperm-specific lactate dehydrogenase results in high antibody titers but does not reduce fertility. Mol Reprod Dev. 2002;62:257–64.

Wang XL, Zhao XR, Yu M, Yuan MM, Yao XY, Li DJ. Gene conjugation of molecular adjuvant C3d to hCG-beta increased the anti-hCGbeta Th2 and humoral immune response in DNA immunization. J Gene Med. 2006;8:498–505.

Wood DM, Liu C, Dunbar BS. Effect of alloimmunization and heteroimmunization with zonae pellucidae on fertility in rabbits. Biol Reprod. 1981;25:439–50.

Xiang RL, Zhou F, Yang Y, Peng JP. Construction of the plasmid pCMV4-rZPC'DNA vaccine and analysis of its contraceptive potential. Biol Reprod. 2003;68:1518–24.

Zeng XY, Turkstra JA, Tsigos A, Meloen RH, Liu XY, Chen FQ, Schaaper WM, Oonk HB, Guo DZ, Van de Wiel DF. Effects of active immunization against GnRH on serum LH, inhibin A, sexual development and growth rate in Chinese female pigs. Theriogenology. 2002;58:1315–26.

Index

E.R. Weissenbacher et al., *Immunology of the Female Genital Tract*,
DOI 10.1007/978-3-642-14906-1, © Springer-Verlag Berlin Heidelberg 2014

Mucosal immune system
    antigen uptake and processing, 9
    cytokine regulation, gut, 12
    discrete inductive sites, 16
    effector sites, MALT, 11–12
    exogenous stimulants, 8
    female reproductive tract, 1, 2
    inductive sites, GALT, 10–11
    protection, mucosal surfaces, 8, 9
    S-IgA, major Ig subclass (*see* S-IgA, mucosal
        immune system)
    and systemic compartments, 8

N
Nasal immunization
    animal studies, 44
    IgG antibodies, 44–45
    prevention, STDs, 45
    and vaginal vaccination, 44
    viral/bacterial antigens, 44
Natural killer (NK) cells
    apoptosis, 172
    CD56+ cells, 196, 197
    CD56 NK and dim cells, 30
    cell surface receptors, 32
    chemokine receptors, 30–31
    Chlamydia trachomatis, 113
    cytotoxicity, 172
    DC-derived IL-2, 33
    decidual, 171
    description, 29
    distribution and characteristics, 30
    endometrium, menstruation, 48, 196
    functions, 29, 31
    healthy and abnormal, 32
    HLA-C interactions, 171–172
    and HLA-G polymorphisms, 197
    and IFN, 197
    in vitro studies, 172
    and IL-15, 69
    innate immune responses against HSV-2, 69
    ITAM, 33
    lymphocyte-deficient mice, 70
    maternal immune cells, 171
    membrane-bound HLA-G, 33
    MHC I-binding inhibitory receptors, 33
    mucosal tissues, 29–30
    phenotypes, 30
    PIBF, 172
    placental tissue, 196
    recognition and interactions, 32–33
    regulation, sex hormones, 32
    regulation through cytokines, 32
    and RSA, 196, 197
    spiral artery transformation, 172
    and TLRs, 33
    trophoblasts, 171
    uterus, 171
Neutrophils
    cervix, 35

    characteristics and functions, 36
    Chlamydia trachomatis, 113
    commensal microorganisms, 34
    cytokines, 34
    description, 33
    E-and P-selectins, 34
    endogenous and bacterial chemoattractant signals, 34
    endometrium, menstruation, 47
    fallopian tube, 35
    IL-8, 34
    inflammatory signals, 33
    innate immune responses, HSV, 70
    innate immune responses, trichomoniasis, 134–135
    ovary, 35–36
    T cells and macrophages, 34
    uterus, 35
    vaginal lavage fluid, women, 34–35
Nitric oxide and RNIs, 135–136
NK. *See* Natural killer (NK) cells
Non-organ-specific autoantibodies
    ACA, 213
    APAs, 212, 213
    aPS, 213
    IVF, 212
    pathogenetic role, 213
    pathological assay, 213
    SMA, 212

O
Opa proteins, 107–108
Open reading frames (ORFs), 95
ORFs. *See* Open reading frames (ORFs)
Ovary, neutrophils
    corpus luteum, 36
    follicles, 35
    FSH and LH, 35–36
    menstrual cycle, 35
    tissue remodeling, 35

P
PAMPs. *See* Pathogen-associated molecular patterns
        (PAMPs)
Pathogen-associated molecular patterns (PAMPs)
    germline-encoded receptors, 4
    and TLRs, 4
PIBF. *See* Progesterone-induced blocking factor
        (PIBF)
PIF. *See* Preimplantation factor (PIF)
POF. *See* Premature ovarian failure (POF)
PPROM. *See* Premature rupture of membranes
        (PPROM)
Preeclampsia
    autoantibodies, 189
    cytokines
        endothelial dysfunction, 188
        IFN, 188
        IL, 188
        leptin, 188
        MMP, 189